Syndromic Neurosurgery

Editors

JAMES A. STADLER III
MARI L. GROVES

NEUROSURGERY
CLINICS OF NORTH AMERICA

www.neurosurgery.theclinics.com

Consulting Editors
RUSSELL R. LONSER
DANIEL K. RESNICK

January 2022 • Volume 33 • Number 1

ELSEVIER

1600 John F. Kennedy Boulevard • Suite 1800 • Philadelphia, Pennsylvania, 19103-2899

http://www.theclinics.com

NEUROSURGERY CLINICS OF NORTH AMERICA Volume 33, Number 1
January 2022 ISSN 1042-3680, ISBN-13: 978-0-323-83532-9

Editor: Stacy Eastman
Developmental Editor: Ann Gielou Posedio

Neurosurgery Clinics of North America (ISSN 1042-3680) is published quarterly by Elsevier Inc., 360 Park Avenue South, New York, NY 10010-1710. Months of issue are January, April, July, and October. Business and Editorial Offices: 1600 John F. Kennedy Blvd., Suite 1800, Philadelphia, PA 19103-2899. Customer Service Office: 11830 Westline Industrial Drive, St. Louis, MO 63146. Periodicals postage paid at New York, NY, and additional mailing offices. Subscription prices are $447.00 per year (US individuals), $1,043.00 per year (US institutions), $479.00 per year (Canadian individuals), $1,074.00 per year (Canadian institutions), $556.00 per year (international individuals), $1,074.00 per year (international institutions), $100.00 per year (US students), $255.00 per year (international students), and $100.00 per year (Canadian students). International air speed delivery is included in all *Clinics* subscription prices. All prices are subject to change without notice. **POSTMASTER:** Send address changes to *Neurosurgery Clinics of North America*, Elsevier Periodicals Customer Service, 11830 Westline Industrial Drive, St. Louis, MO 63146. **Customer Service: 1-800-654-2452 (US and Canada). From outside the US and Canada, call: 1-314-453-7041. Fax: 1-314-453-5170. E-mail: JournalsCustomerService-usa@elsevier.com (for print support) and journalsonlinesupport-usa@elsevier.com (for online support).**

Reprints. For copies of 100 or more, of articles in this publication, please contact the Commercial Reprints Department, Elsevier Inc., 360 Park Avenue South, New York, NY 10010-1710. Tel. 212-633-3874; Fax: 212-633-3820; E-mail: reprints@elsevier.com.

Neurosurgery Clinics of North America is covered in *MEDLINE/PubMed (Index Medicus), EMBASE/Excerpta Medica, and Current Contents/Clinical Medicine (CC/CM).*

Contributors

CONSULTING EDITORS

RUSSELL R. LONSER, MD
Professor and Chair, Department of
Neurological Surgery, The Ohio State
University Wexner Medical Center, Columbus,
Ohio, USA

DANIEL K. RESNICK, MD, MS
Professor and Vice Chairman, Program
Director, Department of Neurosurgery,
University of Wisconsin-Madison School of
Medicine and Public Health, Madison,
Wisconsin, USA

EDITORS

JAMES A. STADLER III, MD
Assistant Professor (CHS) of Neurosurgery and
Pediatrics, Department of Neurological
Surgery, University of Wisconsin-Madison
School of Medicine and Public Health,
Madison, Wisconsin, USA

MARI L. GROVES, MD
Assistant Professor of Neurosurgery, Division
of Pediatric Neurosurgery, Johns Hopkins
Hospital, Baltimore, Maryland, USA

AUTHORS

RAHEEL AHMED, MD, PhD
Department of Neurosurgery, University of
Wisconsin-Madison School of Medicine
and Public Health, Madison, Wisconsin, USA

MICHAEL B. BOBER, MD, PhD
Professor of Pediatrics, Nemours/A.I. duPont
Hospital for Children, Wilmington, Delaware,
USA

JEFFREY W. CAMPBELL, MD, MS, MBA
Division of Pediatric Neurosurgery, Nemours/
A.I. duPont Hospital for Children, Wilmington,
Delaware, USA

JUSTIN T. COLEMAN
South Georgia Medical Center, Valdosta,
Georgia, USA

MOISE DANIELPOUR, MD
Associate Professor and The Paul and
Vera Guerin Family Chair in Pediatric
Neurosurgery, Department of Neurological
Surgery, Cedars-Sinai Medical Center, Los
Angeles, California, USA

ELIZABETH JUAREZ DIAZ, BS
Washington University School of Medicine,
St Louis, Missouri, USA

ANGELA DUKER, MS
Masters of Genetic Counseling, Nemours/A.I.
duPont Hospital for Children, Wilmington,
Delaware, USA

ARAVINDA GANAPATHY, BS, MS
Washington University School of Medicine,
St Louis, Missouri, USA

MARI L. GROVES, MD
Assistant Professor of Neurosurgery,
Division of Pediatric Neurosurgery, Johns
Hopkins Hospital, Baltimore, Maryland,
USA

DAVID S. HERSH, MD
Division of Neurosurgery, Connecticut
Children's, Hartford, Connecticut, USA;
Assistant Professor of Surgery, UConn
School of Medicine, Farmington, Connecticut,
USA

JULIE HOOVER-FONG, MD, PhD
Professor of Genetic Medicine and Pediatrics, Greenberg Center for Skeletal Dysplasias, McKusick Nathans Department of Genetic Medicine, Johns Hopkins University, Baltimore, Maryland, USA

CHRISTOPHER D. HUGHES, MD, MPH
Divisions of Plastic Surgery and Craniofacial Surgery, Connecticut Children's, Hartford, Connecticut, USA; Assistant Professor of Surgery, UConn School of Medicine, Farmington, Connecticut, USA

IJEZIE A. IKWUEZUNMA, BA, BS
Fellow, Department of Orthopaedic Surgery, Johns Hopkins Medical Institutions, Baltimore, Maryland, USA

RAJIV R. IYER, MD
Assistant Professor, Department of Neurosurgery, Division of Pediatric Neurosurgery, University of Utah/Primary Children's Hospital, Salt Lake City, Utah, USA

ALON KASHANIAN, BS
Maxine Dunitz Neurosurgical Institute, Cedars-Sinai Medical Center, Los Angeles, California, USA

KRISTIN A. KEITH, DO
Resident Physician, Temple, Texas, USA

JANET M. LEGARE, MD, Clinical Professor of Pediatrics, University of Wisconsin-Madison School of Medicine and Public Health, Madison, Wisconsin, USA

KIMBERLY A. MACKEY, MD
South Georgia Medical Center, Valdosta, Georgia, USA; Staff Neurosurgeon, Department of Neurosurgery, Children's Hospital of the King's Daughters, Norfolk, Virginia, USA

ANTHONY NGUYEN, MD
Resident Physician, Temple, Texas, USA

ERICKA OKENFUSS, MS
Genetic Counselor, Department of Genetics, Kaiser Permanente of Northern California, Sacramento, California, USA

RABIA QAISER, MD
Assistant Professor, Texas A & M University, Director of Pediatric Neurosurgery; Temple, Texas, USA

LAURA K. REED, MD
Resident Physician, Temple, Texas, USA

SAI ANUSHA SANKA, BA, MPH
Medical Student, Division of Pediatric Neurosurgery, Department of Neurosurgery, Washington University School of Medicine, Washington University in St. Louis, St Louis, Missouri, USA

RAVI SAVARIRAYAN, MBBS, MD
Professor, Victorian Clinical Genetics Services, Murdoch Children's Research Institute, University of Melbourne, Parkville, Victoria, Australia

PAUL D. SPONSELLER, MD, MBA
Professor and Head, Pediatric Orthopaedics, Johns Hopkins Medical Institutions, Baltimore, Maryland, USA

JAMES A. STADLER III, MD
Assistant Professor (CHS) of Neurosurgery and Pediatrics, Department of Neurological Surgery, University of Wisconsin-Madison School of Medicine and Public Health, Madison, Wisconsin, USA

JENNIFER M. STRAHLE, MD
Associate Professor of Neurosurgery, Orthopedic Surgery and Pediatrics, Department of Neurosurgery, Washington University School of Medicine, St Louis, Missouri, USA

LAURA C. SWANSON, MD, PhD
Department of Pediatrics, Ann & Robert H. Lurie Children's Hospital of Chicago, Chicago, Illinois, USA

MARY C THEROUX, MD
Professor of Anesthesiology and Pediatrics, Department of Anesthesia, Nemours/A.I.

duPont Hospital for Children, Wilmington,
Delaware, USA

KAAMYA VARAGUR, BA, MPhil
Medical Student, Division of Pediatric
Neurosurgery, Department of Neurosurgery,
Washington University School of Medicine,
Washington University in St. Louis, St Louis,
Missouri, USA

MELISSA A. VILLEGAS, MD
Assistant Professor of Pediatrics and
Rehabilitation Medicine, University of
Wisconsin-Madison School of Medicine
and Public Health, Madison, Wisconsin, USA

KLANE WHITE, MS, MD
Professor of Orthopaedic Surgery,
Seattle Children's, Seattle, Washington, USA

duPont Hospital for Children, Wilmington, Delaware, USA.

KAAMYA VARAGUR, BA, MPhil
Medical Student, Division of Pediatric Neurosurgery, Department of Neurosurgery, Washington University, School of Medicine, Washington University in St. Louis, St Louis, Missouri, USA.

MELISSA A. VILLEGAS, MD
Assistant Professor of Pediatrics and Rehabilitation Medicine, University of Wisconsin-Madison School of Medicine and Public Health, Madison, Wisconsin, USA.

KLANE WHITE, MS, MD
Professor, Orthopaedic Surgery, Seattle Children's, Seattle, Washington, USA.

Contents

The developing field of syndromic neurosurgery has significant challenges and opportunities in quality and safety. Quality care must be safe, effective, patient-centered, timely, efficient, and equitable; the Donabedian model focused on system structures, processes, and outcomes is a helpful framework to guide improvement in these areas. Ultimately, a successful syndromic neurosurgery program will bring together an interested multidisciplinary team of experts who will grow care through open communication and steady improvement efforts.

Neurosurgical patients with genetic syndromes often receive care from multidisciplinary teams. Successful models range from multiple providers in one clinic space seeing a patient together to specialists located at different institutions working together. Collaboration and bidirectional communication are key. Multidisciplinary care improves outcomes and patient satisfaction. Choosing the goal of the clinic, using ancillary staff, and obtaining institutional buy-in are important initial first steps to establishing a multidisciplinary team clinic. Multidisciplinary teams can leverage technology to expand care via telehealth in multidisciplinary clinics and more vitally communication between providers on the team.

Achondroplasia is the most common of skeletal dysplasias and is caused by a defect in endochondral bone formation. In addition to skeletal deformities, patients with achondroplasia possess significant abnormalities of the axial skeleton, including small skull base with a narrowed foramen magnum and small vertebral bodies with shortened pedicles. Consequently, patients with achondroplasia are at risk of several severe neurologic conditions, such as cervicomedullary compression, spinal stenosis, and hydrocephalus, which frequently require the attention of a neurosurgeon. This article provides an updated review on the neurosurgical evaluation and care of children with Achondroplasia.

Current medical discussion for patients with skeletal dysplasia, specifically achondroplasia, focuses on infancy and early childhood within high volume multidisciplinary centers. Most neurosurgical concerns arising from a defect in the endochondral ossification results in early fusion of the synchondrosis and may impact patients early in life. As patients age, the neurosurgical focus shifts from primarily cranial to spinal concerns. Often pediatric neurosurgeons may continue to follow their patients with skeletal dysplasia. However, general adult neurosurgeons and orthopedic surgeons may see these graduated adults in their practice. This article provides a review of the common neurosurgical concerns for patients with achondroplasia.

Anesthetic Concerns of Children With Skeletal Dysplasia   37

Mary C. Theroux and Jeffrey W. Campbell

Children with skeletal dysplasia present unique challenges for safe anesthetic care including differences in the anatomy of the respiratory system, possibility of cervical spine instability or spinal stenosis, and a unique body habitus. Even seemingly routine anesthesia can result in respiratory arrest or spinal cord injury. These complications can largely be avoided by proper planning such as appropriate techniques for the intubation of difficult airways, recognition of cervical instability, neuromonitoring for any anesthesia over an hour in patients with severe spinal stenosis, and preoperative assessment of the trachea and avoidance of neuraxial anesthesia in children with Morquio syndrome and other MPS.

Surgical Evaluation and Management of Spinal Pathology in Patients with Connective Tissue Disorders   49

Ijezie A. Ikwuezunma and Paul D. Sponseller

Connective tissue disorders represent a varied spectrum of syndromes that have important implications for the spine deformity surgeon. Spine surgeons must be aware of these diverse and global manifestations of disease because they have significant impact on perioperative and postoperative outcomes.

Neurosurgical Evaluation and Management of Patients with Chromosomal Abnormalities   61

James A. Stadler III

Patients with chromosomal abnormalities are at risk for numerous neurosurgical pathologies, given the broad impact and multisystem involvement of these disorders. Down syndrome (trisomy 21), Edwards syndrome (trisomy 18), Patau syndrome (trisomy 13), Klinefelter syndrome (47,XXY), and velocardiofacial or DiGeorge syndrome (22q11.2 deletion) are particularly associated with neurosurgical concerns. Given the heterogeneity of concerns and presentations, these patients benefit from multidisciplinary care provided by teams familiar with their specific syndrome.

Syndromic Hydrocephalus   67

Kaamya Varagur, Sai Anusha Sanka, and Jennifer M. Strahle

Hydrocephalus, the abnormal accumulation and impaired circulation/clearance of cerebrospinal fluid, occurs as a common phenotypic feature of a diverse group of genetic syndromes. In this review, we outline the genetic mutations, pathogenesis, and accompanying symptoms underlying syndromic hydrocephalus in the context of: L1 syndrome, syndromic craniosynostoses, achondroplasia, NF 1/2, Down's syndrome, tuberous sclerosis, Walker–Warburg syndrome, primary ciliary dyskinesia, and osteogenesis imperfecta. Further, we discuss emerging genetic variants associated with syndromic hydrocephalus.

The phakomatoses are a group of genetic and acquired disorders characterized by neurologic, cutaneous, and often ocular manifestations, thus commonly referred to as neurocutaneous syndromes. In several of these conditions the underlying genetic pathophysiology has been elucidated, which will continue to play an important role in advancing therapeutic techniques. This article focuses on several examples of such neurocutaneous syndromes, with special attention to the relevant neurosurgical considerations of these patients.

There are multiple syndromes associated with tumors of the central nervous system (CNS). The most common CNS tumor syndrome is neurofibromatosis-1, with well-defined major and minor criteria needed for diagnosis. Other syndromes with variable degree of CNS and extra-CNS involvement that the neurosurgeon should be aware of include neurofibromatosis-2; Turcot syndrome; Cowden syndrome; Gorlin syndrome; Li-Fraumeni syndrome; ataxia-telangiectasia; multiple endocrine neoplasia type 1; von Hippel-Lindau syndrome; and tuberous sclerosis complex. Although most CNS tumor syndromes follow an autosomal dominant pattern of inheritance, the genetic underpinnings of each disease are complex and increasingly better understood.

Craniosynostosis involves the premature fusion of 1 or more cranial sutures and commonly presents as an isolated, nonsyndromic diagnosis. A subset of patients have syndromic craniosynostosis. Several unique considerations must be taken into account when managing patients with syndromic craniosynostosis. A multidisciplinary craniofacial team with a central coordinator is particularly useful for coordinating care among various specialists, and close monitoring is mandatory owing to the increased risk of intracranial hypertension. Surgical management varies among centers, but core options include fronto-orbital advancement with cranial vault remodeling, posterior vault expansion, endoscopic-assisted suturectomy with postoperative orthotic therapy, and midface advancement.

This review describes the clinical presentations and treatment options for commonly recognized epilepsy syndromes in the pediatric age group, based on the 2017 International League Against Epilepsy classification. Structural epilepsies that are amenable to surgical intervention are discussed. Lastly, emerging technologies are reviewed that are expanding our knowledge of underlying epilepsy pathologies and will guide future syndromic classification systems including genetic testing and tissue repositories.

There is a wide range of cerebrovascular conditions that afflict patients, some that are associated with particular syndromes. Multidisciplinary care is necessary to ensure comprehensive evaluation and management. The possible consequences of these neurovascular diseases can be devastating, and as such, early recognition and accurate diagnosis are crucial. This text aims to increase clinician awareness of these diseases by focusing on a variety of neurovascular diseases, including rarer clinical entities, with a focus on underlying pathophysiology and associated genetics, presentation, diagnosis, and management of each disease.

NEUROSURGERY CLINICS OF NORTH AMERICA

SERIES OF RELATED INTEREST

Neurologic Clinics
https://www.neurologic.theclinics.com/
Neuroimaging Clinics
https://www.neuroimaging.theclinics.com/

THE CLINICS ARE AVAILABLE ONLINE!
Access your subscription at:
www.theclinics.com

Preface

Syndromic Neurosurgery: Pulling It Together

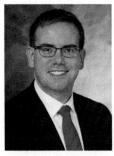

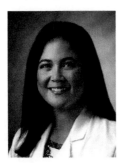

James A. Stadler III, MD   Mari L. Groves, MD

Editors

In this issue of *Neurosurgery Clinics of North America*, we are excited to explore the growing field of syndromic neurosurgery. While neurosurgeons have long cared for patients with cranial and spinal syndromes, we increasingly see organization of the specialty within and across institutions. One of the primary challenges, both in clinical practice and in reviewing these topics, is the shear breadth of a field defined by such divergent syndromes. However, several unifying themes have emerged as this resource came together.

The first, and perhaps most important, message from all the following reviews is the importance of true multidisciplinary care. No population benefits more from genuinely interested providers with such divergent backgrounds as seen on focused clinical teams for rare, syndromic conditions. Across the spectrum of disorders and concerns,

these teams are critical for safe, effective, patient-centered care.

We also see the value of experience. Many cranial and spinal syndromes are quite rare and are not encountered in routine practice. Combined with anatomic, pathologic, perioperative, anesthetic, and surgical nuances, management of these patients can be daunting and carries significant risk. Consultation with experts in a given diagnosis, even informally, is a valuable tool for any neurosurgeon.

Last, we appreciate the optimism for the future in caring for patients with complex syndromic concerns. Increasing collaboration across institutions is helping to level clinical and research silos. Experts across the field are bringing the best technologies to bear—genetically, medically, and surgically—and rapidly organizing previously scattered patterns of care and opinions.

Neurosurg Clin N Am 33 (2022) xiii–xiv
https://doi.org/10.1016/j.nec.2021.09.014
1042-3680/22/© 2021 Published by Elsevier Inc.

Caring for patients with complex cranial and spinal syndromes will always have challenges and opportunities for improvement. This growth will continue as a result of increasing awareness of the unique considerations for patients with neurosurgical syndromes and collaboration between providers dedicated to their care. We would like to particularly thank each of the authors in this issue not only for their excellent articles here but also for their broader expertise and contributions to the field. This is an exciting time for a growing field within our specialty, and we are grateful for the help bringing together these discussions.

James A. Stadler III, MD
Department of Neurological Surgery
University of Wisconsin School of Medicine
and Public Health
University of Wisconsin-Madison
600 Highland Avenue
Madison, WI 53792, USA

Mari L. Groves, MD
Division of Pediatric Neurosurgery
Johns Hopkins Hospital
600 North Wolfe Street, Phipps #556
Baltimore, MD 21287, USA

E-mail addresses:
stadler@neurosurgery.wisc.edu (J.A. Stadler)
mgroves2@jhmi.edu (M.L. Groves)

Safety and Quality in Syndromic Neurosurgery

James A. Stadler III, MD[a],*, Mari L. Groves, MD[b]

KEYWORDS

- Syndromic neurosurgery • Patient safety • Health care quality

KEY POINTS

- Quality care needs to be safe, effective, patient-centered, timely, efficient, and equitable.
- Improvement efforts can focus on the structures, processes, and/or outcomes of care.
- Establishing true multidisciplinary or interdisciplinary care is the start of most programs in syndromic neurosurgery.
- Good communication is critical for patients with complex cranial and spinal syndromic concerns.

INTRODUCTION

In 2001, the Institute of Medicine released the landmark report *Crossing the Quality Chasm: A New Health System for the 21st Century*. This report advanced the simple idea that "the ultimate test of the quality of a health care system is whether it helps the people it intends to help" and that this is best accomplished by ensuring that health care is safe, effective, patient-centered, timely, efficient, and equitable.[1] Although many efforts have sought to implement improvements, an early framework by Avedis Donabedian continues to form the basis of subsequent safety and quality research. The Donabedian model, with a focus on fundamental *Structures* ("how is care organized?"), *Processes* ("what is actually done?"), and *Outcomes* ("what was the result?"), is particularly relevant for the new and complex field of syndromic neurosurgery.[2–4]

Neurosurgeons focused on the care of patients with complex congenital syndromes face significant challenges in quality and safety. Immensely varied syndromes with frequently individualized presentations, rapidly advancing technologies in the broader field of neurosurgery, and limited research to define benchmark performance in these patient populations all preclude simple and universal solutions. However, the field also benefits from improved collaborations within and across multidisciplinary teams, growing appreciation for safety and quality improvement efforts in health care systems, and advancing data and research initiatives. For interested teams, focusing development on the structure, processes, and outcomes in their system is a powerful investment to improve the safety and quality of care for these challenging populations.

DISCUSSION
Characteristics of Quality Care

The ideal characteristics of a health care system (safe, effective, patient-centered, timely, efficient, and equitable) help shape goals for teams developing syndromic neurosurgery. All program development and quality improvement efforts are based on advancing one or more of these characteristics, and in practices with minimal universal standards or benchmarks, it is important for growth to be guided by more fundamental principles.

Patient safety is central to quality. Specific to syndromic neurosurgery, varied presentations of relatively rare conditions, dispersed expertise, and perioperative risks unique to the patient populations create concerns regarding the safety and efficacy of surgery. Clear communication

[a] Department of Neurological Surgery, University of Wisconsin School of Medicine and Public Health, University of Wisconsin-Madison, 600 Highland Avenue, Madison, WI 53792, USA; [b] Division of Pediatric Neurosurgery, Johns Hopkins University, 600 N. Wolfe Street, Phipps #556, Baltimore, MD 21287, USA
* Corresponding author.
E-mail address: stadler@neurosurgery.wisc.edu

Neurosurg Clin N Am 33 (2022) 1–5
https://doi.org/10.1016/j.nec.2021.09.001

within multidisciplinary teams and consultation with providers familiar with the management of patients with complex cranial and spinal syndromes mitigate these risks.[5–12]

Improving the efficiency of care while maintaining a patient-centered focus is also challenging in patients with complex neurosurgical syndromes. Given the general absence of population-level evidence and guidelines, care is often dependent on individual teams determining specific indications for management. Basic principles of obtaining careful histories and examinations and hypothesis-driven testing currently drive the standard of care, and this will hopefully be increasingly advanced by shared data and experiences.[13]

Perhaps the most significant risk to quality care in syndromic neurosurgery, however, comes ensuring timely and equitable care. Currently, many patients with neurosurgical syndromes lack access to true multidisciplinary or interdisciplinary care with surgeons and teams specialized in these areas.[14–16] This inherently creates quality gaps that are difficult to fill by these consolidated programs. Although opportunities such as expanded telemedicine access and cross-institutional collaborations should be aggressively pursued, even simple efforts such as discussing complex cases with colleagues who have managed patients with similar concerns can help as well.[17–21]

Structure

In developing syndromic neurosurgery programs, a focus on the structure of care is critical. These specialized programs are currently most concentrated at medical centers with existing representation and interest from relevant subspecialties; depending on the patient population served, this may include neurosurgery, interventional neuroradiology, plastic surgery, orthopedic surgery, otolaryngology, urology, ophthalmology, genetics, developmental pediatrics, nephrology, cardiology, pulmonology, rehabilitation medicine, and the full range of therapy teams. Larger centers may benefit from multiple independent interdisciplinary clinic teams to accommodate patients with specific syndromes or concerns.[7,22–25]

Most patient care, however, is driven by the broader health care system, which should also be considered and improved when possible. It is helpful to envision the path of a patient starting at the point of diagnosis or referral and extending throughout their care. Matured programs will streamline appointments and consultations, diagnostics, surgical planning, and longitudinal care. Increasingly, this includes the coordination of care for patients traveling regionally or nationally for subspecialized care, and both telemedicine options and dedicated care coordinators are invaluable for these efforts.

Within a hospital system, structural considerations include patient capacity, hospital staffing and training, provider availability and interest, existing technologies and the need for acquisitions, referral patterns, and the potential for growth. Specific structural needs are heavily dependent on program size and goals, the population served and their needs, and existing resources.

Processes

Improving processes within a health care system and the team often provides the greatest yield once the larger structure components are established. Often, the most important processes to install are centered on team communication and mechanisms for continuous monitoring and improvement.

Most complex care starts with organized communication. This is particularly true in syndromic neurosurgery, whereby no individual provider is likely to completely understand every aspect of a patient's care. Although open communication is important throughout a patient's course, this is perhaps most critical in the perioperative period. For patients undergoing complex cranial and spinal procedures, it is often helpful to use structured communication of preoperative, intraoperative, and postoperative plans, expectations, concerns, and needs.[12,23–27] This can be shared through standardized documents showing a surgical plan, interdisciplinary meetings, or both. A sample plan for a patient planned for multilevel thoracolumbar decompression and correction of syndromic scoliosis secondary to achondroplasia shows information that may be helpful to the intraoperative surgical, anesthesia, nursing, and neuromonitoring teams, and these can be routinely shared among all involved teams along with similar pre and postoperative notes (**Fig. 1**).

Dedicated quality improvement mechanisms form the basis for subsequent efforts. Many frameworks can be used for process improvement; rapid-cycle plan-do-study-act (PDSA) methods may be particularly well-suited to the needs of specialized surgical programs, but the quality improvement approach should be tailored to specific improvement goals.[28,29] Regardless of the method, the goal of these efforts is to identify and measure a core aspect of providing care that is desired for the population, find opportunities to improve the consistency of delivery and assess success. When fruitful, this measure should then be reinforced and monitored to provide a new

Adult Congenital Neurosurgery Spine Plan: Day-of-Surgery
Patient Name: ▮
Surgery Date: ▮

Intraoperative Plan:

Safety Stop

Anesthesia: GETA, arterial line, IVs, Foley, MAINTAIN MAPS, transfuse prn for hgb 9-10

Neuromonitoring: MEP / SSEP, LE EMG

Positioning: pins/Mayfield, open Jackson, arms up

Medications: Antibiotics, TXA, Ondansetron, NMB for exposure

Skin prep: Alcohol, scrub brushes, chlorhexidine

Local anesthetic

Expose T4 – ilium, XR confirmation after partial exposure

Note prior T12 – L3 laminectomies

T12 – L3 decompressions with facetectomies/PCO

T9 – T11 PCOs

T4 – ilium instrumentation: O-arm → Nav/screws → O-arm (x ?)

Rods / correction (Elevate MAPs)

Additional TL rods

Finalize instrumentation

Pulse lavage / antibiotic irrigation

Arthrodesis T4 – ilium

Grafting / vancomycin powder

JP x 2 (Flat #7 clotstop)

Closure – 0 vicryls, 2-0 vicryls, staples

Dressings: Mepilex Ag

Additional equipment/notes:

Jackson table, pins/mayfield

Smoke evacuator

Drill x 1, bone mill

Monopolar x 2, bipolar x 2, Suction x 2, Aquamantys

CellSaver

Stealth arm at feet

Grafts: crushed cancellous chips 60cc x 4 in room

Vancomycin powder

Pulse lavage

Anticipated Instrumentation		
Left		Right
	C1	
	C2	
	C3	
	C4	
	C5	
	C6	
	C7	
	T1	
	T2	
	T3	
5.5 x 30	T4	5.5 x 30
5.5 x 35	T5	5.5 x 35
5.5 x 35	T6	5.5 x 35
5.5 x 35	T7	5.5 x 35
5.5 x 40	T8	5.5 x 40
5.5 x 40	T9	5.5 x 40
6.5 x 40	T10	6.5 x 40
6.5 x 40	T11	6.5 x 40
6.5 x 45	T12	6.5 x 45
6.5 x 45	L1	6.5 x 45
6.5 x 50	L2	6.5 x 50
6.5 x 45	L3	6.5 x 45
7.5 x 40	L4	7.5 x 40
7.5 x 40	L5	7.5 x 40
Nav	S1	Nav
Nav	Iliac	Nav

Fig. 1. A sample intraoperative plan for a patient with achondroplasia undergoing a multilevel thoracolumbar decompression for stenosis and correction of syndromic scoliosis. This plan is shared with all intraoperative teams, and similarly, structured documents facilitate preoperative and postoperative communication for complex surgeries.

benchmark and further improvement should be sought.

Outcomes

Although improving patient outcomes is the ultimate goal of all health care safety and quality work, this is frequently the most difficult aspect to meaningfully measure. Individual patient factors heavily skew traditional outcome measures in small populations and validated outcome measures specific to patients undergoing neurosurgical procedures for syndromic concerns are lacking.

Variations in outcome measures across centers are currently unlikely to reflect the true quality of delivered care but may allow for reflective improvement in the structures and processes of individual programs. Outcome measures such as surgical complication rates and patient-reported outcomes should be collected and, when possible, this data should be pooled to help expand the understanding of appropriate case-mix adjustments and baseline expectations. Although this understandably takes years to realize even individual outcomes, such efforts will ultimately improve both direct patient care and broader appreciation for the value provided in these populations.

SUMMARY

Many researchers in patient safety and health care quality have provided frameworks and models for quality care. Each offers insights into important aspects of care, but ultimately most systems are best served by focusing on fundamental ideas. In the developing field of syndromic neurosurgery, core principles include bringing together interested teams with subspecialty experience and expertise in the care of patients with complex cranial and spinal syndromes, facilitating open communication, and growing through steady improvement efforts.

CLINICS CARE POINTS

- Any syndromic neurosurgery program should undertake a regular and genuinely self-critical assessment of their opportunities for improvement and growth
- Open communication between teams is critical, particularly in the perioperative period for patients with complex syndromic concerns
- Sharing structured perioperative plans with all teams involved in a patient's care, ideally well in advance of an intervention to allow for input and adjustment, is particularly helpful

DISCLOSURE

The authors have nothing to disclose.

REFERENCES

1. Crossing the quality Chasm: a new health system for the 21st century.
2. Donabedian A. Evaluating the quality of medical care. Milbank Mem Fund Q 1966;44(3).
3. Ayanian J, Markel H. Donabedian's lasting framework for health care quality. N Engl J Med 2016; 375(3):205–7.
4. Shojania K, Showstack J, Wachter R. Assessing hospital quality: a review for clinicians. Eff Clin Pract 2001;4(2):82–90.
5. Sacks G, Shannon E, Dawes A, et al. Teamwork, communication and safety climate: a systematic review of interventions to improve surgical culture. BMJ Qual Saf 2015;24(7):458–67.
6. Russ S, Rout S, Sevdalis N, et al. Do safety checklists improve teamwork and communication in the operating room? A systematic review. Ann Surg 2013;258(6):856–71.
7. Steelman VM, Stratton MD. The leadership role: designing perioperative surgical services for safety and efficiency. In: Surgical patient care: improving safety, quality and value. Springer International Publishing; 2017. p. 297–311.
8. Treadwell JR, Lucas S, Tsou AY. Surgical checklists: A systematic review of impacts and implementation. BMJ Qual Saf 2014;23(4):299–318.
9. Vetter TR, Paiste J, Chu DI. The perioperative surgical home: the new frontier. In: Surgical patient care: improving safety, quality and value. Springer International Publishing; 2017. p. 785–97.
10. Westman M, Takala R, Rahi M, et al. The need for surgical safety checklists in neurosurgery now and in the future-a systematic review. World Neurosurg 2020;134:614–28.e3.
11. Zuckerman SL, Green CS, Carr KR, et al. Neurosurgical checklists: a review. Neurosurg Focus 2012;33(5).
12. Sedra F, Shafafy R, Sadek AR, et al. Perioperative optimization of patients with neuromuscular disorders undergoing scoliosis corrective surgery: a multidisciplinary team approach. Glob Spine J 2021;11(2):240–8.
13. Carlson BC, Milbrandt TA, Larson AN. Quality, safety, and value in pediatric spine surgery. Orthop Clin North Am 2018;49(4):491–501.
14. Ahmed AK, Duhaime AC, Smith TR. Geographic proximity to specialized pediatric neurosurgical care in the contiguous United States. J Neurosurg Pediatr 2018;21(4):434–8.
15. Austin MT, Hamilton E, Zebda D, et al. Health disparities and impact on outcomes in children with primary central nervous system solid tumors. J Neurosurg Pediatr 2016;18(5):585–93.
16. Punchak M, Mukhopadhyay S, Sachdev S, et al. Neurosurgical care: availability and access in low-income and middle-income countries. World Neurosurg 2018;112:e240–54.
17. Kahn EN, La Marca F, Mazzola CA. Neurosurgery and telemedicine in the united states: assessment of the risks and opportunities. World Neurosurg 2016;89:133–8.
18. Hayward K, Han SH, Simko A, et al. Socioeconomic patient benefits of a pediatric neurosurgery telemedicine clinic. J Neurosurg Pediatr 2020;25(2):204–8.
19. Simko A, Han SH, Aldana PR. Telemedicine: providing access to care in pediatric neurosurgery to underserved communities. World Neurosurg 2020;138:556–7.
20. Eichberg DG, Basil GW, Di L, et al. Telemedicine in neurosurgery: lessons learned from a systematic review of the literature for the COVID-19 era and beyond. Neurosurgery 2020.
21. Paul JC, Lonner BS, Toombs CS. Greater operative volume is associated with lower complication rates in adolescent spinal deformity surgery. Spine (Phila Pa 1976) 2015;40(3):162–70.
22. Allen D, Gillen E, Rixson L. The effectiveness of integrated care pathways for adults and children in health care settings: a systematic review. JBI Database Syst Rev 2009;7(3):80–129.
23. Friedman GN, Benton JA, Echt M, et al. Multidisciplinary approaches to complication reduction in complex spine surgery: a systematic review. Spine J 2020;20(8):1248–60.
24. Johnston C. Preoperative medical and surgical planning for early onset scoliosis. Spine (Phila Pa 1976) 2010;35(25):2239–44.
25. Miyanji F, Greer B, Desai S, et al. Improving quality and safety in paediatric spinal surgery: the team approach. Bone Joint J 2018;100B(4):493–8.

26. Buchlak QD, Yanamadala V, Leveque JC, et al. Complication avoidance with pre-operative screening: insights from the Seattle spine team. Curr Rev Musculoskelet Med 2016;9(3):316–26.

27. Lepänluoma M, Takala R, Kotkansalo A, et al. Surgical safety checklist is associated with improved operating room safety culture, reduced wound complications, and unplanned readmissions in a pilot study in neurosurgery. Scand J Surg 2014;103(1):66–72.

28. Taylor M, McNicholas C, Nicolay C, et al. Systematic review of the application of the plan-do-study-act method to improve quality in healthcare. BMJ Qual Saf 2014;23(4):290–8.

29. Knudsen SV, Laursen HVB, Johnsen SP, et al. Can quality improvement improve the quality of care? A systematic review of reported effects and methodological rigor in plan-do-study-act projects. BMC Health Serv Res 2019;19(1).

Multidisciplinary Care of Neurosurgical Patients with Genetic Syndromes

Melissa A. Villegas, MD[a], Ericka Okenfuss, MS[b], Ravi Savarirayan, MBBS, MD[c],
Klane White, MS, MD[d], Julie Hoover-Fong, MD, PhD[e],
Michael B. Bober, MD, PhD[f], Angela Duker, MS[f], Janet M. Legare, MD[a],*

KEYWORDS
• Multidisciplinary • Interdisciplinary • Team-based care • Genetic syndromes • Skeletal dysplasia

KEY POINTS

- Multidisciplinary care improves outcomes for neurosurgical patients
- Communication, consistent personnel, and unified treatment goals are vital.
- Multidisciplinary care can be provided in a multitude of clinical settings as long as good 2-way communication is present.
- Technology increases the reach of multidisciplinary care for neurosurgical patients.

INTRODUCTION

Multidisciplinary is a term often broadly applied in medicine today. This term is used to describe care teams, interventions, methods for patient evaluation, and research. Despite this, the term multidisciplinary is relatively new in the long history of medicine,[1] and although a loose overarching definition involving a group of multiple medical specialists or allied health professions remains consistent, the methods for implementation of multidisciplinary care are vast.

Within these various interpretations adapted for specific disease processes, there is evidence for the benefits of multidisciplinary care. Multidisciplinary care has been shown to improve patient outcomes for diseases including heart failure, diabetes, and cancer.[2–7] Case management and nurse educators are often central to chronic disease interventions.[2–4] Other methods focus on team-based care with multiple allied health professionals providing a variety of evidence-based treatments. This type of team-based multidisciplinary intervention has demonstrated symptom improvement for patients with functional gastrointestinal disorders compared with usual care[8] and increased remission of depression.[9] Multidisciplinary teams are the norm for treating patients with orofacial clefts, a practice that dates back to the 1930s in the United States.[10,11] Cancer care has perhaps one of the longest and most multifaceted uses of multidisciplinary care from care conferences or tumor boards to clinics with resulting improvement in diagnosis, changes in management decisions, and increased patient and provider satisfaction.[6,7,12,13]

Multidisciplinary care brings together specialists with varying areas of knowledge to address parts of the patient's disease process or treatment plan. It is no surprise that this is often the

[a] University of Wisconsin School of Medicine and Public Health, 1500 Highland Avenue, Madison, WI 53705, USA; [b] Department of Genetics, Kaiser Permanente of Northern California, 1650 Response Road Kaiser, Sacramento, CA 95815, USA; [c] Victorian Clinical Genetics Services, Murdoch Children's Research Institute and University of Melbourne, Parkville, Victoria 3052, Australia; [d] Seattle Children's, 4800 Sand Point Way, OA.9. 120, Seattle, WA 98105, USA; [e] Greenberg Center for Skeletal Dysplasias, McKusick Nathans Department of Genetic Medicine, Johns Hopkins University, 600 N. Wolfe Street, Blalock 1008, Baltimore, MD 21287, USA; [f] A.I. duPont Hospital for Children, 1600 Rockland Road, Wilmington, DE 19803, USA
* Corresponding author.
E-mail address: jmlegare@pediatrics.wisc.edu

Neurosurg Clin N Am 33 (2022) 7–15
https://doi.org/10.1016/j.nec.2021.09.002

recommended type of care for patients with many complex medical conditions such as Duchenne muscular dystrophy[14] and tuberous sclerosis[15] and has been implemented in the care of patients with diagnoses such as nonsyndromic[16] and syndromic craniosynostosis.[17] Patients with genetic syndromes often have multisystem involvement with some also having developmental delay and functional deficits, all of which cannot be addressed by any single discipline.[18–20] At a minimum, multidisciplinary clinics provide patient convenience with multiple appointments occurring on the same day decreasing the need for multiple trips to clinic, time spent, cost of transport,[21] opportunity costs,[22] and facility fees. Although patients could, and often do, see each specialist individually, multidisciplinary care within a unified team or with communication between providers is ideal.

It is within these multidisciplinary teams that neurosurgical patients with genetic syndromes are most likely to receive care. This article explores multiple models of multidisciplinary care for neurosurgical patients with genetic syndromes using established skeletal dysplasia clinics as an example to illuminate positives, potential challenges, and future directions.

DEFINITIONS

Although often used interchangeably, multidisciplinary and interdisciplinary represent 2 distinct models of care.[1,23] Multidisciplinary care often involves each specialist seeing the patient separately whether in a dedicated multidisciplinary clinic or with separate appointments in the specialty's home clinic. In giving recommendations, each specialist stays within their own area.[1,24] There is often one specialty that serves as a lead for the clinic and the team. Recommendations from all specialties are combined to provide the plan for the patient. This model provides the benefit of flexibility with the potential for specialists to be housed at various locations (clinic or institution); however, this can lead to care wherein all specialties are not aware of other care goals (**Fig. 1**).

With interdisciplinary care, specialists work together to create recommendations based on the synthesis of information and expertise from all.[1,24,25] Discussion between specialists is had before, during, and after visits. Teams may even see the patient together, and some argue that this is true interdisciplinary care.[23] Such care creates the advantage of all goals being known by all team members with the ability to create a more unified plan for the patient; however, this usually

requires all providers to be at the same location, which limits this model to large centers with multi-specialty groups. It can also be challenging to fit these clinics into schedules because of potentially lower clinic volume (see **Fig. 1**).

Although these definitions remain distinct, in reality, team-based care likely occurs somewhere along a spectrum between the true definitions of multidisciplinary and interdisciplinary care with increasing communication and collaboration seeming to define movement along the spectrum (**Fig. 2**). A team's care style likely falls into various places for each individual patient under their care. With this in mind and for ease of use, multidisciplinary will be used to define care that falls anywhere within this spectrum throughout the remainder of this article.

CURRENT MODELS OF MULTIDISCIPLINARY CARE

There are many models for multidisciplinary care. Successful examples range from multidisciplinary clinics with all providers present in clinic to clinics where patients are scheduled separately with all providers with coordinated appointments over one to several days. Most institutions use a combination of traditional visits and multidisciplinary teams to provide appropriate care. Not every patient or encounter requires multidisciplinary care. A sample of existing multidisciplinary clinics and teams, predominantly for patients with skeletal dysplasia and other genetic skeletal disorders, was surveyed to exemplify currently successful models (**Table 1**).

Team and clinic structure of those surveyed include:

- All specialists scheduled with their full day dedicated to the clinic and team conference or huddle
- A primary subset of specialists in clinic with additional specialists pulled in or scheduled with patients as needed
- Separate provider schedules that are blocked for patients with skeletal dysplasia to be seen by all necessary specialists over a series of 1 to 3 days
- One coordinating provider and various subspecialists at other institutions within the broader regional area

Each clinic has some form of care coordination that is integral to clinic function. Clinic coordinator responsibilities can include:

- Controlling the clinic or providers' schedules to best schedule patients efficiently
- Completing preclinic phone calls to gather information and triage concerns before the visit

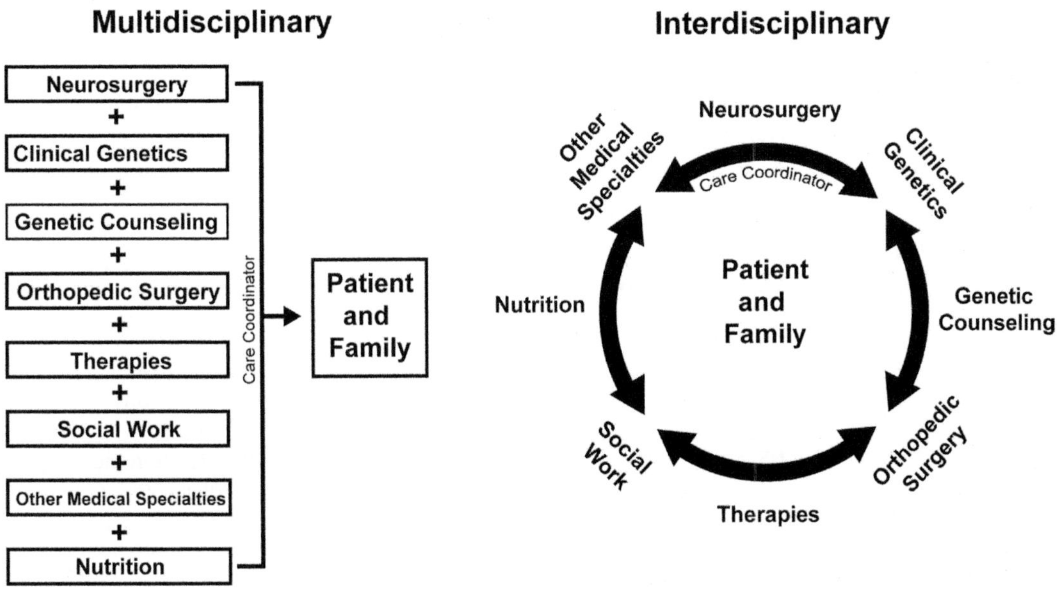

Multidisciplinary

Neurosurgery
+
Clinical Genetics
+
Genetic Counseling
+
Orthopedic Surgery
+
Therapies
+
Social Work
+
Other Medical Specialties
+
Nutrition

Care Coordinator → Patient and Family

Interdisciplinary

Neurosurgery

Other Medical Specialties

Clinical Genetics

Care Coordinator

Nutrition

Patient and Family

Genetic Counseling

Social Work

Orthopedic Surgery

Therapies

Fig. 1. Illustration of differences in composition and approach between multidisciplinary and interdisciplinary care with team members remaining separated and adding recommendations in sequence to give to the patient with multidisciplinary care contrasting with bidirectional communication between team members centered around the patient with interdisciplinary care.

- Summarizing recommendations, coordinating follow-up care, serving as contact person for concerns between visits

Communication is another key feature of each clinic. Examples of methods used by teams include:

- Preclinic team meetings
- Synchronous communication during clinic
- Virtual conversation through e-mail or the electronic medical record
- Telephone communication
- Postclinic team meetings

Although most of the previous examples are housed within individual institutions, multidisciplinary care is not limited to this structure. In some locations, the specialists in a specific condition are not present at the same institution. In these situations, a "consortium" can form with providers from a variety of institutions working together for patient care. For example, providing care to patients with skeletal dysplasia in the Midwest region of the United States can include neurosurgery, specialized orthopedics, otolaryngology, and

genetics separated institutionally and geographically across the region. These providers share patients across the area but communicate to discuss goals and treatment to provide multidisciplinary care.

No one model is best for every institution or location. Each institution develops their care method based on local factors, specialists available, and precedents from already existing clinics and teams. In essence, scheduled team meetings and huddles are important as a baseline, but the goal is to ultimately have a smooth flow of information bidirectionally between all specialists and the patient. The patient is the most valuable member of the team and helps lead the team in the direction preferred. Multidisciplinary care may look different between patients, even at the same institution.

ESTABLISHING A MULTIDISCIPLINARY TEAM
Initial Considerations

When starting a multidisciplinary clinic, the goal should be assessed. Is it one stop for all medical specialists? Is it to discuss the function and

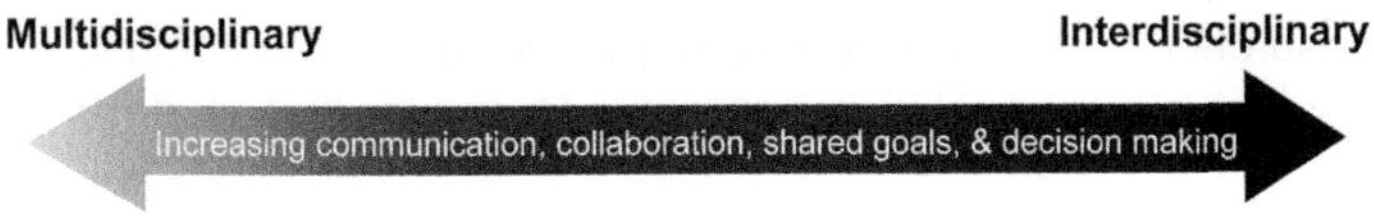

Multidisciplinary   Interdisciplinary

Increasing communication, collaboration, shared goals, & decision making →

Fig. 2. Multidisciplinary/interdisciplinary care spectrum illustration with increasing communication, collaboration, and shared goals and decision making moving teams toward interdisciplinary care and increasing separation of providers and specialty-specific goals moving teams toward multidisciplinary care.

Table 1
Examples of multidisciplinary clinics and multidisciplinary care provided from teams surveyed

Disciplines in Same Location	Team Disciplines in Home Clinic	Frequency of MDT Clinic	Communication Modalities
Genetics, GC, NS, Ortho, ENT, PM&R, OT, PT, SLP, Nutrition, SW, Neuro		Monthly	Team meeting after clinic
Genetics, GC, Ortho, OT, Nutrition	NS, Endo, Radiology	Monthly	Preclinic team meeting, synchronous discussions
Genetics, GC, Ortho	NS, Card, Pulm	Every other week	Weekly team meetings, synchronous discussions
Genetics, GC, Ortho, Endo, Metabolic bone disease NP	NS, Card, Pulm	Every other week	Weekly team meetings, synchronous discussions
Genetics, GC	NS, ENT, Sleep, Pulm, Audiology, Eye	Weekly	Weekly team meetings, electronic, phone, face to face with other disciplines
Genetics, GC, Renal, Ortho, nutrition	NS, ENT, Eye	Every other week	Preclinic team meeting
Genetics, Development, SLP, OT, PT, Audiology, SW	NS, Ortho, Neuro, ENT,	Weekly	Preclinic team meeting, synchronous discussions
Genetics, GC	NS, Ped CC, PT, research, Ortho anesthesia, SW	Weekly	Team meeting weekly. Informal daily communication.
Genetics, GC, Ped CC, APN, Ortho, PT, SW	Sleep, Pulm	Weekly	Team meeting before clinic, informal communication
Genetics	NS, Ortho, ENT	1 week, coordinated per month	Electronic communication after visits; lead provider determines overall goals.

Abbreviations: APN, Advanced practice nurse; Card, cardiology; Endo, endocrinology; ENT, otolaryngology; Eye, ophthalmology; GC, genetic counseling; MDT, multidisciplinary team; Neuro, Neurology; NS, neurosurgery, Ortho, Orthopedics; OT, occupational therapy; Ped CC, pediatric complex care; PM&R, physical medicine and rehab; PT, physical therapy; Pulm, pulmonology; Renal, nephrology; SLP, speech language pathologist; Sleep, sleep medicine; SW, social work.

medical issues of the patient? Is it to discuss one particular management issue that is common in a certain group of patients? There is no single right answer. Once the goal is established, planning for the best method for goal attainment can occur. Choosing which providers to include in clinic or team composition is foundational.[26] Some clinics are structured with providers from multiple different medical specialties (neurosurgery, neurology, pulmonary, cardiology, orthopedic surgery), whereas other clinics are structured with allied health professionals including speech and language pathology (SLP), physical therapy, occupational therapy (OT), case management, social

work, and nutrition. For example, neurosurgery, plastic surgery, and OT may create the team for a brachial plexus clinic, whereas neurosurgery, ENT, SLP, dentistry/orthodontia, ophthalmology, and genetics may participate in a craniofacial clinic.

Care should be taken when choosing providers to include because too many people in the clinic can be disorienting resulting in miscommunication.[27] It is necessary to ensure that all desired specialties are available and willing to participate. Once the team members are identified, the structure for visits within the clinic can be further defined. Some clinics function best with every provider seeing every patient. In some, only the necessary providers see the patient; however, this decision should be made by expert team members because it is difficult for the patient to know whom they need to see for evaluation.

Ancillary staff who can effectively triage, schedule, and assess insurance coverage for patients are of utmost importance. This staff keeps providers functioning at the top of their ability and not bogged down with other duties. Case management and social work can help patients and families follow through with recommendations, especially for patients with complex medical needs. Clinic coordinators who can field questions between appointments also help streamline care with less waste and inefficiency. Identification of a patient care coordinator was the most highly agreed upon need for implementing a multidisciplinary tuberous sclerosis team based on expert consensus.[28] Clinic coordinators can also serve as a point of contact with the patient's primary care provider to ensure continuity and open communication.

Multidisciplinary care does not require a multidisciplinary clinic. Patients can be coordinated to see multiple specialties over the course of several days with the providers collaborating via back-and-forth electronic communication. If this is the case, one provider or specialty must take the lead in coordinating the appointments and reaching out to specialties for recommendations after the patient is seen. Flexibility is also key; if one provider can join another provider's appointment that is true interdisciplinary care because both providers can work together with the patient to decide the next steps. This approach improves patient satisfaction and medical decision making. Collaboration needs to include physicians, advanced providers, and allied health professionals.

The institution or health care corporation needs to be in support of multidisciplinary care and specific clinic goals for a multidisciplinary clinic to be successful. Collaboration takes time and can decrease patient volume initially; however, the care is more comprehensive and may provide better visibility and marketing to the institution thus increasing the overall patient volumes over time.

Factors Contributing to Ideal Team Function

Having a unified purpose, mutual respect for other members of the team, and good communication are top promoters of good clinic function.[1,27] Each team member must value the outcomes as a whole over individual opinions or productivity with time spent discussing the patient necessary to create unified goals. Communication can take

multiple forms as previously detailed with a key being true discussion. Communication and unified recommendations are key so that the patient and the family, as well as the primary care provider, know and understand the next steps. It can be disorienting and frustrating when patients hear different messages from different specialties, whereas effective multidisciplinary communication in the hospital has been associated with improved patient perceived quality of care.[29]

Multidisciplinary teams should ideally have consistent team members[28]; this was considered of utmost importance for clinics surveyed because it allows each specialist to learn the nuances of their system in relation to rare diagnoses therefore increasing comfort and expertise among team members. This consistency also facilitates communication and promotes true collaboration because the entire team is invested in the population. Teams do grow and change with time, for example, with the addition of therapy disciplines. Although team members' contributions should be considered of equal value, it is helpful, especially when establishing a team, to have a designated team leader.[28,30] This leader could be the coordinator but is more likely a designated medical professional who works to help organize the team, promote goals, and elucidate feedback for improved teamwork. Pearls and pitfalls for multidisciplinary care are summarized in **Table 2**.

BENEFITS OF MULTIDISCIPLINARY CARE

Multidisciplinary care and corresponding increased communication between team members has multiple potential benefits including improved outcomes for surgical patients with decreased adverse events,[31,32] decreased length of stay,[29,31] and decreased postoperative pain.[29] Time to surgery was decreased following the creation of a multidisciplinary craniofacial clinic for patients with genetic syndromes at one center.[17] Multidisciplinary care results in improved patient satisfaction[17,31] decreased perioperative complications,[33] and improved quality of care. Patients benefit indirectly as well with decreased time away from work or school. In addition to these tangible benefits, multidisciplinary teams create an environment for learning with knowledge sharing between team members and the opportunity for incorporation of learners.

Despite these known benefits, cost of multidisciplinary care can remain a potential barrier to institutional buy-in; however, several recent studies have shown that multidisciplinary clinics are financially feasible.[34,35] With Centers for Medicare and Medicaid services movement toward

Table 2
Potential pearls and pitfalls with multidisciplinary clinics and teams from those surveyed

	Pearls	Pitfalls
Personnel	• Consistent personnel from each specialty so that they learn the nuances of their system with relation to the disorder	• Rotation of providers scheduled in clinic resulting in less knowledge of care related to a specific diagnosis
Communication	• Preclinic meeting to discuss patients and provide an opportunity for teaching • Effective communication including discussion between all the providers • Team meetings to facilitate communication between providers after patient visits to agree on care plan (in person vs electronic)	• Limited or unilateral communication • Plan communicated to family without discussion or synthesis into cohesive and consistent recommendations
Growth	• Addition of specialists over time as clinic evolves and needs are identified	• Increased demands on providers resulting in some specialties being intermittently pulled without additional coverage • Inability to add desired specialties
Partnerships	• Flexibility with use of regional specialists with condition-specific knowledge	• Loss of ability to partner with other health care organizations
Time utilization	• Dedicated scheduler, coordinator, case management, and social work	• Lack of unified coordination resulting in fragmented care and poor utilization of provider time
Insurance	• Dedicated personnel obtaining insurance clearance, ideally working with scheduler and clinic coordinator	• Difficulty with insurance authorization with patients coming from multiple locations/states with some patients unable to be seen

value-based care,[36] institutions will likely also have increased interest in decreasing patient-related costs, one of the core components of value-based care,[36] with possible savings associated with multidisciplinary care. One study showed a potential for 20% to 40% cost savings for patients with laryngeal clefts with multidisciplinary care in aerodigestive centers.[37] Costs of patient hospitalization can be decreased with multidisciplinary neurosurgical care.[31,32] Effective multidisciplinary clinics also ultimately increase surgical volume for the institution, thereby increasing surgical relative value units. A second key feature of value-based care is "better patient care,"[36] attainment of which can affect reimbursement for hospitalizations.[36] Multidisciplinary care is a potential method for targeting this aim.

FURTHER DIRECTIONS FOR MULTIDISCIPLINARY CARE

Although the aforementioned models have traditionally involved face-to-face visits, the coronavirus disease 2019 (COVID-19) pandemic has created unique challenges and led to an opportunity to rapidly pivot to telehealth platforms for completion of medical visits. Although thorough coverage of this topic is outside the scope of this article, given the recent temporary regulative changes and future potential, this is covered briefly here. Multidisciplinary care via telehealth occurred with growing use before the COVID-19 pandemic to increase patient access to care in particular for patients living in remote areas for conditions such as stroke[38] and to improve access to pediatric neurosurgical consultation.[39] In addition to increased access, telehealth can decrease patient burden with elimination of travel time and associated direct and indirect costs as well as decreased time away from work.[22]

Many more teams are now using telehealth to provide multidisciplinary care. Similar to in-person care, the format is tailored to the institution, patient population, and overall goals; this can range from care that closely resembles in-person care except that it is conducted via video (synchronous) to prerecorded assessments that are then reviewed by all members of the team separately to evaluate and provide recommendations (asynchronous).[40,41] Evaluation of neurosurgical patients via telehealth is feasible in selected patients[39,42] and results in patient satisfaction with the method of care.[43]

Although this represents a potential option for expansion of multidisciplinary care of patients with genetic syndromes, there are also barriers. All specialists likely need to be within a single institution or health care system to access the technology platform. The dedicated time required can also be greater as providers join visits in combination with other team members for longer total appointment duration leading to decreased efficiency and fewer patients able to be seen. Although it is possible to have providers rotate between virtual patients similar to movement through an in-person clinic, this requires significant coordination to function smoothly. Beyond this, state licensure laws often require the practitioner to be licensed in the state where the patient is located at the time of the encounter, which significantly limits who can be seen remotely[44] in patients with rare diagnoses who often travel across state lines to access specialized care. Reimbursement for telehealth is also limiting,[45,46] although this has expanded, again related to COVID-19.[36,45,47] It is unclear if this will be sustained long term. Patients previously could not be seen within their home for care to be reimbursed[36,47]; this would certainly create a significant barrier if that rule were reestablished. In addition to logistical, licensure, and reimbursement challenges, not all patients have access to the necessary technology to successfully complete a remote visit.[40]

Beyond these limitations, telehealth can offer a more accessible avenue to create diverse teams across institutions to provide care for patients with genetic syndromes. Virtual applications facilitate communication between specialists, whether at the same or separate institutions, which is necessary to achieve collaborative care.

SUMMARY

Care for complex neurosurgical patients with genetic syndromes will often involve multidisciplinary teams to target all facets of the disorder. Although the structure of these teams can take many forms, bidirectional communication and collaboration are unifying characteristics and core elements of successful multidisciplinary teams. The goal of this care is to not only address all patient problem areas related to their diagnosis but also provide recommendations that are cohesive and consistent rather than disparate or contradictory while always maintaining the patient and family at the center of decision making. Multidisciplinary care is feasible based on cost but requires institutional buy-in related to infrastructure and time required. If implemented successfully, this type of care can result in improved patient outcomes and patient satisfaction. Knowing this, it is certainly plausible that improved overall patient care and self-advocacy may translate into improved outcomes for neurosurgical patients with genetic syndromes both preoperatively and postoperatively.

CLINICS CARE POINTS

- Ideal multidisciplinary care of patients with genetic syndromes involves a consistent team that has developed specific knowledge of the condition.

- Communication with true back-and-forth discussion (verbal or electronic) between providers is vital so that all knowledge and evaluations can be brought together to create cohesive recommendations for the patient and their family.

- Multidisciplinary teams can take many forms from all providers in one space at one time to appointments with multiple providers in their home clinics over a few days with discussion and communication after the appointments.

- Openness and the willingness to work with and learn from colleagues is key. Constant reevaluation of the team and growth as knowledge emerges is necessary.

DISCLOSURE

The following is a list of grants and funding. There are no conflicts of interest related to this article.

R. Savarirayan is a paid consultant to BioMarin, Pfizer, QED, Ascendis. J. Hoover-Fong is a paid advisor to Biomarin, Pfizer, and Ascendis and receives grants from Biomarin. K. White is a paid consultant for BioMarin and receives grants from BioMarin, Ultragenyx, Pfizer, and Ascendis. M.B. Bober is a paid consultant for Biomarin, Pfizer, Ascendis, QED, Medlife Discoveries, and Alexion and receives research funding from Biomarin, Shire, Pfizer, Ascendis, QED, and Medlife Discoveries. A. Duker receives research funding from Potentials Foundation and Walking with Giants Foundation. J.M. Legare is a paid consultant for BioMarin and Ascendis and receives research funding from BioMarin and Ascendis.

REFERENCES

1. Choi BC, Pak AW. Multidisciplinarity, interdisciplinarity and transdisciplinarity in health research, services, education and policy: 1. Definitions, objectives, and evidence of effectiveness. Clin Invest Med 2006;29(6):351–64.

2. Roccaforte R, Demers C, Baldassarre F, et al. Effectiveness of comprehensive disease management programmes in improving clinical outcomes in heart failure patients. A meta-analysis. Eur J Heart Fail 2005;7(7):1133–44.

3. Gwadry-Sridhar FH, Flintoft V, Lee DS, et al. A systematic review and meta-analysis of studies comparing readmission rates and mortality rates in patients with heart failure. Arch Intern Med 2004; 164(21):2315–20.

4. Norris SL, Nichols PJ, Caspersen CJ, et al. The effectiveness of disease and case management for people with diabetes. A systematic review. Am J Prev Med 2002;22(4 Suppl):15–38.

5. Renders CM, Valk GD, Griffin S, et al. Interventions to improve the management of diabetes mellitus in primary care, outpatient and community settings. Cochrane Database Syst Rev 2001;2000(1): Cd001481.

6. Brar SS, Hong NL, Wright FC. Multidisciplinary cancer care: does it improve outcomes? J Surg Oncol 2014;110(5):494–9.

7. Pillay B, Wootten AC, Crowe H, et al. The impact of multidisciplinary team meetings on patient assessment, management and outcomes in oncology settings: a systematic review of the literature. Cancer Treat Rev 2016;42:56–72.

8. Basnayake C, Kamm MA, Stanley A, et al. Standard gastroenterologist versus multidisciplinary treatment for functional gastrointestinal disorders (MANTRA): an open-label, single-centre, randomised controlled trial. Lancet Gastroenterol Hepatol 2020;5(10): 890–9.

9. Murray G, Michalak EE, Axler A, et al. Relief of chronic or resistant depression (Re-ChORD): a pragmatic, randomized, open-treatment trial of an integrative program intervention for chronic depression. J Affect Disord 2010;123(1–3):243–8.

10. American cleft palate-craniofacial association. Available at: https://acpa-cpf.org/. Accessed February 15, 2021.

11. Long RE. Improving outcomes for the patient with cleft lip and palate: the team concept and 70 years of experience in cleft care. J Lancaster Gen Hosp 2009;4(2):5.

12. Basta YL, Baur OL, van Dieren S, et al. Is there a benefit of multidisciplinary cancer team meetings for patients with gastrointestinal malignancies? Ann Surg Oncol 2016;23(8):2430–7.

13. Taylor C, Munro AJ, Glynne-Jones R, et al. Multidisciplinary team working in cancer: what is the evidence? BMJ 2010;340:c951.

14. Birnkrant DJ, Bushby K, Bann CM, et al. Diagnosis and management of Duchenne muscular dystrophy, part 1: diagnosis, and neuromuscular, rehabilitation, endocrine, and gastrointestinal and nutritional management. Lancet Neurol 2018;17(3):251–67.

15. Krueger DA, Northrup H. Tuberous sclerosis complex surveillance and management: recommendations of the 2012 International Tuberous Sclerosis Complex Consensus Conference. Pediatr Neurol 2013;49(4):255–65.

16. Birgfeld CB, Dufton L, Naumann H, et al. Safety of open cranial vault surgery for single-suture craniosynostosis: a case for the multidisciplinary team. J Craniofac Surg 2015;26(7):2052–8.

17. Hoffman C, Yuan M, Boyke A, et al. Impact of a multidisciplinary craniofacial clinic for patients with craniofacial syndromes on patient satisfaction and outcome. Cleft Palate Craniofac J 2020;57(12): 1357–61.

18. Amudhavalli SM, Gadea R, Gripp K. Aymé-Gripp syndrome. In: Adam MP, Ardinger HH, Pagon RA, et al, editors. GeneReviews(®). Seattle (WA): University of Washington, Seattle Copyright © 1993-2021, University of Washington, Seattle. GeneReviews is a registered trademark of the University of Washington, Seattle. All rights reserved; 1993.

19. Emanuel BS, Zackai EH, Medne L. Emanuel syndrome. In: Adam MP, Ardinger HH, Pagon RA, et al, editors. GeneReviews(®). Seattle (WA): University of Washington, Seattle Copyright © 1993-2020, University of Washington, Seattle. GeneReviews is a registered trademark of the University of Washington, Seattle. All rights reserved; 1993.

20. Kartalias K, Gillies AP, Peña MT, et al. Fourteen-year follow-up of a child with acroscyphodysplasia with emphasis on the need for multidisciplinary management: a case report. BMC Med Genet 2020;21(1): 189.

21. Ray KN, Chari AV, Engberg J, et al. Disparities in time spent seeking medical care in the United States. JAMA Intern Med 2015;175(12):1983–6.

22. Ray KN, Chari AV, Engberg J, et al. Opportunity costs of ambulatory medical care in the United States. Am J Manag Care 2015;21(8):567–74.

23. Jessup RL. Interdisciplinary versus multidisciplinary care teams: do we understand the difference? Aust Health Rev 2007;31(3):330–1.

24. Körner M. Interprofessional teamwork in medical rehabilitation: a comparison of multidisciplinary and interdisciplinary team approach. Clin Rehabil 2010;24(8):745–55.

25. Saxena N, Rizk DV. The interdisciplinary team: the whole is larger than the parts. Adv Chronic Kidney Dis 2014;21(4):333–7.

26. Rosen MA, DiazGranados D, Dietz AS, et al. Teamwork in healthcare: key discoveries enabling safer, high-quality care. Am Psychol 2018;73(4):433–50.

27. Nancarrow SA, Booth A, Ariss S, et al. Ten principles of good interdisciplinary team work. Hum Resour Health 2013;11:19.

28. Auvin S, Bissler JJ, Cottin V, et al. A step-wise approach for establishing a multidisciplinary team for the management of tuberous sclerosis complex: a Delphi consensus report. Orphanet J Rare Dis 2019;14(1):91.

29. Gittell JH, Fairfield KM, Bierbaum B, et al. Impact of relational coordination on quality of care, postoperative pain and functioning, and length of stay: a nine-hospital study of surgical patients. Med Care 2000; 38(8):807–19.

30. Choi BC, Pak AW. Multidisciplinarity, interdisciplinarity, and transdisciplinarity in health research, services, education and policy: 2. Promotors, barriers, and strategies of enhancement. Clin Invest Med 2007;30(6):E224–32.

31. Chan AY, Vadera S. Implementation of interdisciplinary neurosurgery morning huddle: cost-effectiveness and increased patient satisfaction. J Neurosurg 2018;128(1):258–61.

32. Weant KA, Armitstead JA, Ladha AM, et al. Cost effectiveness of a clinical pharmacist on a neurosurgical team. Neurosurgery 2009;65(5):946–50 [discussion 941–50].

33. Sethi R, Buchlak QD, Yanamadala V, et al. A systematic multidisciplinary initiative for reducing the risk of complications in adult scoliosis surgery. J Neurosurg Spine 2017;26(6):744–50.

34. Mudd PA, Silva AL, Callicott SS, et al. Cost analysis of a multidisciplinary aerodigestive clinic: are such clinics financially feasible? Ann Otol Rhinol Laryngol 2017;126(5):401–6.

35. Straughan AJ, Mudd PA, Silva AL, et al. Cost analysis of a multidisciplinary vascular anomaly clinic. Ann Otol Rhinol Laryngol 2019;128(5):401–5.

36. Value-based programs. Available at: https://www.cms. gov/Medicare/Quality-Initiatives-Patient-Assessment-Instruments/Value-Based-Programs/Value-Based-Programs. Accessed February 1, 2021.

37. Garcia JA, Mistry B, Hardy S, et al. Time-driven activity-based costing to estimate cost of care at multidisciplinary aerodigestive centers. Laryngoscope 2017;127(9):2152–8.

38. Müller-Barna P, Hubert GJ, Boy S, et al. TeleStroke units serving as a model of care in rural areas: 10-year experience of the TeleMedical project for integrative stroke care. Stroke 2014;45(9):2739–44.

39. James HE. Pediatric neurosurgery telemedicine clinics: a model to provide care to geographically underserved areas of the United States and its territories. J Neurosurg Pediatr 2016;25(6):753–7.

40. Haulman A, Geronimo A, Chahwala A, et al. The use of telehealth to enhance care in ALS and other neuromuscular disorders. Muscle Nerve 2020; 61(6):682–91.

41. Pulley MT, Brittain R, Hodges W, et al. Multidisciplinary amyotrophic lateral sclerosis telemedicine care: the store and forward method. Muscle Nerve 2019;59(1):34–9.

42. Basil GW, Eichberg DG, Perez-Dickens M, et al. Letter: implementation of a neurosurgery telehealth program amid the COVID-19 crisis-challenges, lessons learned, and a way forward. Neurosurgery 2020; 87(2):E260–2.

43. Mohanty A, Srinivasan VM, Burkhardt JK, et al. Ambulatory neurosurgery in the COVID-19 era: patient and provider satisfaction with telemedicine. Neurosurg Focus 2020;49(6):E13.

44. Becker CD, Dandy K, Gaujean M, et al. Legal perspectives on telemedicine part 1: legal and regulatory issues. Perm J 2019;23:18–293.

45. Klein BC, Busis NA. COVID-19 is catalyzing the adoption of teleneurology. Neurology 2020;94: 903–4.

46. Blue R, Yang AI, Zhou C, et al. Telemedicine in the era of coronavirus disease 2019 (COVID-19): a neurosurgical perspective. World Neurosurg 2020; 139:549–57.

47. Telehealth. Available at: https://www.medicare.gov/ coverage/telehealth. Accessed January 31, 2021.

Neurosurgical Evaluation and Management of Children with Achondroplasia

Alon Kashanian, BS[a], James A. Stadler III, MD[b], Moise Danielpour, MD[a],*

KEYWORDS

- Achondroplasia • Cervicomedullary compression • Foramen magnum stenosis • Hydrocephalus
- Spinal stenosis • Ventriculomegaly

KEY POINTS

- Children with achondroplasia are at risk of several serious neurologic conditions, including cervicomedullary compression, spinal stenosis, hydrocephalus, and sudden death.
- Patients require an early comprehensive evaluation and proactive management by a multidisciplinary team familiar with this genetic disorder.
- Increasing knowledge of the natural history of these conditions, greater surgical experience, as well advancements in imaging protocol, have led to more refined indications for neurosurgery in this population.
- Surgical interventions, including foramen magnum decompression, can be performed safely and are effective in the treatment of cervicomedullary compression.
- In children with symptomatic foramen magnum stenosis and progressive hydrocephalus, a cervicomedullary decompression may lead to the stabilization of hydrocephalus.
- Future clinical trials, such as the evaluation of endoscopic third ventriculostomy for hydrocephalus, will be valuable for determining the most efficacious treatment strategies in these children.

INTRODUCTION

Achondroplasia (OMIM: 100,800) is the most common of the skeletal dysplasias, arising in about 1 out of every 25,000 to 30,000 individuals, with more than 250,000 affected people worldwide.[1–4] It is caused by gain-of-function mutations in fibroblast growth factor receptor 3 (FGFR3) and is inherited in an autosomal dominant pattern, although about 80% of cases are due to new mutations in the FGFR3 gene.[1] The molecular defect in achondroplasia results in a quantitative decrease in the rate of endochondral ossification, which, in conjunction with undisturbed periosteal bone formation, leads to a short, squat shape of the tubular bones.[5]

Patients with achondroplasia possess significant abnormalities of the axial skeleton including a relatively small skull base and narrowed foramen magnum, venous outflow obstruction due to skull base foraminal stenosis, small and narrow vertebral bodies with shortened pedicles, and finally, ligamentous hypertrophy. Consequently, neurosurgical complications of achondroplasia in children include cervicomedullary compression, spinal stenosis, and hydrocephalus (**Fig. 1**). The following review provides an update on the neurosurgical evaluation and management of these conditions in children with achondroplasia.

[a] Maxine Dunitz Neurosurgical Institute, Cedars-Sinai Medical Center, 127 S. San Vicente Boulevard, 6th Floor #A6600, Los Angeles, CA 90048, USA; [b] Department of Neurological Surgery, University of Wisconsin School of Medicine and Public Health, 600 Highland Avenue, Madison, WI 53792, USA
* Corresponding author. Department of Neurosurgery, Maxine Dunitz Neurosurgical Institute, Cedars-Sinai Medical Center, 127 S. San Vicente Boulevard, 6th Floor #A6600, Los Angeles, CA 90048.
E-mail address: Moise.Danielpour@cshs.org
Twitter: @AlonKashanian (A.K.); @stadler_md (J.A.S.); @m_danielpour (M.D.)

Neurosurg Clin N Am 33 (2022) 17–23
https://doi.org/10.1016/j.nec.2021.09.003
1042-3680/22/© 2021 Elsevier Inc. All rights reserved.

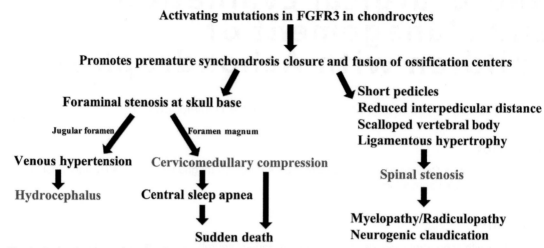

Fig. 1. Activating mutations in FGFR3 within chondrocytes can lead to cervicomedullary compression, spinal ste-nosis, or hydrocephalus by decreasing the relative rate of endochondral bone formation. (*Adapted from* Mukher-jee D, Pressman BD, Krakow D, et al. Dynamic cervicomedullary cord compression and alterations in cerebrospinal fluid dynamics in children with achondroplasia: review of an 11-year surgical case series. *J Neurosurg Pediatr.* 2014;14(3):238–244; with permission.)

DISCUSSION
Cervicomedullary Compression

Cervicomedullary compression is a significant contributor to morbidity and mortality in children with achondroplasia.[6–8] The skull base is formed by endochondral ossification and is therefore dysplastic in children with achondroplasia. The resulting foramen magnum stenosis (FMS) poses a major risk of compression to several vital struc-tures at the cervicomedullary junction. Acute or chronic compression at the level of the foramen magnum may lead to apnea and sudden unex-pected death.[8] Although sudden death is less likely to occur after the age of 1 year,[8,9] FMS can persist and result in neurologic dysfunction due to brainstem compression or upper cervical myelopathy.

Evaluation

Given that almost all infants with achondroplasia have some degree of foramen magnum narrow-ing,[10] it is important that these infants undergo careful evaluation. The consensus among the Skeletal Dysplasia Management Consortium (SDMC) is that infants with achondroplasia require a comprehensive history and physical examination every 2 months as part of screening for FMS.[6] This evaluation involves a careful neurologic examina-tion focusing on the signs and symptoms of cervi-comedullary compression including, but not limited to, weakness, lack of overall movement, asymmetric limb motion, weak suck with feeding, sustained clonus, asymmetric reflexes, and failure to meet developmental milestones for infants with

achondroplasia.[11] The treating physician, frequently a geneticist, should continue to be vigi-lant for signs of brainstem compression or cervical myelopathy in these children in both early and late childhood.[12] Overnight sleep studies that assess for central and obstructive sleep apneas, hypoxia, and hypercapnia with EEG are recommended in all infants with achondroplasia and should be used in combination with other modalities, such as history and physical examination, to assess for FMS.[6] The American Academy of Pediatrics Guideline on Health Supervision for children with achondro-plasia suggests that the care of every infant with achondroplasia should include neuroimaging assessment.[13] In a more targeted approach, the SDMC recommends that magnetic resonance im-aging (MRI) studies should be used more spar-ingly, and only in the presence of abnormalities in screening tests (history, physical examination, and overnight sleep study) to assess for FMS. Of course, these recommendations need to be adjusted to the availability of specialists comfort-able with assessing patients with achondroplasia and FMS, and in the absence of access to subspe-cialists, MRI can be a very important screening modality.

Surgical management

Fortunately, despite having a narrow foramen magnum, most children with achondroplasia achieve normal motor and intellectual develop-ment, and do not require neurosurgical interven-tion.[14,15] However, for a select group of children with symptomatic FMS, cervicomedullary decom-pression (CMD) is an effective procedure to widen the foramen magnum and relieve pressure at the cervicomedullary junction.[16–18] The criteria for CMD have previously been described in large surgical case series, and generally include clinical and imaging findings consistent with symptomatic FMS.[19,20] The SDMC recommends surgical decompression for 2 scenarios of MRI-defined FMS in infants with achondroplasia: FMS with cord signal change and FMS with the indentation of the spinal cord combined with abnormal neurologic findings.[6] At our institution, patients undergo MRI that incorporates cerebrospinal fluid (CSF) flow studies with the cervical spine in neutral, flexed, and extended positions to assess for the obstruction of CSF flow anterior to the spinal cord. In total, patients meet the criteria for decompressive surgery if they either have evidence on MRI of lack of CSF flow anterior to the spinal cord on neutral or flexed position or intracord lesions on T2-weighted imaging with either: (a) evidence of central sleep apnea or (b) other signs and/or symptoms of cervicomedullary compression, such as difficulty swallowing, hypertonia, paresis, or clonus. In a previous case series, we observed the restoration of CSF flow after CMD in all children with FMS who had diminished or obliterated CSF flow at the craniocervical junction on preoperative imaging.[16] Additionally, some

children with normal anterior CSF flow on neutral studies were found to have cervicomedullary compression and obliteration of CSF flow on flexion-extension MRI. Not all of these patients were found to have T2 changes that would predict cervicomedullary compression on dynamic studies. We, therefore, recommend flexion-extension sagittal imaging on all symptomatic patients being evaluated for FMS unless there is already complete obliteration of CSF flow and cervicomedullary compression present on a neutral study. Based on these findings, we believe that there may be a role for the use of dynamic cervical flexion and extension MRI (**Fig. 2**) and CSF flow studies in the evaluation of cervicomedullary compression in symptomatic patients with achondroplasia.

Spinal Stenosis

Individuals with achondroplasia have significantly compromised caliber of the spinal canal due to the early fusion of the pedicles to the vertebral bodies at the neurocentral synchondrosis.[21] Consequently, the pedicles are shortened in the anteroposterior length and the interpedicular distance is decreased, commonly leading to segmental spinal stenosis.[22] Additionally, many individuals are affected by thoracolumbar kyphosis

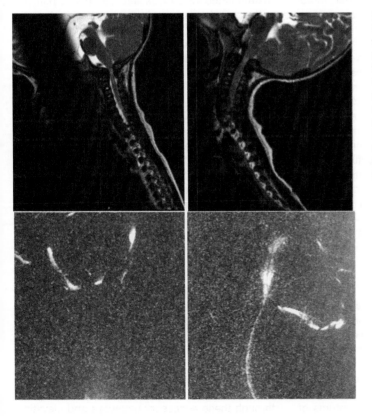

Fig. 2. Preoperative dynamic sagittal MR imaging in a 5-year-old child with achondroplasia. The cervical canal was significantly narrowed in flexion (*top left*) compared with extension (*top right*) and neutral studies on T2-weighted MRI. Cervical spine cine CSF flow studies demonstrated near-complete cessation of flow with the neck in the flexed position (*bottom left*) and minimal flow anterior to the spinal cord when in the extended position (*bottom right*).

and lumbar hyperlordosis, which are thought to increase the likelihood of stenosis.[23–25] Whereas complications related to cervicomedullary compression tend to resolve during childhood because the foramen magnum grows in size relative to the size of the spinal cord,[19] the complications from spinal stenosis increase with age.[15] Almost 10% of children with achondroplasia have neurologic signs of stenosis by the age of 10 years, and about 80% have these signs by the age of 60 years.[15] Interestingly, intraoperative evaluation suggests that there is a significant overgrowth of ligamentum even at a young age, contributing to the segmental nature of spinal stenosis in these patients.

Evaluation

Symptomatic spinal stenosis can occur at any level throughout the spine in patients with achondroplasia.[26] Therefore, signs and symptoms of spinal stenosis may differ depending on the area of spinal compression, requiring careful attention to history and physical examination. Lumbar stenosis can result in lower motor symptoms of neurogenic claudication, such as lower limb weakness, tingling, and pain or cramping in the back, buttocks and legs, which is usually relieved by leaning forward or squatting.[27] Stenosis of the thoracic spine can present with upper motor neuron symptoms such as hyperreflexia, urinary incontinence, bowel dysfunction, gait disturbance, Babinski reflex, and clonus.[27] Furthermore, pain and stiffness in the neck, as well as symptoms such as weakness, numbness, and loss of dexterity, can occur in the upper extremities with compression or injury to the cervical spine.[26] Correlating clinical presentation with neuroimaging of the spine is valuable for achieving a correct diagnosis and appropriate management. Flexion-extension MRI can be particularly useful for evaluating cervical instability in these patients, but there is very little evidence of the presence of instability without a prior history of multilevel laminectomies.[27] In fact, the presence of significant ligamentous laxity and overgrowth may lead the uninitiated to diagnose a child with ligamentous laxity as having cervical instability.

Surgical management

Approximately one-third of patients with achondroplasia will develop symptomatic spinal stenosis requiring surgical intervention in their lifetime.[28] However, the need for surgery in the pediatric population is less common.[29] In their "Best Practice Guidelines for Management of Spinal Disorders in Skeletal Dysplasia," White and colleagues agreed that progressive signs and symptoms of spinal stenosis causing reduced physical function in achondroplasia should be treated surgically by decompression when appropriate nonoperative measures are ineffective.[30] More specifically, Sciubba and colleagues used the following criteria for selecting patients for spinal decompressive surgery in the largest series to date on spinal stenosis surgery in pediatric patients with achondroplasia[26]: 1. The presence of progressive signs or symptoms of chronic spinal cord compression (weakness, bowel or bladder dysfunction, hyper-reflexia or hypertonia, spastic gait, or clonus) or chronic nerve root compression (neurogenic claudication, weakness or sensory disturbance in a radicular pattern, or hyporeflexia) and 2. neuroimaging evidence of spinal stenosis. Spinal procedures in children with achondroplasia may be technically challenging and require that the neurosurgeon be comfortable with the care of complications related to this patient cohort. In particular, the dura mater is especially thin and fragile in these patients, which increases the chance of inadvertent durotomy and subsequent CSF leak during surgical decompression.[31] Furthermore, skeletally immature patients are at high risk for developing postlaminectomy thoracolumbar kyphosis.[32] Indeed, the consensus is that surgical multilevel decompression over 2 levels be accompanied by instrumented fusion in skeletally immature patients with achondroplasia and progressive symptomatic spinal stenosis.[30] It is also important to follow these patients for progressive deformity, screw failure, or fractures that can result from seemingly trivial falls.

Hydrocephalus

One-hundred years ago, Walter Dandy observed hydrocephalus in a patient with chondrodysplasia and discussed its etiology as secondary to the obstruction of CSF flow in the posterior fossa.[33] Since then, most evidence indicates that children with achondroplasia develop hydrocephalus primarily due to venous sinus hypertension secondary to stenosis of the jugular foramen and in some cases, the jugular vein at the thoracic inlet.[34–36] This increase in intracranial venous pressure can limit venous CSF absorption through the superior sagittal sinus, resulting in possible increased intracranial pulse pressure and ventriculomegaly.[35] Additionally, obstruction to blood outflow through the jugular veins can promote collateral venous circulation through the emissary veins,[37,38] leading to the prominence of superficial veins of the scalp and skull in these children. We think that the balance between venous outflow through these accessory pathways and elevation of intracranial venous pressure resulting from jugular foraminal stenosis and the resultant intracranial pressure wave and CSF reabsorption (through pressure gated mechanism at the arachnoid granulations) will ultimately dictate the likelihood of progressive ventriculomegaly.

More recent evidence suggests that children with achondroplasia may also suffer from noncommunicating hydrocephalus.[16,39–41] We previously observed improvement in CSF flow on cine MRI studies in several children with FMS after CMD surgery, suggesting the possibility that at least in some patients, a relative impediment to CSF flow at the craniocervical junction may lead to hydrocephalus.[16,39] In a follow-up to this study, we demonstrated that many of these patients with progressive ventriculomegaly and FMS a have an improvement in their signs of ventriculomegaly after CMD and did not require a ventriculoperitoneal shunt (VPS).[40] Furthermore, Swift and colleagues described successful stabilization in ventriculomegaly following endoscopic third ventriculostomy (ETV) in 3 patients with achondroplasia and FMS.[41] In total, multiple etiologies may play a role in the development of hydrocephalus in these children.

Evaluation

When evaluating for hydrocephalus in children with achondroplasia, it is important to differentiate between macrocephaly with ventriculomegaly under normal pressure and clinically significant progressive ventriculomegaly. All children with achondroplasia should have head growth monitored with serial head circumference measurements, plotted on head circumference charts specific for children with achondroplasia.[42] Additionally, children should be evaluated for the signs and symptoms of increased intracranial pressure. Given that there is a delay in sutural maturation in achondroplasia, head circumference and fontanelle measurements should continue to at least 5 to 6 years of age.[12] Hydrocephalus in these children most often presents insidiously with mild symptoms such as lethargy, irritability, and headache. Patients with enlarging head circumference as well as signs or symptoms of increased intracranial pressure should be investigated with intracranial imaging, either ultrasonography or MR imaging. Although cranial ultrasonography is thought to be an adequate screening test in a child with an open fontanelle, MRI allows for the assessment of ventricular size, presence of jugular foraminal stenosis, CSF outflow obstruction, presence of a stenotic foramen magnum, as well as the evidence of transependymal CSF flow.

Surgical management

Most of the children with achondroplasia and mild to moderately enlarged ventricles have spontaneous arrestment of their ventriculomegaly and do not require treatment.[19,43] Rather, ventriculoperitoneal shunting should be reserved for symptomatic patients with enlarging ventricles. King and colleagues reported that 4.3% of children with achondroplasia under their care required shunting.[29] Determining which patients need intervention can be challenging and should be selected judicially, especially given the high rate of VPS complications and revisions in this patient population. Although an Evans ratio (maximum ventricular width divided by the maximum internal diameter of the skull) of at least 0.30 has been used to diagnose hydrocephalus in individuals of average stature, results from our recent case series suggest that children with a ratio of at least 0.50 may be more likely to be symptomatic and potentially require surgical intervention.[40]

Placement of a VPS may not always be necessary to treat symptomatic progressive hydrocephalus in children with achondroplasia. In a specific subgroup of patients with both progressive ventriculomegaly and symptomatic FMS, we previously showed that CMD can improve or arrest progressive ventriculomegaly and decrease the need for VPS placement.[16,40] ETV has also successfully been used to improve ventriculomegaly in a few patients with FMS.[41] Future clinical trials will be valuable for assessing the role of ETV for the treatment of progressive ventriculomegaly and raised intracranial pressure in patients without symptomatic FMS.

SUMMARY

Achondroplasia is associated with several serious neurologic conditions that require an early comprehensive evaluation and proactive management by a pediatric neurosurgeon and multidisciplinary team. Increasing knowledge of the natural history of these conditions, greater surgical experience, as well advancements in imaging protocol, have led to more refined indications for neurosurgery in children with achondroplasia.

Nevertheless, there are many nuanced characteristics to consider when deliberating surgery in these children, and these need to be assessed carefully minimizing unnecessary procedures and operative morbidity. Future clinical trials, such as the evaluation of ETV for hydrocephalus, will be valuable for determining the most efficacious treatment strategies in these children.

CLINICS CARE POINTS

- Cervicomedullary decompression is a safe and effective procedure in patients with symptomatic FMS.

- Patients with symptomatic FMS are best evaluated with flexion-extension CINE-gated MRI studies.

- Many patients with achondroplasia will have stable arrested hydrocephalus or asymptomatic ventriculomegaly that do not require a CSF diversion procedure.

ACKNOWLEDGEMENTS

This work was partially supported by the Vera and Paul Guerin Family Chair in Pediatric Neurosurgery and the Smidt Family Foundation.

DISCLOSURE

The authors have nothing to disclose.

REFERENCES

1. Horton WA, Hall JG, Hecht JT. Achondroplasia. Lancet 2007;370(9582):162–72.
2. Moffitt KB, Abiri OO, Scheuerle AE, et al. Descriptive epidemiology of selected heritable birth defects in Texas. Birth Defects Res A Clin Mol Teratol 2011; 91(12):990–4.
3. Waller DK, Correa A, Vo TM, et al. The population-based prevalence of achondroplasia and thanatophoric dysplasia in selected regions of the US. Am J Med Genet A 2008;146(18):2385–9.
4. Coi A, Santoro M, Garne E, et al. Epidemiology of achondroplasia: a population-based study in Europe. Am J Med Genet A 2019;179(9). ajmg.a. 61289.
5. Rimoin DL, Hughes GN, Kaufman RL, et al. Endochondral ossification in Achondroplastic Dwarfism. N Engl J Med 1970;283(14):728–35.
6. White KK, Bompadre V, Goldberg MJ, et al. Best practices in the evaluation and treatment of foramen magnum stenosis in achondroplasia during infancy. Am J Med Genet A 2016;170(1):42–51.
7. Hecht JT, Butler IJ. Neurologic morbidity associated with achondroplasia. J Child Neurol 1990;5(2):84–97.
8. Pauli RM, Scott CI, Wassman ER, et al. Apnea and sudden unexpected death in infants with achondroplasia. J Pediatr 1984;104(3):342–8.
9. Hecht JT, Francomano CA, Horton WA, et al. Mortality in achondroplasia. Am J Hum Genet 1987;41(3): 454–64.
10. Hecht JT, Horton WA, Reid CS, et al. Growth of the foramen magnum in achondroplasia. Am J Med Genet 1989;32(4):528–35.
11. Simmons K, Hashmi SS, Scheuerle A, et al. Mortality in babies with achondroplasia: revisited. Birth Defects Res A Clin Mol Teratol 2014;100(4):247–9.
12. Pauli RM. Achondroplasia: a comprehensive clinical review. Orphanet J Rare Dis 2019;14(1):1.
13. Trotter TL, Hall JG. Health supervision for children with achondroplasia. Pediatrics 2005;116(3):771–83.
14. Reid CS, Pyeritz RE, Kopits SE, et al. Cervicomedullary compression in young patients with achondroplasia: value of comprehensive neurologic and respiratory evaluation. J Pediatr 1987;110(4):522–30.
15. Hunter AGW, Bankier A, Rogers JG, et al. Medical complications of achondroplasia: a multicentre patient review. J Med Genet 1998;35(9):705–12.
16. Mukherjee D, Pressman BD, Krakow D, et al. Dynamic cervicomedullary cord compression and alterations in cerebrospinal fluid dynamics in children with achondroplasia: review of an 11-year surgical case series. J Neurosurg Pediatr 2014; 14(3):238–44.
17. Bagley CA, Pindrik JA, Bookland MJ, et al. Cervicomedullary decompression for foramen magnum stenosis in achondroplasia. J Neurosurg Pediatr 2006; 104(3):166–72.
18. Shimony N, Ben-Sira L, Sivan Y, et al. Surgical treatment for cervicomedullary compression among infants with achondroplasia. Child's Nerv Syst 2015; 31(5):743–50.
19. Rimoin DL. Invited editorial: cervicomedullary junction compression in infants with achondroplasia: when to perform neurosurgical decompression. Am J Hum Genet 1995;56:824–7.
20. Pauli RM, Horton VK, Glinski LP, et al. Prospective assessment of risks for cervicomedullary-junction compression in infants with achondroplasia. Am J Hum Genet 1995;56(3):732–44.
21. Nelson MA. Kyphosis and lumbar stenosis in achondroplasia. Basic Life Sci 1988;48:305–11.
22. Srikumaran U, Woodard EJ, Leet AI, et al. Pedicle and spinal canal parameters of the lower thoracic and lumbar vertebrae in the achondroplast population. Spine (Phila Pa 1976) 2007;32(22):2423–31.
23. Siebens AA, Hungerford DS, Kirby NA. Curves of the achondroplastic spine: a new hypothesis. Johns Hopkins Med J 1978;142(6):205–10.
24. Schkrohowsky JG, Hoernschemeyer DG, Carson BS, et al. Early presentation of spinal stenosis in achondroplasia. J Pediatr Orthop 2007;27(2):119–22.
25. Kopits SE. Thoracolumbar kyphosis and lumbosacral hyperlordosis in achondroplastic children. Basic Life Sci 1988;48:241–55.
26. Sciubba DM, Noggle JC, Marupudi NI, et al. Spinal stenosis surgery in pediatric patients with achondroplasia. J Neurosurg 2007;106(5 SUPPL):372–8.

27. White KK, Sucato DJ. Spinal deformity in the skeletal dysplasias. Curr Opin Orthop 2006;17(6):499–510.

28. Hecht JT, Butler IJ, Scott CI. Long-term neurological sequelae in achondroplasia. Eur J Pediatr 1984; 143(1):58–60.

29. King JAJ, Vachhrajani S, Drake JM, et al. Neurosurgical implications of achondroplasia: A review. J Neurosurg Pediatr 2009;4(4):297–306.

30. White KK, White KK, Bober MB, et al. Best practice guidelines for management of spinal disorders in skeletal dysplasia. Orphanet J Rare Dis 2020; 15(1):161.

31. Morgan DF, Young RF. Spinal neurological complications of achondroplasia. Results of surgical treatment. J Neurosurg 1980;52(4):463–72.

32. Ain MC, Shirley ED, Pirouzmanesh A, et al. Postlaminectomy kyphosis in the skeletally immature achondroplast. Spine (Phila Pa 1976) 2006;31(2):197–201.

33. Dandy WE. Hydrocephalus in Chondrodystrophy. Johns Hopkins Hosp Bull 1921;32:5–10.

34. Brühl K, Stoeter P, Wietek B, et al. Cerebral spinal fluid flow, venous drainage and spinal cord compression in achondroplastic children: Impact of magnetic resonance findings for decompressive surgery at the cranio-cervical junction. Eur J Pediatr 2001;160(1):10–20.

35. Steinbok P, Hall J, Flodmark O. Hydrocephalus in achondroplasia: the possible role of intracranial venous hypertension. J Neurosurg 1989;71(C):42–8.

36. Pierre-Kahn A, Hirsch JF, Renier D, et al. Hydrocephalus and achondroplasia: a study of 25 observations. Pediatr Neurosurg 1980;7(4):205–19.

37. Mueller SM, Reinertson JE. Reversal of emissary vein blood flow in achondroplastic dwarfs. Neurology 1980;30(7):769–72.

38. Moritani T, Aihara T, Oguma E, et al. Magnetic resonance venography of achondroplasia: correlation of venous narrowing at the jugular foramen with hydrocephalus. Clin Imaging 2006;30(3):195–200.

39. Danielpour M, Wilcox WR, Alanay Y, et al. Dynamic cervicomedullary cord compression and alterations in cerebrospinal fluid dynamics in children with achondroplasia: Report of four cases. J Neurosurg Pediatr 2007;107(6):504–7.

40. Kashanian A, Chan J, Mukherjee D, et al. Improvement in ventriculomegaly following cervicomedullary decompressive surgery in children with achondroplasia and foramen magnum stenosis. Am J Med Genet A 2020;8. ajmg.a.61640.

41. Swift D, Nagy L, Robertson B. Endoscopic third ventriculostomy in hydrocephalus associated with achondroplasia. J Neurosurg Pediatr 2011; 9(January):73–81.

42. Horton WA, Rotter JI, Rimoin DL, et al. Standard growth curves for achondroplasia. J Pediatr 2009; 93(3):435–8.

43. Yamada H, Nakamura S, Tajima M, et al. Neurological manifestations of pediatric achondroplasia. J Neurosurg 1981;54:49–57.

Neurosurgical Evaluation and Management of Adults with Achondroplasia

Mari L. Groves, MD[a],*, Alon Kashanian, BS[b], Moise Danielpour, MD[b],
James A. Stadler III, MD[c]

KEYWORDS

- Achondroplasia • Spinal stenosis • Cervicomedullary compression • Foramen magnum stenosis
- Hydrocephalus

KEY POINTS

- Incidence of spinal stenosis has been estimated as high as nearly 90% in patients with achondroplasia with 10% to 40% of patients requiring surgery throughout their lifetime.
- Although most children outgrow and improve their thoracolumbar kyphosis, 10% to 15% of patients will develop a fixed, rigid spinal deformity that may lead to spinal cord compression with progressive clinical decline over the course of their life
- Neurologic sequelae from prior foramen magnum decompression and CSF diversion procedures should be considered when patients present with new-onset neurologic signs or symptoms.

INTRODUCTION

Skeletal dysplasias encompass more than 400 conditions that affect bone development, neurologic function, and growth of the cartilage, of which achondroplasia is the most common. Achondroplasia affects approximately 1 in 25,000 to 30,000 individuals, with more than 250,000 people affected worldwide.[1–3] Changes within the fibroblast growth factor receptor 3 (FGFR3) are inherited through an autosomal dominant pattern, but approximately 80% of cases are due to new sporadic mutations in the FGFR3 gene.[2]

Patients with achondroplasia may present with a variety of neurologic concerns during early childhood, including ventriculomegaly and hydrocephalus, foramen magnum compression, and thoracolumbar kyphosis. This review provides an update on the neurosurgical evaluation and management of these conditions in adults with achondroplasia.

DISCUSSION

Cervical, Thoracic, and Lumbar Stenosis

Understanding spinal development is important in the contextual understanding of why patients with achondroplasia develop spinal stenosis. Spinal growth and development occurs through ossification of synchondroses, or "growth plates"; these are cartilaginous joints primarily found in the developing skeleton and have the potential for growth until ossification occurs. Spinal growth first starts at the thoracolumbar region in the developing fetus and then progresses in a cranial and caudal direction during early development. The spine has both primary and secondary ossification centers that are oblique in nature. Growth along these

[a] Division of Pediatric Neurosurgery, Johns Hopkins Hospital, 600 N Wolfe Street, Phipps 556, Baltimore, MD 21287, USA; [b] Maxine Dunitz Neurosurgical Institute, Cedars-Sinai Medical Center, 127 South San Vicente Boulevard, 6th Floor #A6600, Los Angeles, CA 90048, USA; [c] Department of Neurological Surgery, University of Wisconsin School of Medicine and Public Health, 600 Highland Avenue, Madison, WI 53792, USA
* Corresponding author.
E-mail address: mgroves2@jhmi.edu
Twitter: @AlonKashanian (A.K.); @m_danielpour (M.D.); @stadler_md (J.A.S.)

Neurosurg Clin N Am 33 (2022) 25–35
https://doi.org/10.1016/j.nec.2021.09.011
1042-3680/22/© 2021 Elsevier Inc. All rights reserved.

centers allows for increase in the spinal canal in all dimensions as well as pedicle growth.[4–6] Typical maturation occurs until the synchondroses fuse at around 6 to 8 years of age, at which point the spine has reached its maximal neural canal width. Accelerated maturation of the synchondrosis leads to early ossification with resultant shortened pedicles and an overall narrowed spinal canal.[6] Vertebral body height, or longitudinal growth, continues to occur along the epiphyseal plates until around 18 to 20 years of age.

For patients with achondroplasia, spinal stenosis may occur in widespread fashion. Adult spinal disease differs from that of adolescents in that congenital spinal stenosis is exacerbated by degenerative changes of the spine. Hypertrophic changes within the discoligamentous complex further constrict the already narrowed diameter of the spinal canal. For purposes of the discussion we discuss regional spinal stenosis and specific implications for management and care.

Evaluation

Incidence of spinal stenosis has been estimated between 20% and 89% in patients with achondroplasia with 10% to 40% of patients requiring surgery throughout their lifetime.[7–11] Spinal stenosis may occur at any level and can be seen due to concurrent degenerative spondylosis and ligamentum flavum hypertrophy, which further tightens an already stenotic canal.[12] In addition, in the thoracolumbar spine, any residual focal kyphosis and compensatory lumbar hyperlordosis may exacerbate symptoms seen in this population.[8,13] To address the symptomatic level, careful attention must be given to localizing signs and symptoms as radiographically the entire spine may look quite stenotic.

Stenosis of the cervical spine may present with cervical myelopathy such as upper motor neuron symptoms such as gait disturbance, proximal weakness of the lower extremities, hyperreflexia, sphincter dysfunction, clonus, and a positive Babinski reflex.[14] In addition, focal signs and symptoms may arise within the neck such as pain and stiffness, radicular symptoms in the upper extremities with pain and numbness, distal weakness in the hand intrinsic musculature, and loss of hand dexterity. Thoracic stenosis may present with similar symptoms such as claudication, lower extremity weakness, and sensory changes that typically occur within the truncal area and diffusely extend into the lower extremities. Unlike cervical stenosis, thoracic stenosis does not have associated neck or upper extremity symptoms. Lumbar stenosis most commonly presents with signs of neurogenic claudication, such as lower limb weakness (proximal weakness greater than distal) or cramping in the back, buttock, or legs, which is typically relieved with forward leaning or squatting.[14]

If spinal stenosis is suspected, whole neuroaxis imaging including the cervical, thoracic, and lumbar spine should be considered given the propensity for widespread stenosis. Standard MRI protocols should provide relevant information regarding degree of stenosis and loss of cerebrospinal space (CSF) space. Up to two-thirds of patients may have some degree of T2 signal change and myelomalacia without concurrent stenosis at the level of the foramen magnum or upper cervical spine[15]; this might indicate prior compression, and the clinical significance is not well understood. MRI also helps assess facet hypertrophy, thickening of the ligamentum flavum, and concurrent disk herniation or protrusion. Imaging may show progression of degenerative processes including disk narrowing, bulging, enfolding and thickening of the ligamentum flavum, as well as facet osteoarthritis (**Fig. 1**). With progressive disease there can be a combination of disk protrusion, ligamentum flavum, and facet joints that encroach on the spinal canal that exacerbates the already narrowed bony canal. The further progressive narrowing and obliteration of CSF space may lead to quicker compromise of the neural elements and clinical symptoms.[12]

For patients who have had prior CSF diversion or foramen magnum decompression, cranial imaging can also help rule out any insidious disorders or other neurologic areas of concern. Computed tomography (CT) helps provide information on bony anatomy. In general, pedicle morphologies are generous and provide favorable targets for posterior instrumentation if indicated. In patients who have had previous instrumentation, metal artifact may obstruct areas of possible stenosis, and as such, CT myelography may help supplement information on adjacent segment disease or recurrent stenosis through areas of prior decompression and fusion. In patients with prior surgical decompression and fusion, CT imaging will also help determine any areas of pseudoarthrosis that may act as a pain generator.

Upright radiographs help give an overall assessment of the patient's global spinal alignment and as such, Posterior/Anterior (PA) and lateral scoliosis films should be obtained. In the past few decades, the correlation between sagittal spinal and pelvic parameters and the physiology and pathophysiology of disease in the average stature population has been well described.[16–19] Briefly for review, overall sagittal balance relies on equilibrium between thoracic kyphosis (TK), lumbar

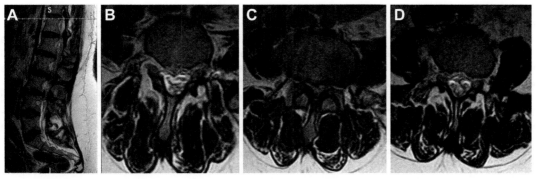

Fig. 1. Patient with Achondroplasia and multilevel spinal stenosis (A). Axial images show preserved CSF space above and below the diskoligamentous level (B & D). However, at the level of the disk and facet (C), overgrowth is seen that significantly constricts and narrows the already stenotic neural canal width; this may occur at multiple levels leading to progressive neurologic symptoms.

lordosis (LL), and pelvic anatomy leading to the minimum energy expenditure. Spinal and pelvic balance and gross orientation are important for spinal biomechanics and disease progression in the average stature population. In the average stature population, normal TK ranges between 20° and 50°, thoracolumbar junction is 0° and 10°, LL is on average 40° to 60°, and pelvic tilt is less than 20°. There are significant differences in sagittal parameters when comparing patients of average stature and patients with achondroplasia. In general, patients with achondroplasia showed thoracolumbar hyperkyphosis and lumbar hyperlordosis.[20] In addition, they have a more horizontal sacrum with posterior deviation of the hip joint that is likely compensatory for hip flexion contractures. Hong and colleagues[20] also showed that both lumbar hyperlordosis and thoracolumbar kyphosis were found to be related to increased pain scores.

Surgical management

Approximately one-third of patients with achondroplasia will develop symptomatic spinal stenosis requiring surgical intervention in their lifetime.[7,8,21] Patients with skeletal dysplasia often have multiple medical comorbidities and have increased perioperative complications. White and colleagues discussed in their "Best Practice Guidelines for Management of Spinal Disorders in Skeletal Dysplasia" that progressive signs and symptoms of spinal stenosis may cause reduced physical function (2006). In these instances, surgical decompression should be considered where nonoperative measures have failed to prevent progressive disease.

Surgical indications for adults are similar to those in the pediatric population. Neurologic imaging will often show some degree of significant spinal stenosis throughout the neuraxis. Localization

can be challenging to identify the appropriate area of stenosis. Surgeons should pay attention to areas of stenosis with underlying cord signal change, indicating some degree of edema or vascular compromise, because these typically will indicate areas that require decompression. Obliteration or loss of CSF space surrounding the spinal cord or nerve roots may be seen in some patients with achondroplasia. However, widespread decompression should be avoided in favor of targeted decompression for areas of clinical concern.

A comprehensive examination is necessary to evaluate the appropriate level of stenosis. Presence of progressive signs or symptoms of chronic spinal cord compression such as weakness, bowel or bladder dysfunction, hyperreflexia or hypertonia, spastic gait, or clonus are important markers of stenosis. In addition, chronic nerve root compression with neurogenic claudication, weakness or sensory disturbance in a radicular pattern, or hyporeflexia may also help point the examiner to the appropriate level of symptomatic spinal compression.

Surgical techniques Spinal procedures should take into consideration any prior surgeries, overall alignment, and number of spinal levels involved. Decompression alone may be considered in patients with relatively normal sagittal and pelvic alignment if only a few spinal levels are involved. However, posterior instrumentation and fusion should be considered if more than 5 spinal levels are involved, if the decompression spans the cervicothoracic junction or thoracolumbar junction, or if the global alignment is such that posterior destabilization may lead to worsening kyphosis and subsequent anterior compression. Without stabilization, those patients will be at high risk for progression or adjacent segment disease requiring revision surgery with fusion and stabilization (**Fig. 2**).

Surgical techniques for patients with achondroplasia largely mirror that of the average stature population. Given the congenital narrowing of the canal, posterior approaches have been favored for multilevel decompression over anterior approaches. Although there are no contraindications for anterior approaches, care should be taken to fully assess the levels needed for decompression. Laminectomies over multiple levels may be accomplished through either the ultrasonic bone curette (BoneScalpel) or high-speed drill. Care must be taken to incise the bone only, and if no fusion or arthrodesis is planned, to take less than 50% of the facet joints. In addition, ensuring adequate decompression without compromising the pars articularis must be planned carefully to avoid destabilization. Given the very thin dura, care should be taken to avoid entering the dura during decompression. Use of the bone scalpel has been shown to have improved outcomes with lower incidences of durotomy.[22] Hypertrophic joints and calcified ligamentous flavum may be fused to the dura, and care should be taken when dissecting this area.

In those cases in which internal fixation and fusion are needed, lateral mass screws are placed within the cervical facets and pedicle screws are used in the thoracic and lumbar spine. Typical external landmarks are comparable to the average stature population and can be confirmed on fluoroscopy or radiography. Although the overall pedicle length is shortened, in general, the pedicles are typically generous in width and can accommodate larger-diameter screws. Intraoperative neuromonitoring including somatosensory evoked potentials and transcranial electrical simulation-induced motor evoked potentials are used to monitor cord function throughout the duration of surgery. In cases in which patients have underlying neurologic dysfunction or significant cervical stenosis, prepositioning and postpositioning monitoring should be used to ensure stability.

Surgical complications Several series have reported increased rates of complications as high as 48% to 61%.[23–26] In addition, revision surgical rates have been reported as high as 36%. Patients with achondroplasia may have atypical collagen formation, which can lead to friable connective tissues, thus predisposing patients to dural tears and

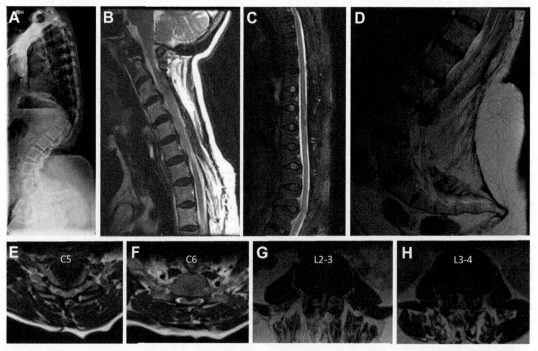

Fig. 2. A 52-year-old woman with achondroplasia who first underwent pan-spinal laminectomies at the ages 30 and 32 years now presented with some mild claudication-type symptoms, but still was fairly active at 30 minutes per day. Despite laminectomies from C3 through L5, she has had relatively little progressive thoracolumbar kyphosis on standing scoliosis films (A) or through pan-spinal MRI (B–D). Given progressive mechanical pain as well as worsening cervical (E, F) and thoracolumbar (G, H) stenosis. She ultimately underwent both cervical stabilization and facet overgrowth thoracolumbar fusion.

wound healing complications.[27–29] Dural tears are one of the most common complications seen following surgery, as commonly as 36% to 55%.[23–25,27,29,30] The dura is typically thin and transparent and may be densely adherent to the overlying ligamentum flavum and periosteum.[31] In addition, hyperplastic intervertebral disks and ligamentum flavum are associated with decreased epidural fat leading to less protection for the neural elements than normal. In multiple series, dural tears are consistently the most common complication and should be anticipated. In patients with prior surgery primary repair of the dural tear may not be possible. As such, this complication should be anticipated and involvement with a plastic surgery team can augment closure with rotational myofascial flaps to help contain development of a pseudomeningocele.[32,33]

Other complications include neurologic changes or loss (12%–23%) and infection (8%–9%).[23–25,27] Patients with achondroplasia may be more susceptible to variability in nonanatomical factors such as blood pressure management or anesthetic technique that can augment perfusion to the spinal cord during surgery.[34] Other medical complications should be anticipated but are less common and include deep venous thrombosis and pulmonary embolism, urinary tract infections, and gastrointestinal complications.

Thoracolumbar Kyphosis

Thoracolumbar kyphosis is commonly seen during infancy as discussed in elsewhere in this issue. However, although seen in 90% in children younger than 1 year, there is improvement in most children by 3 years of age.[35–38] However, some degree of kyphosis may persist in up to 30% of children and adolescents.[39,40] If the kyphosis is significant enough, abnormal physiologic forces can be placed on the outer epiphyseal ring, which can progress to decrease the growth of the anterior column. Over time this may lead to a fixed deformity in approximately 10% to 15% of adults.[38] If not corrected, progressive forces may lead to worsening kyphosis and spinal compression due to diskoligamentous and bony compression. The degree of severity of thoracolumbar deformity and spinal stenosis influences the incidence of neurologic symptoms.[8,38,41–43] Bailey[44] reported that 72% of achondroplastic patients with neurologic symptoms had sagittal kyphosis or spinal stenosis. Patients who present with acute angular thoracolumbar kyphosis, progressive kyphosis, or a kyphotic deformity greater than 60° to 70° should be considered for surgical decompression and deformity correction.[45,46]

Clinical presentation of thoracolumbar kyphosis is similar to that of patients with stenosis of the thoracolumbar spine and can result from draping or tethering of the spinal cord over the kyphotic apex.[32,33] Persistent compression may lead to ongoing damage of the spinal cord and can cause progressive clinical symptoms; these may include worsening claudication, difficulty walking, heaviness of the legs, and paraplegia, numbness, or tingling. These symptoms may improve initially with rest, but they will typically become progressive and permanent.

Iatrogenic causes for progressive sagittal deformity and ongoing kyphosis can be considered due to destabilization of the vertebral column. However, postlaminectomy kyphosis is not typically seen in skeletally mature patients who have undergone decompression alone and is more commonly described in skeletally immature patients who have undergone decompression. Patients who have had a greater length or involvement of spinal levels requiring decompression as well as laminectomies in the lower thoracic or lumbar spine may also have a higher incidence of progressive kyphosis development.[47] This higher incidence is hypothesized to occur due to loss of the posterior ligamentous tension band thus reducing posterior stability and exacerbating the anterior stressors. These forces are also likely worse if patients already have an underlying thoracolumbar kyphosis.[45]

Evaluation

Overall global alignment and pelvic parameters should be considered when evaluating patients with thoracolumbar kyphosis. Standing radiographs should be obtained to help characterize the patient's sacral slope, pelvic tilt (PT), and pelvic incidence. Furthermore, pelvic parameters can influence global spinal alignment with changes in LL, TK, as well as cervical alignment (**Fig. 3**). Several studies have shown that in the average stature population spinopelvic parameters are important contributors to back pain. Glassman and colleagues[48] first reported the relationship between global alignment of the sagittal vertical axis and pain. Patients may also undergo lateral thoracolumbar film taken in hyperextension over a bolster to help predict the degree the flexibility of the curve and predicted degree of correction (**Fig. 4**).

Patients with achondroplasia have a lower pelvic incidence than an average stature population. A lower PT indicates a more horizontal sacrum with posterior deviation of the hip joint. Patients may also be prone to flexion contractures of their hamstrings.[20] Pelvic orientation is also effected

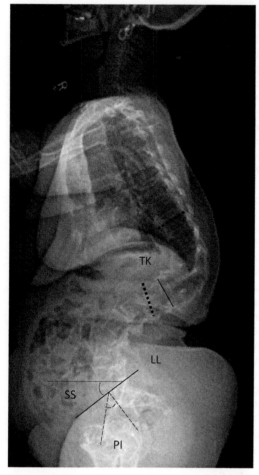

Fig. 3. Standing radiographs should be obtained to help characterize the patient's sacral slope (SS), pelvic tilt (PT), and pelvic incidence (PI). Sacral slope (*narrow dash*) is defined as the angle between the sacral end plate and the horizontal. Pelvic incidence (*wide dash*) is defined as the angle between a line perpendicular to the sacral end plate and the line joining the middle of the sacral plate and hip axis. Pelvic tilt is defined as the angle between the vertical and the line joining the middle of the sacral end plate and hip axis. Pelvic parameters can influence global spinal alignment with changes in lumbar lordosis (*solid line*), thoracic kyphosis (*dotted line*), as well as cervical alignment. Patients with achondroplasia have a lower pelvic incidence than an average stature population. A lower PT indicates a more horizontal sacrum with posterior deviation of the hip joint.

by the development of a smaller sacrum. Prior studies have also shown a higher lumbar hyperlordosis in a typically compensatory manner to compensate for the pelvic orientation.[20,41] When considering spinal deformity correction, care should be taken to not change the global sagittal balance significantly because studies have also

shown that less LL may lead to spinal imbalance and increased pain severity.[20,41]

Radiographic imaging should include pan-spinal MRI to fully evaluate any additional areas of spinal stenosis and for surgical planning of the decompression and spinal fusion. Additional evaluation is comparable to workup for patients with spinal stenosis.

Surgical management

Surgical deformity correction and decompression for patients with achondroplasia and may be approached in a variety of ways. Deformity correction may be attempted either through a 2-stage, anterior/posterior correction or a single-stage, posterior correction alone. Spinal cord monitoring should be used for all spinal deformity surgeries. If there is a concern that the surgical procedure will be lengthy with the potential for significant blood loss, staging the procedure should be considered. Staging will allow adequate anesthesia resuscitation because intravascular volume may be underestimated due to small body size.[14] The thoracolumbar kyphosis is often rigid in nature and correction can carry higher risk, so a conservative approach may be prudent in certain patient populations.

The decision for the amount of correction should take into consideration the sagittal balance of the patient as well as other comorbidities that may make tolerating a longer, high-risk surgery less desirable. Sagittal balance is influenced, while standing, by thoracolumbar kyphosis, lumbar hyperlordosis, and contracture of the hip joints. In older patients, the lumbar hyperlordosis and hip flexion with relation to the pelvis are fixed, and so overcorrection of the kyphosis may not be compensated by the remaining lumbar spine.[20] If complete correction is not the goal, surgery may be tailored to optimize and weigh goals of neurologic decompression versus spinal deformity correction.

A staged procedure that considers direct correction of the anterior column allows for maximum deformity correction as well as access for anterior arthrodesis. Anterior-only approaches were historically favored with diskectomies and fibular strut grafts. As a stand-alone construct, these have fallen out of favor because they do not improve the superimposed spinal stenosis and can promote junctional disease if the kyphosis is not adequately corrected. Anterior approaches through the retroperitoneal space are now used to access to the anterior column and may include diskectomies alone or full resection of the wedged vertebrae. Anterior diskectomies or releases are performed for arthrodesis as well as deformity correction because they allow for greater

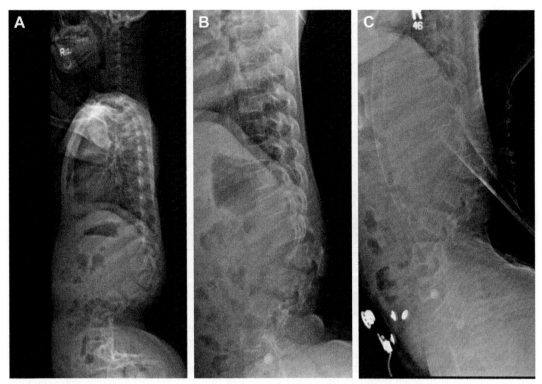

Fig. 4. Lateral standing scoliosis films should be obtained to evaluate the degree of kyphosis. Dynamic or provocative imaging may be helpful in assessing flexibility across thoracolumbar kyphosis and to help guide surgical planning; This may be done through either hyperextension films while lying prone (*B*) or hyperextending across a bolster (*C*) to determine the amount of correction possible without osteotomies. Often, wedged vertebrae are stiff and fixed deformities with minimal correction through positioning.

restoration of anterior column height. Releasing maneuvers also allow for indirect decompression and restoration of the anterior column through grafts placement. When planning a surgical deformity correction, restoration of height minimizes any additional forces on the spinal construct that would impair long-term rates of arthrodesis. Access may be more challenging due to relatively large iliac crests that may limit access to the retroperitoneal space, and this should be fully evaluated in person before surgical planning.

Staged approaches are then followed with a posterior approach that allows posterior decompression of the central and lateral recesses as well as supplementation with instrumentation. For patients with significant, fixed deformities, a staged procedure may allow for better access of a wedged vertebrae. One disadvantage of a staged technique is the potential morbidity of 2 procedures. With modern pedicle screw instrumentation, the enhanced rigidity of fixation in combination with a posterior arthrodesis alone may result in successful fusion without an anterior procedure.[41,49]

For posterior approaches to the spine, corrective maneuvers through posterior osteotomies can give access to the anterior spine and disk spaces, although this is generally more challenging because the shape of the laminae can make this access higher risk (**Fig. 5**). There is very little space to maneuver around the narrowed neural canal width, and so care must be taken to not excessively manipulate the thin dura. If the spinal cord is significantly draped over the anterior vertebrae, the risk of neurologic injury is also quite high.[32,33,41] Posterior decompression should extend to any areas of CSF obliteration both above and below the apical vertebrae because these areas have accelerated stenosis over time due to junctional changes. Surgical techniques are otherwise similar to those used for decompression and fusion as described earlier.

Surgical complication A recent analysis of syndromic scoliosis cases showed that rates of major complications were almost 3 times higher in patients with syndromic causes of scoliosis when compared with patients with idiopathic disease.[27]

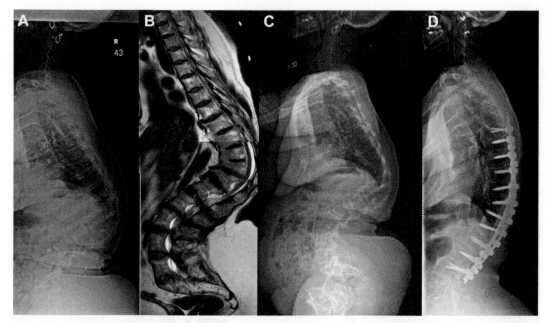

Fig. 5. Preoperative and postoperative imaging of 56-year-old patient with achondroplasia. She originally presented in 2005 with longstanding back and leg pain, numbness and tingling, and significant claudication over the previous several years; this had gradually worsened with time, and in 2016 both MRI and standing scoliosis films (*A, B*) demonstrated some progression of her kyphosis with early autofusion across the apex. Patient delayed surgery until 2020 when symptoms progressively worsened to where she had difficulty ambulating and had worsening bowel and bladder incontinence. Preoperative radiograph showed overall stable deformity. Standing scoliosis film demonstrates her acute angulation across the T10-T12 levels with compensatory hyperlordosis of her lumbar spine (*C*). Single-stage surgery using a posterior-only approach was used for decompression, correction, and spinal fusion (*D*).

Neurologic injury and pulmonary embolism were 2 more commonly observed major complications. Procedural and device-related complications were also more common. Although this patient population at large included other forms of syndromic spinal deformity, patients with achondroplasia comprised a total of 148 patients within the cohort.

Wang and colleagues[49] also described their series of patients who underwent posterior-only vertebral column resection for thoracolumbar kyphosis. Five patients (71%) had preoperative neurologic symptoms and improved postoperatively. However, surgical complications were quite high (%) and included rod breakages (43%), neurologic complications (28%), dural tears (14%), CSF leaks (14%), and proximal junction kyphosis (14%).

Recurrent Disorders

Hydrocephalus

Hydrocephalus development and cause in patients with achondroplasia is described in more detail elsewhere in this issue. Rates of shunting have decreased because stricter criteria have been used to differentiate ventriculomegaly from overt hydrocephalus. More contemporary series have seen shunting rates of 4.3% to 5.1%[50] compared with historical averages of 10% to 20%.[51] If hydrocephalus was treated with a shunt or endoscopic third ventriculostomy, patients should have routine follow-up with their neurosurgeons. Timing of follow-up imaging and clinical follow-up may vary depending on the age and clinical stability. As patients age, generally follow-up becomes more spread out on an as-needed basis. Adult patients should be aware of symptoms that may represent a shunt malfunction. Typical signs and symptoms may present with lethargy or tiredness, progressive headaches sometimes worse in the morning, swelling along the shunt tubing site, nausea or emesis, or difficulty with double vision. If patients have borderline significant stenosis at the foramen magnum or throughout their spine they may have progressive worsening neck or back pain as well. Patients should have a basic understanding of their shunt system in the event they travel from their home institution. In the modern era, a variety of devices and smart phone apps exist to consolidate shunt information including type of shunt, shunt setting if applicable, distal tubing location, prior surgeries, and representative imaging. Having this information may be helpful if there are questions or issues that arise during travel.

Patients who have required shunting in the past may be at risk for a variety of shunt-related issues as they age. Proximal or distal shunt malfunction may occur at any time, and vigilance should be maintained throughout a patient's life. Treating teams should never assume that the shunt is nonfunctional without first undergoing comprehensive assessment of the shunt system. Shunt systems should never be removed unless a stepwise approach has been completed to ensure safety that may include having a clamped system with normal intracranial pressures and lack of clinical symptoms.

Foramen magnum stenosis

Cervicomedullary stenosis remains a significant contributor to morbidity and mortality for children with achondroplasia.[52] The cause and full evaluation for compression has been further described elsewhere in this issue. Recurrence of foramen magnum stenosis may be seen at any time and should be fully evaluated in patients presenting with concerns of new neurologic symptoms. Rates of restenosis have been well described in the pediatric population at around 10% but have not been well defined for adults.[53] Signs and symptoms of cervicomedullary compression may include signs similar to cervical myelopathy such as weakness, lack of overall movement, asymmetric limb motion, as well as brainstem compression. Brainstem compression may manifest with gagging, coughing, worsening obstructive apnea, or central apneic events. Overnight sleep studies that assess for central and obstructive sleep apneas, hypoxia, and hypercapnia with electroencephalography should be considered for patients presenting with new neurologic signs or symptoms concerning for upper cervical or brainstem compression.

Surgical management of restenosis is challenging. As in the index case, patients have a significantly horizontal orientation of their foramen magnum.[53] Recurrent cases may have regrowth of the fibrous band at the base of the foramen magnum and calcification of this scar tissue. The risk and rate of CSF leak remain high. Care should be taken to evaluate for enough lateral decompression and to ensure that fibrous bands that may jut into the skull base are fully removed. Intraoperative monitoring should be considered because monitoring can provide critical feedback throughout both the positioning and surgical procedure. Ultrasonography may also be used as an adjunct to evaluate for adequate decompression via CSF pulsations surrounding the brainstem.

SUMMARY

In conclusion, neurosurgical concerns for patients with achondroplasia shift toward spinal stenosis disorders. However, common pediatric disorders including CSF diversion procedures as well as foramen magnum stenosis should be considered in the workup for global neurologic decline and localization of significant spinal stenosis may be challenging given widespread stenosis seen on typical imaging. When progressive neurologic symptoms are seen, surgical timing should be considered and weighed carefully with the severity of clinical presentation. Surgical risks remain higher across the board for patients with achondroplasia and are a significant concern for many patients. Preoperative planning should take into consideration unique anatomic factors to help anticipate and minimize complications when possible. A multidisciplinary approach is helpful to ensure the best patient outcomes.

CLINICS CARE POINTS

- Congenital stenosis may be significant throughout the cervical, thoracic, and/or lumbar spine. Imaging findings should be taken in context of clinical symptoms and presentation.
- Localization of clinical symptoms will help neurosurgeons identify the most symptomatic area of constriction in patients with significant pan-spinal stenosis.
- Thoracolumbar kyphosis spontaneously resolves in most infants. However, if persistent and nonresponsive to bracing, persistent kyphosis may become symptomatic into adulthood. Decompression and correction of this deformity should be considered in these patients who meet surgical criteria.
- Patients who have shunted hydrocephalus should have their shunt evaluated if presenting with insidious symptoms such as headaches or neck pain. Shunt malfunction should always be considered as part of the evaluation for new clinical decline and should be ruled out.
- Foramen magnum restenosis may occur in a delayed fashion, and decompression should be considered when patients present with cervical myelopathy with corollary imaging stenosis.

DISCLOSURE

The authors have nothing to disclose.

REFERENCES

1. Coi A, Santoro M, Garne E, et al. Epidemiology of achondroplasia: a population based study in Europe. Am J Med Genet A 2019;179(9):1791–8.
2. Horton WA, Hall JG, Hecht JT. Achondroplasia. Lancet 2007;370(9582):162–72.
3. Waller DK, Correa A, Vo TM, et al. The population-based prevalence of achondroplasia and thanatophoric dysplasia in selected regions of the US. Am J Med Genet A 2008;146(18):2385–9.
4. Nelson MA. Kyphosis and lumbar stenosis in achondroplasia. Basic Life Sci 1988;48:305–11.
5. O'Brien JP, Mehdian H. Relevant principles in the management of spinal disorders in achondroplasia. Basic Life Sci 1988;48:293–8.
6. Ponseti IV. Skeletal growth in achondroplasia. J Bone Joint Surg Am 1970;52:701–16.
7. Agabegi SS, Antekeier DP, Crawford AH, et al. Post-laminectomy kyphosis in an achondroplastic adolescent treated for spinal stenosis. Orthopedics 2008; 31:168.
8. Ain MC, Shirley ED, Pirouzmanesh A, et al. Postlaminectomy kyphosis in the skeletally immature achondroplast. Spine (Phila Pa 1976) 2006;31:197–201.
9. Hall G. New York: human achondroplasia. In: The natural history of achondroplasiavol. 3. New York, NY: Plenum Press; 1988. p. 3–9.
10. Hunter AG, Bankier A, Rogers JG, et al. Medical complications of achondroplasia: a multicentre patient review. J Med Genet 1998;35:705–12.
11. Streeten E, Uematsu S, Hurko O, et al. Extended laminectomy for spinal stenosis in achondroplasia. Basic Life Sci 1988;48:261–73.
12. Huet T, Cohen-Solal M, Laredo JD, et al. Lumbar spinal stenosis and disc alterations affect the upper lumbar spine in adults with achondroplasia. Sci Rep 2020;10(1):4699.
13. Thomeer RT, van Dijk JM. Surgical treatment of lumbar stenosis in achondroplasia. J Neurosurg 2002; 96(3 Suppl):292–7.
14. White KK, Sucato DJ. Spinal deformity in the skeletal dysplasias. Curr Opin Orthop 2006;17(6):499–510.
15. van Dijk JMC, Lubout CMA, Brouwer PA. Cervical high-intensity intramedullary lesions without spinal cord compression in achondroplasia. J Neurosurg Spine SPI 2007;6(4):304–8.
16. Boulay C, Tardieu C, Hecquet J, et al. Sagittal alignment of spine and pelvis regulated by pelvic incidence: standard values and prediction of lordosis. Eur Spine J 2006;15:415–22.
17. During J, Goudfrooij H, Keessen W, et al. Toward standards for posture. Postural characteristics of the lower back system in normal and pathologic conditions. Spine (Phila Pa 1976) 1985;10:83–7.
18. Farfan HF. The biomechanical advantage of lordosis and hip extension for upright activity. Man as compared with other anthropoids. Spine (Phila Pa 1976) 1978;3:336–42.
19. Giglio GC, Passariello R, Pagnotta G, et al. Anatomy of the lumbar spine in achondroplasia. Basic Life Sci 1988;48:227–39.
20. Hong JY, Suh SW, Modi HN, et al. Analysis of sagittal spinopelvic parameters in achondroplasia. Spine (Phila Pa 1976) 2011;36(18):E1233–9.
21. Hecht JT, Butler IJ, Scott CI. Long-term neurological sequelae in achondroplasia. Eur J Pediatr 1984; 143(1):58–60.
22. Bydon M, Macki M, Xu R, et al. Spinal decompression in achondroplastic patients using high-speed drill versus ultrasonic bone curette: technical note and outcomes in 30 cases. J Pediatr Orthop 2014; 34(8):780–6.
23. Ain MC, Chang TL, Schkrohowsky JG, et al. Rates of perioperative complications associated with laminectomies in patients with achondroplasia. J Bone Joint Surg Am 2008;90(2):295–8.
24. Carlisle ES, Ting BL, Abdullah MA, et al. Laminectomy in patients with achondroplasia: the impact of time to surgery on long-term function. Spine (Phila Pa 1976) 2011;36(11):886–92.
25. Vleggeert-Lankamp C, Eul WP. Surgical decompression of thoracic spinal stenosis in achondroplasia: indication and outcome: clinical article. J Neurosurg Spine 2012;17(2):164–72.
26. Wynne-Davies R, Walsh WK, Achondroplasia GJ, et al. Clinical variation and spinal stenosis. J Bone Joint Surg Br 1981;63B(4):508–15.
27. Chung AS, Renfree S, Lockwood DB, et al. Syndromic scoliosis: national trends in surgical management and inpatient hospital outcomes: a 12-year analysis. Spine (Phila Pa 1976) 2019; 44(22):1564–70.
28. Patel H, Cichos KH, Moon AS, et al. Patients with musculoskeletal dysplasia undergoing total joint arthroplasty are at increased risk of surgical site infection. Orthop Traumatol Surg Res 2019;105(7): 1297–301.
29. Shafi K, Lovecchio F, Sava M, et al. Complications and revisions after spine surgery in patients with skeletal dysplasia: have we improved? Glob Spine J 2021. 2192568221994786.
30. Pyeritz RE, Sack GH Jr, Udvarhelyi GB. Thoracolumbosacral laminectomy in achondroplasia: long-term results in 22 patients. Am J Med Genet 1987;28: 433–44.
31. Alexander E Jr. Significance of the small lumbar spinal canal: cauda equina compression syndromes due to spondylosis. 5. Achondroplasia. J Neurosurg 1969;31:513–9.

32. Misra SN, Morgan HW. Thoracolumbar spinal deformity in achondroplasia. Neurosurg Focus 2003; 14(1):e4.

33. Misra SN, Morgan HW, Sedler R. Lumbar myofascial flap for pseudomeningocele repair. Neurosurg Focus 2003;15(3):E13.

34. White KK, Bompadre V, Goldberg MJ, et al. Skeletal dysplasia management consortium. Best practices in peri-operative management of patients with skeletal dysplasia. Am J Med Genet A 2017;173(10): 2584–95.

35. Abousamra O, Shah SA, Heydemann JA, et al. Sagittal spinopelvic parameters in children with achondroplasia. Spine Deform 2019;7(1):163–70.

36. Ahmed M, El-Makhy M, Grevitt M. The natural history of thoracolumbar kyphosis in achondroplasia. Eur Spine J 2019;28(11):2602–7.

37. Borkhuu B, Nagaraju DK, Chan G, et al. Factors related to progression of thoracolumbar kyphosis in children with achondroplasia: a retrospective cohort study of forty-eight children treated in a comprehensive orthopaedic center. Spine (Phila Pa 1976) 2009;34:1699–705.

38. Kopits SE. Thoracolumbar kyphosis and lumbosacral hyperlordosis in achondroplastic children. Basic Life Sci 1988;48:241–55.

39. Hensinger RN. Kyphosis secondary to skeletal dysplasias and metabolic disease. Clin Orthop Relat Res 1977;(128):113–28.

40. Pauli RM, Breed A, Horton VK, et al. Prevention of fixed, angular kyphosis in achondroplasia. J Pediatr Orthop 1997;17:726–33.

41. Ain MC, Browne JA. Spinal arthrodesis with instrumentation for thoracolumbar kyphosis in pediatric achondroplasia. Spine (Phila Pa 1976) 2004;29: 2075–80.

42. Arlet V. Review point of view on the treatment of fixed thoracolumbar kyphosis in immature achondroplastic patient. Eur Spine J 2004;13:462–3.

43. Sarlak AY, Buluc L, Anik Y, et al. Treatment of fixed thoracolumbar kyphosis in immature achondroplastic patient: posterior column resection combined with segmental pedicle screw fixation and posterolateral fusion. Eur Spine J 2004;13:458–61.

44. Bailey JA. II. Orthopaedic aspects of achondroplasia. J Bone Joint Surg Am 1970;52:1285–301.

45. Lonstein JE. Treatment of kyphosis and lumbar stenosis in achondroplasia. Basic Life Sci 1988;48: 283–92.

46. Lutter LD, Longstein JE, Winter RB, et al. Anatomy of the achondroplastic lumbar canal. Clin Orthop Relat Res 1977;126:139–42.

47. Hallan DR, Mrowczynski OD, McNutt S, et al. Post-laminectomy kyphosis in achondroplasia patients: to concurrently fuse or not. Cureus 2020;12(5): e7966.

48. Glassman SD, Bridwell K, Dimar JR, et al. The impact of positive sagittal balance in adult spinal deformity. Spine (Phila Pa 1976) 2005;30:2024–9.

49. Wang H, Wang S, Wu N, et al. Posterior vertebral column resection (pVCR) for severe thoracolumbar kyphosis in patients with achondroplasia. Glob Spine J 2021. 2192568221989291.

50. Okenfuss E, Moghaddam B, Avins AL. Natural history of achondroplasia: a retrospective review of longitudinal clinical data. Am J Med Genet A 2020; 182(11):2540–51.

51. Pauli RM. Achondroplasia: a comprehensive clinical review. Orphanet J Rare Dis 2019;14(1):1.

52. Legare JM, Liu C, Pauli RM, et al. Achondroplasia Natural History Study (CLARITY): 60-year experience in cervicomedullary decompression in achondroplasia from four skeletal dysplasia centers. J Neurosurg Pediatr 2021;1–7.

53. Bagley CA, Pindrik JA, Bookland MJ, et al. Cervicomedullary decompression for foramen magnum stenosis in achondroplasia. J Neurosurg 2006,104(3 Suppl):166–72.

Anesthetic Concerns of Children With Skeletal Dysplasia

Mary C. Theroux, MD[1], Jeffrey W. Campbell, MD, MS, MBA[2],*

KEYWORDS

- Anesthesia • Intubation • Skeletal dysplasia • Morquio • Mucopolysaccharidoses

KEY POINTS

- Safe anesthetic techniques for children with skeletal dysplasia are impacted by the unique anatomy of the respiratory system, spine abnormalities, and unique body habitues of these children.
- Risk of spinal cord injury exists even when the surgical procedure is distant from the spine.
- Children with Morquio syndrome deserve special consideration both in regard to tracheal abnormalities from vascular compression as well as the risk of spinal cord injury from neuraxial anesthesia.

INTRODUCTION

Children with skeletal dysplasia present unique challenges for the anesthesiologist. Many require multiple surgeries, medical imaging, or other procedures that require various levels of anesthesia and the potential complications from the anesthesia itself range from respiratory arrest to spinal cord injury. Over many years of caring for hundreds of these children, we have gained experience to maximize the likelihood of safe, effective anesthesia care. These learnings include proper preoperative evaluations to identify difficult airways, nuances of airway management in the operating room, techniques to minimize spinal cord injury, use of regional anesthesia, and postoperative pain control. Although each skeletal dysplasia has its own nuance in terms of care, Morquio A requires particular attention to vascular compression of the trachea and the worry about the use of spinal or epidural anesthesia.

AIRWAY MANAGEMENT IN THE OPERATING ROOM

Modified induction to enhance safety: In patients who may be difficult to intubate and/or ventilate using a face mask, it is important to enhance safety during the induction of general anesthesia. To prevent losing the airway without an intravenous (IV) line in place, secure an IV with sedative doses of inhalational agents (eg, nitrous oxide and oxygen 50% each with 1%–2% of sevoflurane) rather than full anesthesia. Anticipate faster uptake of inhalational anesthetics and shorter time to loss of consciousness due to decreased functional residual capacity.

Patients with skeletal dysplasia should be carefully positioned on the operating table because of a high incidence of an abnormal cervical spine with or without instability.[1] Muscle relaxation during the Induction of general anesthetic can cause greater ligamentous laxity and worsen cervical spine alignment. Even without documented cervical instability, these patients should be positioned with a small "shoulder roll" such that the external auditory meatus and the clavicles are in alignment[2] (**Fig. 1**).

Children with significant cervical instability should be fused before proceeding with other elective surgeries to avoid complications such as the 18 years old with spondyloepiphyseal dysplasia who developed tetraparesis following a

[1] Department of Anesthesia, Nemours/AI duPont Hospital for Children, 1600 Rockland Road, Wilmington, DE 19803, USA; [2] Division of Pediatric Neurosurgery, Nemours/AI duPont Hospital for Children, 1600 Rockland Road, Wilmington, DE 19803, USA
* Corresponding author.
E-mail address: jeffrey.campbell@nemours.org

Neurosurg Clin N Am 33 (2022) 37–47
https://doi.org/10.1016/j.nec.2021.09.004
1042-3680/22/© 2021 Elsevier Inc. All rights reserved.

general anesthetic for a relatively minor procedure (removal of the hardware placed earlier for the surgical correction of genu valga).[3] If this is not possible, rigid cervical control is required, such as the Ferno vacuum splint (Frontier Medical [NZ] Ltd., Auckland, New Zealand) that was used by Tofield[4] to keep the head and neck alignment in a neutral and immobile position during a palatoplasty for a severe cleft palate in a 4 years old with spondyloepiphyseal dysplasia (**Fig. 2**). Monitoring evoked potentials during elective surgeries is an option we have used in similar situations to ensure the safety of the spinal cord, especially in procedures and imaging lasting more than an hour.

Upper airway management: Airway management is one of the most anxiety-provoking aspects of the perioperative care of children with skeletal dysplasia. This consists of 2 distinct components—upper airway management and intubating the trachea. Upper airway management can be more challenging because of abnormal head and neck morphology, large tongue, thickened oropharyngeal mucosa, and infiltrates originating from the primary disease (especially with mucopolysaccharidoses (MPS)) rendering abnormal shape and structure to laryngeal anatomy. In milder forms of obstruction, using an oral airway and carefully displacing tongue with a tongue blade may be sufficient. More difficult upper airways will need displacement of tongue by retraction using a gauze piece or a Magill Forceps[2] or rarely placing a suture through the tongue to act as a tether.[5] Ventilating the anesthetized patient using a face mask frequently require 2 skilled providers with one person maintaining the position of the mask over an oral airway (which anteriorly displaces tongue) whereas the second person squeezes the breathing bag. The use of an oral airway may not consistently improve the patency of the upper airway in children with skeletal dysplasia[6,7] so maintaining an adequate "jaw thrust" and manually displacing the tongue as described might be the only option. The use of muscle relaxants to improve mask ventilation requires good clinical judgment based on experience and is often aided by the patient's previous anesthetic records if available. Many of these patients have tracheobronchial malacia, especially those with Campomelic and Diastrophic dysplasia,[8] which can cause unexpected difficulty during induction of anesthesia. Careful and slow induction of anesthesia with the early placement of IV access enables the anesthesiologist to better evaluate and manage such difficulties.

Intubation of the trachea: In children with dwarfism, intubation can be particularly challenging.[3,9,10] Classically difficult airways such as in children with Pierre Robin[11] or Treacher Collins[12] feature micrognathia, an anteriorly placed larynx, and a tongue-based obstruction of the upper airway. Children with skeletal dysplasia additionally have narrow nasopharyngeal passages,[7] a large and redundant tongue, thickened mucosa,[13] short neck, and decreased mobility of the neck and temporomandibular joints, large pectus carinatum, and abnormalities of laryngeal, tracheal, and bronchial structures.[14] A further challenge is maintaining the head and neck in a neutral position during laryngoscopy and intubation to minimize the movement of the cervical spine.[3] Many of our patients (eg, metatrophic, Morquio, spondyloepiphyseal dysplasia congenita, and Kniest) have undergone prior cervical spine fusion resulting in varying degrees of difficulty with head and neck motion. Two children with the same type of skeletal dysplasia may present with different degrees of difficulty with their airway, partially related to the extent of cervical spine fusion.

Mucopolysaccharide storage disorders (MPSs) are a group of skeletal dysplasia that pose unique difficulties due to unexpected structural abnormalities encountered during airway management. Upper airway abnormalities and sleep-related airway obstruction are a leading cause of morbidity and mortality in these children.[15,16] The incidence of airway-related problems in patients with mucopolysaccharidosis of all types is 26%[17] with the incidence of obstructive sleep apnea (OSA) is as high as 85% in MPS VI.[18] Children with MPS demonstrate significant respiratory findings related to the accumulation of the deposits, in some instances complicated by respiratory muscle weakness from spinal cord myelopathy.[7] Common findings in this study were a narrow upper airway, enlarged tongue, and enlarged tonsils and adenoids. Diffuse thickening of soft tissues surrounding the larynx was seen in 9 of 21 patients. Baines and Keneally reported that 9 of 16 children with MPS had difficulty with airway management.[19] Similarly, Kempthorne and Brown described 5 of 9 children with MPS who had either difficulty maintaining a patent airway or had failed tracheal intubation.[20] One of the children suffered a hypoxic cardiac arrest whereas another child experienced severe bradycardia resulting from hypoxia but did not have an arrest.

Adolescents and adults with Morquio A are at particular risk because of tracheal obstruction at the thoracic outlet, predominately from a tortuous brachiocephalic artery (**Fig. 3**). Unrecognized, this can cause perioperative respiratory arrest or even sudden death without anesthesia.[21] We routinely

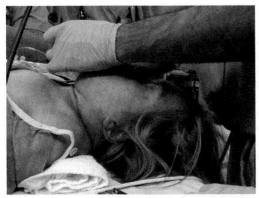

Fig. 1. A small shoulder role is in place to align the external auditory meatus with the clavicle. Note that there is no headrest in place.

image these patients with computed tomography (CT) angiograms of the chest finding most patients with some degree of tracheal narrowing, some severe enough to be symptomatic, or life threatening.[22] We have successfully performed a series of tracheal vascular reconstructions in these patients.[23]

Abnormal airway shape and size have been reported in children with MPS.[24] Shih[14] found abnormal vocal cords on CT in 7 of 13 patients (6 had abnormal shape and 7 had irregular densities). Eight of the 13 tracheas were abnormal, either U-shaped or worm-shaped. MPS patients with the history of OSA are at increased risk for airway emergencies during anesthesia, particularly during the induction of anesthesia and following extubation.[25]

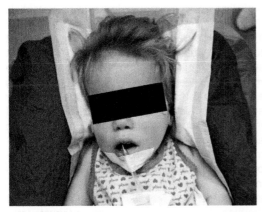

Fig. 2. Ferno vacuum splint (Frontier Medical [NZ] Ltd., Auckland, New Zealand) used to keep head and neck alignment in a neutral position in a child with spondyloepiphyseal dysplasia and unstable cervical spine during palatoplasty.

Cardiac involvement typically starts with valvular involvement of mitral and aortic valves manifesting in regurgitation and/or stenosis.[26] Cardiac lesions were more common with the accumulation of dermatan sulfate.[27] Coronary artery disease including intimal sclerosis[28] and complete obstruction of coronaries may occur as children become older, but has been reported in young children when the disease is severe.[29-31] Significant coronary artery disease may be suspected if the evidence of ischemia is present on a 12 lead electrocardiogram.[32] Myocardial dysfunction and cardiac failure have been reported in multiple studies.[30,31,33,34] Other reported abnormalities include the development of complete atrioventricular block in MPS types II, III, VI.[35-37] Pulmonary hypertension from chronic OSA is common in MPS patients as well.[18,38]

Finally, spinal cord compression and related myelopathy are common in MPS patients especially in Morquio syndrome and Maroteaux–Lamy syndrome (MPS IV A and MPS VI).[39-41] C1-C2 instability is far more common in Morquio syndrome whereas foramen magnum stenosis is more common in MPS VI.[42]

Difficult airway tools: A wide variety of devices and techniques are now available to help intubate tracheas of children who are difficult to intubate using conventional laryngoscopy. Among them, video laryngoscope with angulated blade (eg, GlideScope) and flexible fiberoptic bronchoscope (FOB) are the most likely to succeed consistently and reliably (**Fig. 9**).[43,44] Airway tools such as a light wand or lighted stylet are less useful because of limited ability to displace the soft tissue which obstructs the airway of these patients.

When conventional laryngoscopy is difficult, a GlideScope can be used if the patient's mouth can be opened sufficiently. Adequate displacement of the tongue alone will make the difference between success and failure. **Fig. 4** demonstrates displacing tongue anteriorly simply by using a piece of gauze followed by placement of Glidescope.[2] One disadvantage of GlideScope or similar instruments is the need to have a child either anesthetized or heavily sedated. For children who are not good candidates for deep sedation, FOB can be used with little or no sedation, with local anesthesia to the nasopharyngeal and oropharyngeal mucosa as needed. Sedative agents such as midazolam, dexmetatomidine and fentanyl are frequently used but with cautious titration. Patients remain seemingly awake and spontaneously breathing but tolerate the procedure relatively well. Careful attention to respiratory status when titrating sedation is necessary and should be given by someone other than the

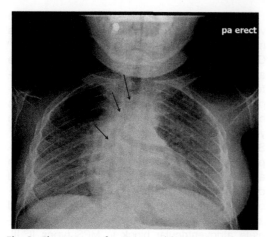

Fig. 3. Chest X-ray of a 15-year-old patient with Morquio Syndrome. Arrows point to the irregular, tortuous shape of the trachea. Narrowing and buckling of the tracheal lumen are evident.

endoscopist. Disadvantages of FOB include the need for greater skill level and the preferred nasal approach when the patient is awake or lightly sedated. The oral approach is only feasible when the patient is anesthetized or deeply sedated. Of note, many of the skeletal dysplasia children have narrow nasopharyngeal space resulting in bleeding and/or failure of intubation.[6,7] The nasopharyngeal path is compromised early during the course of the disease in MPS patients due to the deposits of glycosaminoglycans.[5,7] Laryngeal mask airway (LMA) used as a conduit to perform FOB intubations is another technique that allows oral route for intubations along with maintaining ventilation during the intubation process.[45] This

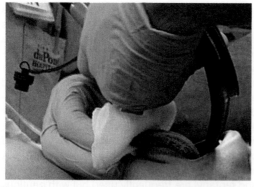

Fig. 4. Anterior retraction of tongue using a piece of gauze followed by placement of GlideScope blade. Note that in this case, the same anesthesiology personnel is doing both; in more difficult cases a second individual may retract the tongue while standing facing the patient.

technique is becoming increasingly popular as LMA designed for such intubation technique is available (eg, air-Q, Mercury Medicals). In severely affected patients, especially in infants, LMA can be placed awake and relief of obstruction can be quite remarkable.[46] We also use a combination of GlideScope and fiberoptic scope (GlideScope assisted Fiberoptic intubations) in situations whereby either one alone does not accomplish successful intubation.[47,48] This combination is usually performed with the placement of Glide-Scope first followed by visualizing a nasally introduced fiberoptic scope which is then guided by the GlideScope view to access laryngeal opening and trachea. The advantage of this technique in patients with skeletal dysplasia is the displacement of soft tissue with the GlideScope allowing easier maneuvering of FOB and entry into the trachea. GlideScope displaces soft tissue efficiently, thus facilitating the placement of fiberoptic scope, which is usually placed nasally.

Tracheostomy is used as a last resort in skeletal dysplasia patients (especially MPS) and can be technically difficult due to the lack of mobility of the head and neck, inability to extend the neck, presence of severe pectus carinatum, and presence of cricoid cartilage below the sternal notch (in older, more advanced cases) necessitating splitting the sternum to access the appropriate anatomic location of the trachea. These are common both in MPS patients and other severe forms of skeletal dysplasia such as metatrophic dysplasia (**Figs. 5** and **6**). Once placed, the management of the tracheostomy may be complicated with difficulty in changing the tracheostomy tube.

Evoked potential monitoring during intubation: When the degree of spinal cord compromise is of sufficient concern, monitoring evoked potentials during the intubation procedure is warranted.[2] This is particularly useful in children who cannot tolerate intubation while awake or under light sedation. Monitoring electrodes are placed once the child is asleep with an IV line in place and using a lower intensity stimulus both motor and sensory evoked potentials are recorded. When the use of muscle relaxant is thought to be necessary to achieve intubation, monitoring will be limited to somatosensory evoked potentials only, an option not preferred by neurophysiologists. To accomplish intubation without the use of muscle relaxants, small amounts of remifentanyl administered at the time of intubation may provide adequate intubating conditions.[49] In a retrospective study of anesthetic management of 28 children with Morquio syndrome at our hospital, we found 7/18 (39%) children who had evoked potentials

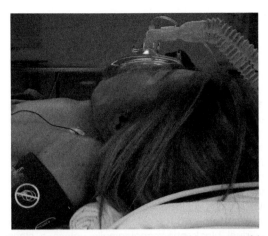

Fig. 5. A 22-year-old patient with metatrophic dysplasia. Due to prior cervical spine fusion limiting mobility compounded by a short neck, she is difficult to ventilate with a face mask and is also difficult to intubate. She has failed intubation as well as traumatic intubation in the past. She is currently managed using awake, sedated fiberoptic bronchoscope assisted intubation.[50]

monitored during their intubation for cervical spine fusion.[2]

Temperature and glycemic control: Little is known about temperature variability and glycemic control of children with skeletal dysplasia under anesthesia. We reported 2 children (1 with a diagnosis of SEDC and the other achondroplasia) who developed intraoperative temperatures of 40 ^{0}C or greater during general anesthesia. Workups for malignant hyperthermia were negative in both patients. Many children with skeletal dysplasia and short-limbed dwarfism have easily elicitable

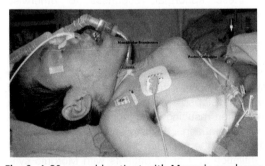

Fig. 6. A 20-year-old patient with Morquio syndrome undergoing tracheostomy. Due to high incidence of instability of C1-C2, motor evoked potentials were monitored during the procedure to ensure the integrity of the spinal cord during the tracheostomy. The obvious pectus carinatum and relative mandibular prominence are also noted.[22]

history of "not able to tolerate heat" and many such patients give a history of excessive sweating and/or having baseline temperatures that are in the upper range of normal (36.5^0 C–37.5^0 C).[51] Careful vigilance and judicious use of warming devices such as forced-air warmers in addition to ensuring adequate hydration will avoid temperatures high enough to be of concern. Related to this, if glucose is not being administered as a part of the intraoperative fluids then glucose levels should be monitored to avoid hypoglycemia in these children. Although to date no studies have been conducted to examine this issue, it would be prudent to exercise caution when solutions without glucose are given to SD children especially if they demonstrate a propensity to have elevated temperatures.

Extubation of trachea: Factors to consider regarding extubation of trachea are: (1) difficulty with intubation, (2) age of the child, (3) type, duration, and the extent of the surgical procedure, (4) blood loss and fluid replacement leading to tissue edema, and (5) history of snoring or OSA.

Difficulty with intubation before surgery predicts that reintubation may be difficult. Compounding the difficulty is the presence of a halo (as is often the case following cervical spine fusion), young age of the patient whereby cooperation is not possible, and blood loss greater than 50% of child's estimated blood volume resulting in fluid administration and generalized edema. These factors also create greater difficulty with managing ventilation via face mask. Clinical judgment and experience in caring for children with skeletal dysplasia play a significant role in deciding when to extubate. Time tested preextubation parameter of checking for a leak around the endotracheal tube by deflating the cuff (of the endotracheal tube) is still practiced by us as an additional measure to check mucosal edema of the trachea. Awake extubation is more commonly used than deep extubation us. It is very helpful to practice "taking a deep breath" with the child before the induction of anesthesia. We go a step further and introduce small amounts of anesthetic during the induction process and practice "taking a deep breath" and "wiggling toes" until the child loses consciousness.[52] We have found this simple step useful and easily reproducible in assessing a patient's cognitive status during emergence as well as assessing spinal cord integrity before extubation.

Position of the head and neck,[53] particularly after cervical spine fusion, is of great importance to ensure optimal airway patency in certain types of skeletal dysplasia. For example, children with

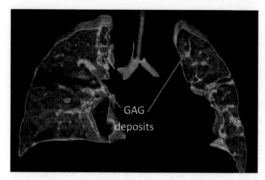

Fig. 7. Three-dimensional reconstruction of the airway with MPS deposits in a patient with Hurler syndrome. Bronchioles with intraluminal deposits of GAG are easily visible.[22]

Morquio frequently demonstrate a "chin-up" or a "looking-up" posture indicative of their optimal position to maintain the patency of their airway.[7,54] If this posture cannot be maintained postoperatively either due to surgical fixation or anesthesia-induced lack of muscle tone, these children may exhibit respiratory distress or respiratory failure. Their airways easily obstruct when the neck is flexed, demonstrated by flow-volume loop, tracheal tomography, and fiberoptic tracheography by Pritzker and colleagues.[55] They noted anterior buckling of the posterior tracheal wall during flexion of the head, which caused a slit-like narrowing of the tracheal lumen. Lack of sufficient tensile integrity of the tracheal walls due to a combination of abnormal hyaline cartilage composition

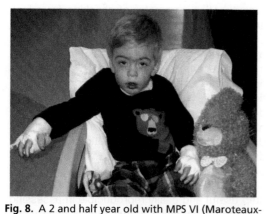

Fig. 8. A 2 and half year old with MPS VI (Maroteaux-Lamy Syndrome). He has undergone the following surgeries already: posterior fossa decompression and C1 laminectomy, bilateral myringotomy tube placement and Auditory brain stem evoked response, a Mediport placement for enzyme therapy, tonsillectomy, and adenoidectomy and carpel tunnel release bilaterally, in addition to anesthesia for MRI.

and GAG deposits in the submucosa may be the causative factors[14] (**Figs. 7** and **8**).

Optimizing other physiologic parameters is important to achieve successful extubation in these otherwise compromised children. Temperature should be close to baseline for the child avoiding hypothermia (leads to difficulty in eliminating anesthetic agents) or hyperthermia (leads to increased metabolic rate and carbon dioxide production requiring greater ventilatory effort). If children have an esophageal temperature of less than 35.5, use a forced-air warmer to prevent heat loss as well as raise core temperature. When using neuromuscular blocking agents, it is prudent to err on the side of caution and reverse residual block pharmacologically unless a clear indication of spontaneous recovery is evident. Children with skeletal dysplasia often have some degree of hypotonia and dose–response studies are not available examining the use of muscle relaxants in children with skeletal dysplasia.

Observe the respiratory pattern closely as the child is emerging from anesthesia for abnormalities such as paradoxic chest wall movements, an indication of the collapse of laryngeal or trachea during inspiration. Several forms of skeletal dysplasia involve connective and cartilaginous tissue abnormalities[53,56–58] that may lead to the loss of normal tone of laryngotracheal structures with anesthetic agents on board. This is possible even when no respiratory abnormalities are present before the anesthetic and will most likely resolve with the elimination of anesthetic over time. We have observed paradoxic breathing in 2 children (1 with metatrophic and the other with Kniest dysplasia) which when examined using FOB via endotracheal tube revealed tracheomalacia which was transient and resolved within the following 12 to 24 hours. Time and patience will resolve much of these abnormal responses to otherwise commonly used anesthetic agents.

Patients with mucopolysaccharidosis (MPS) again pose unique difficulties pertaining to the extubation of their trachea as well. In a study of 21 patients with MPS (6 of whom had Morquio syndrome), Semenza and Pyeritz[7] reported a child who developed adhesions following traumatic intubation resulting in laryngomalacia and stridulous breathing. Ransford and colleagues[59] described the need for postoperative mechanical ventilation in 9 of 17 patients with Morquio syndrome who underwent occipital-cervical fusion, one of whom died due to accidental extubation and failure to reestablish an airway. Emergency tracheostomy could be a significantly more difficult task in such patients due to abnormal

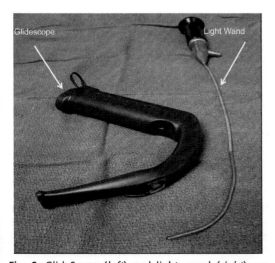

Fig. 9. GlideScope (*left*) and light wand (*right*) are shown here. GlideScope has the ability to displace soft tissue including tongue in children with skeletal dysplasia. It has a video camera which is seen as a whitish structure on the outer surface. Due to its ability to lift and displace soft tissue GlideScope has been successful reliably and consistently in our practice and nationally. Light wand in comparison is flimsy and not able to maneuver around the abundant soft tissue of many of the children with skeletal dysplasia.

anatomy including short neck, inability to extend neck, and pathologic tracheal rings and mucosa.

Intraoperative fluid management: If extubation of trachea is a goal at the end of the surgical procedure then the management of the intraoperative fluids may need to be modified to minimize airway edema. During surgical procedures such as spine fusion involving several vertebral levels, blood loss may be significant (50% of estimated blood volume or greater). Monitoring conventional clotting studies (prothrombin time and partial thromboplastin time) as well as fibrinogen levels may provide additional evidence in deciding to transfuse blood products such as cryoprecipitate. Judicious use of crystalloids and earlier correction of loss of clotting factors and platelets are practiced by us as is the use of thromboelastography to further scrutinize clotting and fibrinolysis.[60] In general, when managing our children with skeletal dysplasia for their scoliosis correction, we allow earlier correction of abnormalities of clotting parameters including fibrinogen and platelets than our management of idiopathic scoliosis patients. Optimizing hematological parameters in the face of the compromised respiratory system (most SD patients have restrictive lung disease especially those in the need of scoliosis correction) is the goal. In addition, we have found this fluid

management regime results in less facial and upper airway mucosal edema.

OTHER MODES OF ANESTHETIC (SPINAL AND EPIDURAL)

In children, there is a limited role for surgical procedures to be performed using regional anesthesia techniques such as spinal or epidural. In adults with achondroplasia, regional techniques have been reported, compelled by the fear of difficulties with airway management.[61] This can be more difficult because of the narrow spinal canal and spinal stenosis in these patients.[62–64] A single-case report of a successful anesthetic achieved as in the case report of a continuous thoracic epidural for nephrectomy[65] should not be mistaken for the safety or the feasibility of the technique in this patient population.

In young children, a caudally placed epidural may be easier if landmarks are palpable and have the theoretical advantage of being away from the spinal cord thus reducing the risk of injury to the spinal cord. A study by Sasaki-Adams et al[66] examining 111 patients' MR images which included 47 different skeletal dysplasia found the mean conus medullaris level at the L-1 vertebral body. The investigators did not find any difference related to the age of the patients or the type of skeletal dysplasia. Only 2 out of 111 patients (1.7%) had a conus level lower than L-2. One patient had Conradi–Hünermann syndrome who had progressive kyphotic deformity to 100° and a conus at the level of sacrum along with a fatty filum. The second patient had diastrophic dystrophy whose conus was found to be at L2-3. He also had progressive kyphosis from 40° to 60°. This patient had a significant loss of evoked potentials during his decompression and fusion surgery.

Lumbar epidural has been placed in spondyloepiphyseal dysplasia patient for caesarian section. Tobias reported the use of a continuous spinal anesthetic in an 8-year-old child with Morquio syndrome to avoid difficulty with intubation.[67] The child was sedated initially with ketamine and later with propofol. Careful titration of the local anesthetic was required as dosing of the local anesthetic subdurally may have unpredictable levels dictated by the compromised spinal canal in different forms of dysplasia.[64] Fewer reports exist for epidural anesthesia in SEDC dwarfs as one would expect as SEDC dwarfism is less common and pregnancy rate for this population even less.

Special note: Neuraxial anesthesia of any type may be contraindicated in patients MPS patients. There have been several cases of spinal cord infarction in the upper thoracic region in patients with Morquio syndrome occurring in the perioperative period. In the first reported case, the patient was undergoing foramen magnum and atlantal decompression[68] and the spinal cord infarction occurred in the thoracic region (C7-T4) of the spinal cord, well away from the operative site. In another case, a 16 years old with Morquio syndrome suffered a severe thoracic spinal cord infarction diagnosed within the first 24 hours following a lower extremity procedure.[69] A lumbar epidural catheter had been placed preoperatively with the patient awake before inducing general anesthesia and a bolus dose of local anesthetic followed by a continuous infusion had been instituted. Patient had excellent analgesia from the epidural route of pain management but the recognition of spinal cord infarction may have been delayed due to the presence of a neuraxial block. We know of 2 other MPS children (personal communication) who have suffered spinal cord infarction under similar circumstances. Even though the relationship between the spinal cord infarction in the upper thoracic region and placement of lumbar epidural is difficult to explain, given the gravity of such devastating complication, we currently recommend that no neuraxial anesthesia, whether epidural or spinal, be performed in children with Morquio syndrome and possibly in other MPS patients with spinal cord compromise. We would like to point out that this contradicts our own publication earlier whereby we discussed placing epidurals in patients with Morquio syndrome successfully.[2]

POSTOPERATIVE PAIN MANAGEMENT

Quite often surgical procedures in children with skeletal dysplasia are extensive in nature. If an epidural is planned for postoperative pain management, careful selection of patients is necessary. As mentioned earlier, we no longer recommend performing epidurals in MPS patients. Due to the inherent abnormalities present in the neuraxial and vertebral column structures in these patients, the use of fluoroscopy is recommended for the placement of epidural catheters. Omnipaque may be injected via the catheter and its spread visualized to document the position of the catheter tip. In children, we often prefer a caudal approach to epidural placement due to the irregularities of the vertebral bodies and the frequently present thoracolumbar kyphosis.[59] In carefully selected patients the successful catheter placement provides satisfactory pain control and may be continued 2 to 3 days postoperatively. Local anesthetic used currently is Bupivacaine 0.125% or ropivacaine .1% with 5 μg/mL of hydromorphone.

Successful use of peripheral nerve blocks and continuous infusion of local anesthetics via catheters placed is becoming increasingly common and may be preferable to neuraxial blocks such as epidural or spinal.

IV opioid (morphine or hydromorphone) are the mainstay of acute postoperative pain management unless a regional technique is in place. Adjutants such as IV acetaminophen, ketorolac (in selective cases), diazepam, and dexmedetomidine are commonly used to decrease the use of opioids and thus minimize their side effects. A continuous, low infusion of the opioid is administered for more extensive procedures such as spine fusion with bolus dosing administered as needed every 2 to 3 hours. When of appropriate age (>6–8 years), patients may be allowed to have PCA (patient-controlled analgesia) which provides greater measure of patient satisfaction.

CLINICS CARE POINTS

- The first priority is maintaining the patency of patient's airway, knowing that face mask bagging may be difficult and inadequate and other MPS.
- Each skeletal dysplasia has its unique impact on the spine and those that impact the cervical spine need special consideration when manipulating the neck for intubation.
- Children with severe thoracic stenosis, especially those with Morquio syndrome, can suffer spinal cord injury from anesthesia alone. For anesthesia lasting over an hour, neuromonitoring is recommended.
- Epidural or spinal anesthesia has been associated with spinal cord injury in children with Morquio syndrome.
- The trachea deviates, buckles and in addition courses over the brachiocephalic artery in children with Morquio syndrome, which can lead to respiratory arrest during anesthesia or sudden death unless reconstructed.

DISCLOSURE

J.W. Campbell – Consultant for BioMarin

REFERENCES

1. McKay SD, Al-Omari A, Tomlinson LA, et al. Review of cervical spine anomalies in genetic syndromes. Spine (Phila Pa 1976) 2012;37(5). https://doi.org/10.1097/BRS.0b013e31823b3ded.

2. Theroux MC, Nerker T, Ditro C, et al. Anesthetic care and perioperative complications of children with Morquio syndrome. Paediatr Anaesth 2012;22(9): 901–7.

3. Redi G. Massive pyramidal tract signs after endotracheal intubation: a case report of spondyloepiphyseal dysplasia congenita. Anesthesiology 1998; 89(5):1262–4.

4. Tofield CE, Mackinnon CA. Cleft Palate Repair in Spondyloepiphyseal Dysplasia Congenita: Minimizing the Risk of Cervical Cord Compression. Cleft Palate Craniofac J 2003;40(6):629–31.

5. Diaz JH, Belani KG. Perioperative management of children with mucopolysaccharidoses. Anesth Analg 1993;77(6):1261–70.

6. Walker RWM, Allen DL, Rothera MR. A fibreoptic intubation technique for children with mucopolysaccharidoses using the laryngeal mask airway. Paediatr Anaesth 1997;7(5):421–6.

7. Semenza GL, Pyeritz RE. Respiratory complications of mucopolysaccharide storage disorders. Med (Baltimore). 1988;67(4):209–19.

8. Nelson ME, Griffin GR, Innis JW, et al. Campomelic dysplasia: Airway management in two patients and an update on clinical-molecular correlations in the head and neck. Ann Otol Rhinol Laryngol 2011; 120(10):682–5.

9. Mather JS. Impossible direct laryngoscopy in achondroplasia: a case report. Anaesthesia 1966; 21(2):244–8.

10. Niwa Y, Hirabayashi Y, Seo N, et al. Use of Parker Flex-Tip® tracheal tube in a patient with Kniest dysplasia. Masui 2011;60(5):631–4.

11. Bookman LB, Melton KR, Pan BS, et al. Neonates with tongue-based airway obstruction: A systematic review. Otolaryngol Head Neck Surg 2012;146(1): 8–18.

12. Hosking J, Zoanetti D, Carlyle A, et al. Anesthesia for Treacher Collins syndrome: A review of airway management in 240 pediatric cases. Paediatr Anaesth 2012;22(8):752–8.

13. Sasaki CT, Richard R, Gaito R, et al. Hunter's syndrome: A study in airway obstruction. Laryngoscope 1987;97(3 Pt 1):280–5. Available at: https://onlinelibrary.wiley.com/doi/epdf/10.1288/00005537-198703000-00005. Accessed June 28, 2021.

14. Shih SL, Lee YJ, Lin SP, et al. Airway changes in children with mucopolysaccharidoses: CT evaluation. Acta Radiol 2002;43(1):40–3.

15. Azevedo ACMM, Schwartz IV, Kalakun L, et al. Clinical and biochemical study of 28 patients with mucopolysaccharides type VI. Clin Genet 2004;66(3): 208–13.

16. Yeung AH, Cowan MJ, Horn B, et al. Airway management in children with mucopolysaccharidoses. Arch Otolaryngol Head Neck Surg 2009;135(1): 73–9.

17. Herrick IA, Rhine EJ. The mucopolysaccharidoses and anaesthesia: a report of clinical experience. Can J Anaesth 1988;35(1):67–73.

18. John Â, Fagondes S, Schwartz I, et al. Sleep abnormalities in untreated patients with mucopolysaccharidosis type VI. Am J Med Genet A 2011;155(7): 1546–51.

19. Baines D, Keneally J. Anaesthetic implications of the mucopolysaccharidoses: a fifteen-year experience in a children's hospital. Anaesth Intensive Care 1983;11(3):198–202.

20. Kempthorne PM, Brown TC. Anaesthesia and the mucopolysaccharidoses: a survey of techniques and problems. Anaesth Intensive Care 1983;11(3): 203–7.

21. Doherty C, Averill LW, Theroux M, et al. Natural history of Morquio A patient with tracheal obstruction from birth to death. Mol Genet Metab Rep 2018;14:59–67.

22. Averill LW, Kecskemethy HH, Theroux MC, et al. Tracheal narrowing in children and adults with mucopolysaccharidosis type IVA: evaluation with computed tomography angiography. Pediatr Radiol 2021;51(7):1202–13.

23. Pizarro C, Davies RR, Theroux M, et al. Surgical Reconstruction for Severe Tracheal Obstruction in Morquio A Syndrome. Ann Thorac Surg 2016; 102(4):e329–31.

24. Simmons MA, Bruce IA, Penney S, et al. Otorhinolaryngological manifestations of the mucopolysaccharidoses. Int J Pediatr Otorhinolaryngol 2005;69(5): 589–95.

25. Belani KG, Krivit W, Carpenter BLM, et al. Children with mucopolysaccharidosis: Perioperative care, morbidity, mortality, and new findings. J Pediatr Surg 1993;28(3):403–10.

26. Wippermann CF, Schranz D, Huth RG. Evaluation of the pulse wave arrival time as a marker for blood pressure changes in critically ill infants and children. J Clin Monit 1995;11(5):324–8.

27. Dangel JH. Cardiovascular changes in children with mucopolysaccharide storage diseases and related disorders- clinical and echocardiographic findings in 64 patients. Eur J Pediatr 1998;157(7):534–8.

28. Factor SM, Biempica L, Goldfischer S. Coronary intimal sclerosis in Morquio's syndrome. Virchows Arch A Pathol Anat Histol 1978;379(1):1–10.

29. Van Den Broek L, Backx APCM, Coolen H, et al. Fatal coronary artery disease in an infant with severe mucopolysaccharidosis type I. Pediatrics 2011; 127(5). https://doi.org/10.1542/peds.2009-2047.

30. Martins AM, Dualibi AP, Norato D, et al. Guidelines for the Management of Mucopolysaccharidosis Type I. J Pediatr 2009;155(4 SUPPL). https://doi.org/10.1016/j.jpeds.2009.07.005.

31. Wraith JE, Beck M, Giugliani R, et al. Initial report from the Hunter Outcome Survey. Genet Med 2008;10(7):508–16.

32. Walker R, Belani KG, Braunlin EA, et al. Anaesthesia and airway management in mucopolysaccharidosis. J Inherit Metab Dis 2013;36(2):211–9.

33. Fesslová V, Corti P, Sersale G, et al. The natural course and the impact of therapies of cardiac involvement in the mucopolysaccharidoses. Cardiol Young 2009;19(2):170–8.

34. Mohan UR, Hay AA, Cleary MA, et al. Cardiovascular changes in children with mucopolysaccharide disorders. Acta Paediatr 2002;91(7):799–804.

35. Misumi I, Chikazawa S, Ishitsu T, et al. Atrioventricular block and diastolic dysfunction in a patient with sanfilippo C. Intern Med 2010;49(21):2313–6.

36. Hishitani T, Wakita S, Isoda T, et al. Sudden death in Hunter syndrome caused by complete atrioventricular block. J Pediatr 2000;136(2):268–9.

37. Dilber E, Çeliker A, Karagöz T, et al. Permanent transfemoral pacemaker implantation in a child with Maroteaux Lamy syndrome. Pacing Clin Electrophysiol 2002;25(12):1784–5.

38. Leal GN, De Paula AC, Leone C, et al. Echocardiographic study of paediatric patients with mucopolysaccharidosis. Cardiol Young 2010;20(3):254–61.

39. Montaño AM, Tomatsu S, Gottesman GS, et al. International Morquio A Registry: Clinical manifestation and natural course of Morquio A disease. J Inherit Metab Dis 2007;30(2):165–74.

40. Solanki GA, Martin KW, Theroux MC, et al. Spinal involvement in mucopolysaccharidosis IVA (Morquio-Brailsford or Morquio A syndrome): presentation, diagnosis and management. J Inherit Metab Dis 2013;36(2):339–55.

41. Linstedt U, Maier C, Joehnk H, et al. Threatening spinal cord compression during anesthesia in a child with mucopolysaccharidosis VI. Anesthesiology 1994;80(1):227–9.

42. Thorne JA, Javadpour M, Hughes DG, et al. Craniovertebral abnormalities in type VI mucopolysaccharidosis (Maroteaux-Lamy syndrome). Neurosurgery 2001;48(4):849–53.

43. Karsli C, Armstrong J, John J. A comparison between the GlideScope® Video Laryngoscope and direct laryngoscope in paediatric patients with difficult airways - a pilot study: Original article. Anaesthesia 2010;65(4):353–7.

44. Aziz MF, Healy D, Kheterpal S, et al. Routine clinical practice effectiveness of the glidescope in difficult airway management: An analysis of 2,004 glidescope intubations, complications, and failures from two institutions. Anesthesiology 2011;114(1):34–41.

45. Inada T, Fujise K, Tachibana K, et al. Orotracheal intubation through the laryngeal mask airway in paediatric patients with Treacher-Collins syndrome. Pediatr Anesth 1995;5(2):129–32.

46. Asai T, Nagata A, Shingu K. Awake tracheal intubation through the laryngeal mask in neonates with upper airway obstruction. Paediatr Anaesth 2008;18(1):77–80.

47. Doyle DJ. GlideScoper®-assisted fiberoptic intubation: a new airway teaching method [12]. Anesthesiology 2004;101(5):1252.

48. Moore MSR, Wong AB. GlideScope® intubation assisted by fiberoptic scope [17]. Anesthesiology 2007;106(4):885.

49. Aouad MT, Yazbeck-Karam VG, Mallat CE, et al. The effect of adjuvant drugs on the quality of tracheal intubation without muscle relaxants in children: a systematic review of randomized trials. Paediatr Anaesth 2012;22(7):616–26.

50. Theroux MC, et al. Metatropic dysplasia-a skeletal dysplasia with challenging airway and other anesthetic concerns. Paediatr Anaesth 2017;27(6):596–603.

51. Sessler DI. Temperature monitoring and perioperative thermoregulation. Anesthesiology 2008;109(2):318–38.

52. DiCindio S, Theroux M, Shah S, et al. Multimodality monitoring of transcranial electric motor and somatosensory-evoked potentials during surgical correction of spinal deformity in patients with cerebral palsy and other neuromuscular disorders. Spine (Phila Pa 1976) 2003;28(16):1851–5.

53. Belik J, Anday EK, Kaplan F, et al. Respiratory complications of metatropic dwarfism. Clin Pediatr (Phila) 1985;24(9):504–11.

54. Walker PP, Rose E, Williams JG. Upper airways abnormalities and tracheal problems in Morquio's disease. Thorax 2003;58(5):458–9.

55. Pritzker MR, King RA, Kronenberg RS. Upper airway obstruction during head flexion in morquio's disease. Am J Med 1980;69(3):467–70.

56. Schwartz NB, Domowicz M. Chondrodysplasias due to proteoglycan defects. Glycobiology 2002;12(4). https://doi.org/10.1093/glycob/12.4.57R.

57. Harding CO, Green CG, Perloff WH, et al. Respiratory complications in children with spondyloepiphyseal dysplasia congenita. Pediatr Pulmonol 1990;9(1):49–54.

58. Hicks J, De Jong A, Barrish J, et al. Tracheomalacia in a neonate with Kniest dysplasia: Histopathologic and ultrastructural features. Ultrastruct Pathol 2001;25(1):79–83.

59. Ransford A, Crockard H, Stevens J, et al. Occipito-atlanto-axial fusion in Morquio-Brailsford syndrome. A ten-year experience - PubMed. J Bone Joint Surg Br 1996;78(2):307–13. Available at: https://pubmed.ncbi.nlm.nih.gov/8666648/. Accessed June 28, 2021.

60. Brenn BR, Theroux MC, Dabney KW, et al. Clotting parameters and thromboelastography in children with neuromuscular and idiopathic scoliosis undergoing posterior spinal fusion. Spine (Phila Pa 1976)

2004;29(15). https://doi.org/10.1097/01.brs.0000132513.88038.64.

61. Wardall GJ, Frame WT. Extradural anaesthesia for caesarean section in achondroplasia. Br J Anaesth 1990;64(3):367–70.

62. Cohen SE. Anesthesia for cesarean section in achondroplastic dwarfs. Anesthesiology 1980;52(3):264–6.

63. Morrow MJ, Black IH. Epidural anaesthesia for Caesarean section in an achondroplastic dwarf. Br J Anaesth 1998;81(4):619–21.

64. DeRenzo JS, Vallejo MC, Ramanathan S. Failed regional anesthesia with reduced spinal bupivacaine dosage in a parturient with achondroplasia presenting for urgent cesarean section. Int J Obstet Anesth 2005;14(2):175–8.

65. Jain A, Bhagat H, Makkar JK, et al. Continuous thoracic epidural analgesia for pain management in achondroplastic patient undergoing unilateral nephrectomy. Saudi J Anaesth 2011;5(2):234–5.

66. Sasaki-Adams DM, Campbell JW, Bajelidze G, et al. Level of the conus in pediatric patients with skeletal dysplasia. J Neurosurg Pediatr 2010;5(5):455–9.

67. Tobias JD. Anesthetic care for the child with Morquio syndrome: General versus regional anesthesia. J Clin Anesth 1999;11(3):242–6.

68. Tong CKW, Chen JCH, Cochrane DD. Spinal cord infarction remote from maximal compression in a patient with Morquio syndrome. J Neurosurg Pediatr 2012;9(6):608–12.

69. Drummond JC, Krane EJ, Tomatsu S, et al. Paraplegia after epidural-general anesthesia in a Morquio patient with moderate thoracic spinal stenosis. Can J Anesth 2015;62(1):45–9.

Surgical Evaluation and Management of Spinal Pathology in Patients with Connective Tissue Disorders

Ijezie A. Ikwuezunma, BA, BS[a], Paul D. Sponseller, MD, MBA[b],*

KEYWORDS

- Marfan syndrome • Ehlers-Danlos syndrome • Loeys-Dietz syndrome • Spine surgery

KEY POINTS

- Heritable connective tissue disorders can affect all the spinal elements.
- Spine surgeons must be aware of broad phenotypic spectrum of connective tissue diseases, because they have significant implication for complications and treatment outcomes.
- Surgical decision-making process should include consideration of the unique challenges including dysplastic changes, osseous abnormalities, and ligamentous laxity.

INTRODUCTION

Connective tissue disorders caused by defects in extracellular matrix elements, such as collagens, elastin, or fibrillin, represent a heterogeneous collection of genetic syndromes characterized by systemic anomalies with important implications for the spine surgeon. Surgeons must be aware of these diverse and global manifestations of disease because they have significant impact on the perioperative and postoperative outcomes. This article provides a general overview of the most common inherited connective tissue disorders, Marfan syndrome (MFS), Ehlers-Danlos syndrome (EDS), and Loeys-Dietz syndrome (LDS), followed by a deeper exploration of the evaluation and management of specific spinal sequelae of disease.

SPECIFIC SYNDROMES

MFS is an autosomal dominant connective tissue disorder caused by a defect in Fibrillin-1, encoded by *FBN1*.[1] MFS is predominantly a clinical diagnosis, relying on major and minor criteria established by the original Ghent nosology[2] (**Table 1**). This diagnostic guideline encompasses the multisystemic breadth of manifestations common to MFS with special emphasis on the cardinal features of disease, of which cardiovascular complications make up the predominant cause of morbidity and mortality.[3] As aortic pathology often remains silent until fatal progression, spine surgeons should be knowledgeable of the characteristic musculoskeletal anomalies, such as pectus excavatum, arachnodactyly, and dolichostenomelia, which are often the first clue to diagnosis[4] (**Fig. 1**).

EDS comprises a group of autosomal dominant, heterogeneous disorders of connective tissue characterized by joint hypermobility, skin extensibility, and tissue friability. Among the 6 subtypes, patients with the classic, vascular, musculocontractural, kyphoscoliotic, and spondylodysplastic forms of EDS have a high risk of aortic, vascular, and musculoskeletal complications, which often require surgical intervention[5] (**Table 2**). Symptoms of chronic, debilitating neuromuscular disease common to all EDS subtypes, including headache,

[a] Department of Orthopaedic Surgery, Johns Hopkins Medical Institutions, Baltimore, MD 21287, USA;
[b] Pediatric Orthopaedics, Johns Hopkins Medical Institutions, Baltimore, MD 21287, USA
* Corresponding author. 1800 Orleans Street, #7359, Baltimore, MD 21287.
E-mail address: psponse@jhmi.edu

Neurosurg Clin N Am 33 (2022) 49–59
https://doi.org/10.1016/j.nec.2021.09.005

Table 1
Revised Ghent criteria for the diagnosis of Marfan syndrome and related conditions

	Diagnostic Scenarios	Systemic Involvement	Points
I	Aortic root diameter (Z≥2) AND ectopia lentis	Wrist AND thumb sign	3
II	Aortic root diameter (Z≥2) AND *FBN1* mutation	Wrist OR thumb sign	1
III	Aortic root diameter (Z≥2) AND systemic score ≥7 points	Pectus carinatum	2
IV	Aortic root diameter[a] AND family history	Pectus excavatum or chest asymmetry	1
V	Ectopia lentis AND *FBN1* mutation	Hindfoot deformity	2
VI	Ectopia lentis AND family history	Plain pes planus	1
VII	Systemic score ≥7 points AND family history	Pneumothorax	2
		Dural ectasia	2
		Protrusio acetabula	2
		Reduced US/LS AND increased AS/H AND no severe scoliosis	1
		Scoliosis or thoracolumbar kyphosis	1
		Reduced elbow extension	1
		3/5 Facial features[b]	1
		Skin striae	1
		Myopia	1
		Mitral valve prolapse	1

Abbreviations: AS/H, arm span/height ratio; FBN1, fibrillin-1 mutation; US/LS, upper segment/lower segment ratio; Z, Z-score.
[a] Z≥2 for those older than 20 years, ≥3 for those younger than 20 years in this scenario.
[b] Dolichocephaly, enophthalmos, downslanting palpebral fissures, malar hypoplasia, retrognathia.
Loeys BL et al., J Med Genet 2010; 47:476-485 https://doi.org/10.1136/jmg.2009.072785

mechanical and myelopathic pain, weakness, motor delay, and impaired sensorium, have been attributed to ligamentous laxity and joint instability.[6]

LDS, characterized by a clinical triad of vascular aneurysms and tortuosity, hypertelorism, and bifid uvula or cleft palate along with neurocognitive and musculoskeletal findings, is caused by heterozygous mutations in the transforming growth factor-beta receptor 1 (*TGF-βR1*) or 2 (*TGF-βR2*) genes.[7,8] Although patients with LDS exhibit a spectrum of aortic pathology as seen in MFS and EDS, they are at higher risk of dissection at younger ages and smaller aortic dimensions, as well as pregnancy-related complications.[9] In short, it is imperative that the surgical community be familiar with the distinct spectrum of phenotypic expression unique to each syndrome to facilitate early detection, minimize complications, and provide optimal care for these patients.[2,10]

DISCUSSION
Dural Ectasia

Dural ectasia (DE), defined as an enlargement, or "ballooning," of the thecal sac anywhere along the spinal column, is common to connective tissue diseases.[11] DE has been theorized to arise secondary to continuous, pulsatile pressure of the cerebrospinal fluid (CSF) on weakened connective tissue, because they commonly occur in the lumbosacral region of the spinal column where the CSF pressure is the highest in the upright position.[4,12] Complications of DE represent the consequences of bony erosion and nerve compression. Erosion of structural lumbosacral elements can result from direct pressure on the surrounding periosteum leading to posterior scalloping of the vertebral body, thinning of the cortex of pedicles and laminae, and widening of the neural foraminae[13,14] (**Fig. 2**). This structural thinning and weakening of the sacrum can

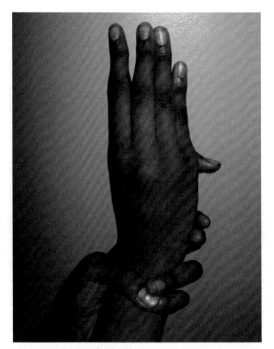

Fig. 1. Thumb and wrist signs: The thumb sign is the ability to pass the entire distal phalanx of the thumb beyond the ulnar border of the clenched fist. The wrist sign is the ability to cover the entire fifth fingernail with the thumb when wrapped around the wrist. Both signs indicate combination of arachnodactyly and laxity.

predispose to microfractures and subsequent instability.[13,15] In addition, DE may cause pain and neurologic deficits secondary to compression, distortion, or traction of neural root sleeves.[11] Among symptomatic patients with radiologically confirmed DE, the most commonly cited complaints include low-back pain, headache, genito-rectal pain, radiculopathy, and sensorimotor deficits of lower extremity.[16–18] Although no correlation has been identified between the volume of the ectasia and the severity of pain, the relief that most patients report when assuming a supine position suggests a direct association between headache and spontaneous CSF leak due to DE.[11] Furthermore, severe DE may lead to anterior meningoceles, which can provoke gastrointestinal issues such as abdominal discomfort, constipation, and incontinence[11] (see **Fig. 2**).

To date there exist no consensus on the imaging method, criteria, and cutoff values for the diagnosis of DE.[16] Böker and colleagues[16] reviewed the benefits and limitations of existing computed tomographic and MRI criteria proposed by

Oosterhof, Habermann, Fattori, Lundby, Ahn, and Pierro and recommended that the diagnosis should be based on the presence of at least one of the following criteria: anterior meningocele or nerve root sleeve herniation, dural sac diameter at S1 or below larger than diameter at L4, or dural sac ratio at S1 greater than 0.64, for the best discrimination between patients with MFS and healthy controls with an 84% sensitivity and 95% specificity.[16,19–24] Alternatively, diagnostic criteria with conventional radiography include interpediculate distance at L4 greater than or equal to 38.0 mm, the sagittal diameter at S1 greater than or equal to 18.0 mm, or scalloping value at L5 greater than or equal to 5.5 mm.[25] However, with a reported sensitivity of 57%, the utility of radiography remains quite limited.[25]

Treatment of symptomatic DE has been variable based on the underlying manifestation. Given the risks of CSF leak with surgery and the relative lack of longitudinal research on spinal stability, we recommend that DE be managed nonoperatively for most cases[11]; this may especially be the case in MFS-associated DE due to potential cardiovascular risks secondary to major hemodynamic changes under anesthesia. Conservative measures such as flat bed rest, hydration, and blood patch, have been variably successful, most likely in light of the postural mechanism of provocation. In the case of persistent symptoms, associated spinal instability or deformity, or cauda equina syndrome, operative intervention is indicated.[26] General methods have revolved around surgical bony decompression with a posterior approach via sacral laminectomy or anteriorly through an open transperitoneal approach, followed by thecal sac reinforcement with mesh and possible lumboperitoneal shunt placement.[11,26,27] Trendelenberg positioning may decrease the expansion of the erratic dura, making surgery easier. More recently, one case series described a laparoscopic approach to treatment as safe and feasible.[28] Surgery for anterior meningocele is cautioned against the given risk of recurrence or harm to surrounding neurovasculature.[29]

Detailed preoperative evaluation with radiographic imaging for selection of anesthetic technique is necessary given the association between failed spinal anesthesia and DE. Epidural anesthesia is relatively contraindicated in DE because of the risk of puncturing the dilated dural sac.[30] It is postulated that excess volume of CSF restricts the spread of intrathecally injected local anesthetic.[30] Furthermore, we advise that patients be closely monitored in the postoperative setting for signs of postdural puncture headache for at least 24 hours.

Table 2
Classification of Ehlers-Danlos syndrome

Number	Descriptive type	Genes	Inheritance	Clinical Features and Notes
I (Gravis)	Classical[a]	COL5A1	AD	Marked joint hypermobility, skin hyperextensibility, bruising, and abnormal scarring
II (Mitis)		COL5A2		
III	Hypermobility[b]	TNXB Largely unknown	AD	Marked joint hypermobility, minor skin findings
IV	Vascular	COL3A1	AD	Thin translucent skin, marked bruising, small joint hypermobility, high risk for rupture of arteries, bowel, and gravid uterus
VIA	Kyphoscoliosis	PLOD1	AR	Joint hypermobility and kyphoscoliosis recalcitrant to surgical intervention, risk for arterial rupture
VIB	Musculocontractural	CHST14	AR	Congenital contractures of digits, dysmorphic features, kyphoscoliosis and hypermobility, hyperextensible thin skin, ocular involvement
VIIA	Arthrochalasia multiplex congenita	COL1A1	AD	Marked joint hypermobility, bilateral congenital hip dislocation
VIIB		COL1A2		
VIIC	Dermatosparaxis	ADAMTS2	AR	Soft, very fragile skin with late-onset skin redundancy, blue sclerae, joint hypermobility
VIII	Periodontitis	Probably heterogeneous; 1 locus at 12p13	AD	Periodontal loss, joint hypermobility, soft skin with characteristic plaque on anterior tibial region
Other	Progeroid	B4GALT7	AR	
	Cardiac valvular	COL1A2	AR (null)	Cardiac valvular insufficiency, joint hypermobility, skin hyperextensibility

(continued on next page)

Table 2
(continued)

Number	Descriptive type	Genes	Inheritance	Clinical Features and Notes
	FKBP14 related	FKBP14	AR	Marked kyphoscoliosis, hearing loss, myopathy, short stature, joint hypermobility
	Spondylocheiro dysplastic	SLC39A13	AR	Spondyloepiphyseal dysplasia with mild short stature, hyperelastic thin skin with easy bruising, protuberant eyes, bluish sclerae, fine wrinkling on palms
	Tenascin-X deficient	TNXB	AR	Joint hypermobility, hyperextensible and sleevelike character to skin, marked bruising, normal scarring
	Periventricular heterotopia	FLNA	XL	Periventricular heterotopia, joint hypermobility

Abbreviations: AD, autosomal dominant; AR, autosomal recessive; XL, X linked.

[a] Specific mutations in *COL1A1* (substitutions of cysteine for arginine residues within the triple helical domain of proα1(I) chains) have been recognized to cause a form of EDS reminiscent of classical type with joint hypermobility, skin hyperextensibility, bruising and abnormal scarring, and predisposition to aortic aneurysm.

[b] One family with a specific mutation in *COL3A1* is said to have only joint hypermobility with none of the other consequences seen in EDS type IV.

Byers PH et al., J Invest Dermatol 2012; 132(E1):6-11. https://doi.org/10.1038/skinbio.2012.3.

Cervical Deformities

Osseous abnormalities of the cervical spine are commonplace in patients with connective tissue disorders. Hobbs and colleagues[31] demonstrated heightened prevalence of focal kyphosis (16%), absent cervical lordosis (35%), and basilar impression (36%) reportedly due to increased odontoid height in patients with connective tissue disorders, such as MFS (**Fig. 3**). Similarly, Fuhrhop and colleagues[32] reported increased rates of cervical deformities in patients with LDS, including atlas and axis malformations, subaxial anomalies, focal cervical kyphosis, anterior/posterior arch defects, and dens elongation. Little evidence has been published on the bony morphology of the cervical spine specifically in patients with EDS.

In addition to abnormalities of the cervical vertebrae, complications of ligamentous deficiencies are commonplace in these patients. Atlantoaxial instability (AAI) due to the characteristic laxity has been widely reported in patients with MFS, EDS, and LDS.[6,31,32] The relative ligamentous incompetence of the atlantoaxial junction leaves it susceptible to instability.[33] As the most mobile joint in the body, the atlantoaxial joint relies heavily on the surrounding ligaments, the transverse and alar ligaments, for mechanical stability.[34] The diagnosis of AAI is predicated on the presence of disabling neck or suboccipital pain, clinical examination findings of cervical medullary syndrome, syncopal episodes, or neurologic deficits and radiographic evidence of instability or neuroaxial compression.[35] Patients may also complain of symptoms related to compromise in vertebral artery blood flow, such as visual disturbances and headaches. Other nonspecific symptoms include nausea, dizziness, facial pain, dysphagia, choking, and respiratory complaints. Physical examination may demonstrate a head tilt, tenderness over the C1 and C2 spinous processes, altered mechanics of neck rotation, hyperreflexia, dysdiadochokinesia, and hypoesthesia to pinprick.[6]

Treatment goals of AAI include stabilization of the spinal column, decompression of neural tissue, and reduction of deformity. First-line treatment typically consists of conservative measures including neck bracing, physical therapy, and avoidance of activities that exacerbate symptoms.

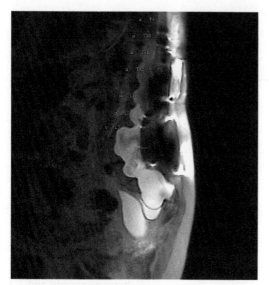

Fig. 2. Dural ectasia: Substantial dural ectasia of lower lumbar in a 26-year-old patient with MFS, resulting in marked bone loss and scalloping of the posterior aspect of the vertebral bodies extending to the sacrum. Imaging also reveals concomitant anterior sacral meningocele.

In light of its unclear natural history, operative treatment for AAI with posterior cervical C1-C2 spinal fusion is only advised in the case of refractory symptoms, severe headache, cervical medullary syndrome, neurologic deficits referable to the

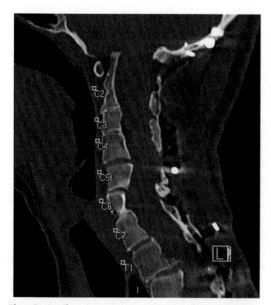

Fig. 3. Basilar impression: computed tomographic scan of 19-year-old patient with LDS demonstrating stable elongation of the C2 vertebral body with basilar impression and mild mass effect on the ventral brainstem at the level of the foramen magnum.

brainstem malformations, or upper spinal cord compression.[36] With ligamentous laxity and dysmorphic cervical spine anatomy detailed earlier, it is likely that these patients are at increased risk of cervical spine injuries, particularly when muscle tone is attenuated by muscle relaxants perioperatively. However, given the infrequency of permanent or debilitating neurologic injury, preoperative imaging for patients undergoing general anesthesia is generally neither necessary nor recommended.[37]

Thoracolumbar Deformities

Connective tissue disorders negatively impact vertebral bony development along the thoracolumbar region of the spine as well. Sponseller and colleagues[38] revealed that pedicle widths and laminar thicknesses were significantly smaller in patients with MFS at all levels, and that patients with MFS-associated DE exhibited significantly greater vertebral scalloping at S1. Furthermore, the skeletal phenotype in patients with EDS and LDS has been associated with low bone mineral density and skeletal fragility confirmed via iliac bone histomorphometry and dual-energy X-ray absorptiometry scan.[39] In concordance, both patients with LDS and EDS experience a higher rate of stress fractures as a result of compromised bone integrity.[40,41]

Spondylolysis is characterized by stress-induced defects in the pars interarticularis, which may result in segmental instability, whereas spondylolisthesis describes the translation, or "slip," of one vertebral body over another.[42] Sponseller and colleagues[43] reported a 6% incidence of spondylolisthesis in patients with MFS, usually of a high grade at the level of the fifth lumbar vertebra. Although the pathogenesis is not well understood, it has been postulated that this spondylotic slip may be the result of underlying connective tissue defects, which impairs ligament and disk strength.[43] This theory is supported by its predilection for women in the general population, given their predisposition for ligamentous laxity secondary to hormonal effects.[44] As a result, the altered properties of the ligaments in patients with connective tissue disorders predisposes to more severe slippage and advanced grade as detailed earlier.[43,45,46]

Clinically, spondylolisthesis is commonly associated with low-back pain and leg symptoms secondary to spinal stenosis or mechanical low-back pain. Patients typically complain of symptoms secondary to neurogenic claudication including radicular lower extremity pain, paresthesia, heaviness or weakness with walking or standing, and acute exacerbation associated with extension of the spine.[47] The diagnoses of spondylolysis and spondylolisthesis are confirmed with standing lateral radiographs. Spondylolisthesis may also exhibit a dynamic component, which may be missed on supine radiographs as displaced segments reduce into anatomic station. Using classification criteria established by Meyerding, increasing grade represents worsening translation with grade V representing spondyloptosis or the complete anterior dislocation of the vertebral body whereby the 2 end plates are no longer congruent[48] (**Fig. 4**). Management typically requires surgical fixation.

Patients with inherited connective tissue disorders experience a higher incidence of thoracic and lumbar spine abnormalities when compared with the general population. Syndromic scoliosis is the term used to refer to scoliosis derived secondarily from systemic disease such as MFS, EDS, and LDS, among other entities. Studies have reported scoliosis in more than half of the individuals with MFS and LDS, and in significant proportion in patients with select subtypes of EDS.[7,43,49] In patients with MFS, Sponseller and colleagues[43] found that the majority had thoracic or thoracolumbar spinal curves, with no reported difference in gender balance. The investigators also noted a higher rate of thoracic kyphosis and triple curves within the MFS cohort, owing to the characteristic ligamentous laxity and bony overgrowth, compared with patients with adolescent idiopathic scoliosis.[43] Likewise, Erkula and colleagues[7] found that most patients with LDS had either thoracic or thoracolumbar curves, with no difference between the sexes. Concerning EDS, although all subtypes possess a high risk for developing scoliosis, the spinal curvature seems to be most severe and aggressive in the kyphoscoliosis subtype.[50,51] Other subtypes commonly associated with scoliosis include the classical,

spondylodysplastic, and musculocontractural forms.[52,53] Spinal deformities can lead to chronic back pain and, in severe cases, restrictive lung disease. Deformity is measured clinically using thoracic and lumbar scoliometer angle on forward bend and radiographically using the Cobb angle.[54,55]

Management of scoliosis has similar themes across the different connective tissue disorders. Curve progression should be closely monitored using the Adam's forward-bending test, scoliometer, and anteroposterior and lateral spine films at regular intervals, particularly during adolescence. Conservative therapy with physical therapy, postural education, and joint stabilization with core strengthening may be of benefit, although long-term benefit has yet to be validated. In addition, although spinal orthosis with bracing has emerged as the mainstay of conservative treatment in patients with Adolescent Idiopathic Scoliosis (AIS), the literature suggests limited utility of bracing in patients with syndromic causes of scoliosis.[49,56] Therefore, the current strategy is to offer bracing at earlier thresholds (approximately 20°).

In the case of severe curvatures, surgical treatment of scoliosis or kyphosis is usually possible with a posterior-only approach. Preoperative traction is rarely needed because of the ligamentous laxity. As bleeding may be somewhat higher in this patient population, antifibrinolytics may represent a helpful adjunct. Correction of lumbar or proximal thoracic curves in response to selective fusion is not predictable, so all curves greater than approximately 25 to 30° with rotational characteristics should usually be fused. If patients have dysplastic lumbar vertebrae or significant preoperative imbalance, fusion may need to include the pelvis.[57] Dissection around the sacrum should be done carefully, because the cortex is often thinned and may be absent in some areas, leading to CSF leaks. Furthermore, pedicle screw fixation is often

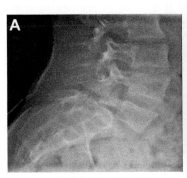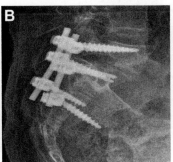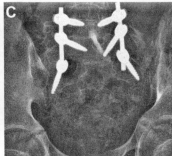

Fig. 4. Spondylolisthesis: Grade V anterior spondylolisthesis of L5 over S1 in a 17-year old with LDS (*A*). Operative management consisted of posterior fusion with L5-S1-S2 ala instrumentation and Bohlman interbody dowel graft (*B, C*).

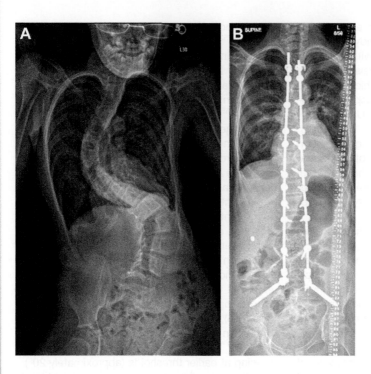

Fig. 5. Surgical correction of scoliosis: Preoperative imaging of 10-year-old patient with MFS and double 90° thoracic and lumbar curves with significant pelvic imbalance (*A*). Spinal fusion extending from the upper thoracic spine to the pelvis joints demonstrated complete deformity correction (*B*).

especially challenging in patients with connective tissue disorders because of the thin pedicles, which often lack a central channel. Intraoperative imaging or navigation and use of an "in-out-in" technique may be needed. Anchors at the ends of the constructs should be carefully assessed for stability, because failure of fixation is more common in patients with connective tissue disorders. Strategies to manage this include supplementing screws with laminar hooks or bands at

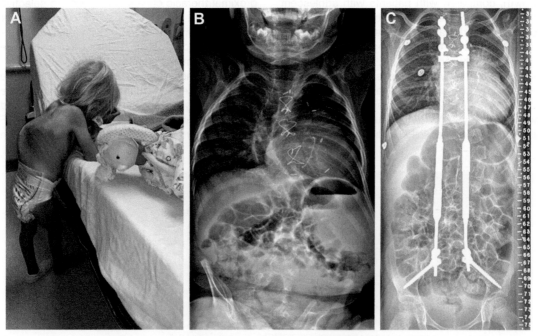

Fig. 6. Magnetically controlled growing rods: 2-year old patient with severe infantile MFS-associated scoliosis as evidenced on preoperative imaging (*A*, *B*). Spinal fusion with magnetic growing rods from T2 to sacrum was indicated due to concerns for respiratory insufficiency secondary to thoracic growth arrest (*C*).

the same level or extension to a lower level (**Fig. 5**). Dissection inside the spinal canal should be limited because of the risk of CSF fluid leakage. Trendelenburg positioning may help to minimize risk. In the event of a CSF leak, management may include direct repair, or use of a patch, sealant, and recumbent positioning.

Given the risk for dramatic progression into adulthood and serious complications, surgery is sometimes required earlier, at younger ages and smaller curves, in patients with syndromic scoliosis compared with those with idiopathic scoliosis. Growing rods can be used to treat progressive spinal deformities if curves become severe before the age of 9 years, because patients with connective tissue disorders do not tend to experience diminishing distractions with time as seen in other deformity types[58,59] (**Fig. 6**).

As the abnormal osseous anatomy and weak connective tissue presents serious complexity to the surgical management of scoliosis in these patients, surgical correction should only be performed by experienced professionals. Rates of major complications, including procedural and device-related ones, have been reported as 3 times higher in patients with syndromic scoliosis compared with idiopathic scoliosis.[60] Proximal and distal junctional kyphosis are common and should be followed closely. In such cases, extension of fusion should be considered to provide added stability. Some patients with LDS have required fusion of the entire spine because of significant deformities, which may evolve separately in the cervical, thoracolumbar, and lumbosacral region.[4] In addition, Levy and colleagues[61] demonstrated that patients with syndromic scoliosis experienced higher rates of postoperative infections, implant failures, and pseudoarthrosis. Patients with MFS are at particular risk given the narrow pedicles, thin lamina, and weakened dural connective tissue, with an estimated dural tear rate of 8% and adjacent segment lamina fracture rate of 8%.[11] Bressner and colleagues[49] reported distinct surgical complications, including greater than typical blood loss and CSF leaks. The investigators also noted that these patients required augmentation of preexisting fusion or repair of fractured rods given failure of fixation.

SUMMARY

In conclusion, heritable connective tissue disorders encompass an array of related syndromes with global manifestations involving the cardiovascular, neurologic, and ocular systems, among others. In particular, patients affected by connective tissue disorders may present with deformities along any or all regions of the spine. Unifying dysplastic changes, including dural abnormalities, bony deformations, and ligamentous laxity, impose additional challenges to surgical care and increased risk for perioperative complications. Therefore, preoperative planning requires careful consideration of these unique complications along with interdisciplinary collaboration to provide patients the best outcomes.

CLINICS CARE POINTS

- Patients with DE are asymptomatic in most cases, because the diagnosis is often an incidental finding. Although a variety of treatments have been reported, none have been consistently effective, making management particularly difficult. Surgical intervention should be cautioned against given risk of injury to nerve roots that course over the dura.

- First-line treatment of cervical abnormalities such as AAI is typically conservative, because patients rarely present with debilitating neurologic injury and the natural history of remains unclear. Posterior cervical spinal fusion is more beneficial in patients with symptoms secondary to ligamentous instability versus osseous instability.

- Surgical correction of thoracolumbar deformities is typically feasible with a posterior-only approach. However, osseous abnormalities and weakened connective tissue present serious complexity to surgical management and increased risk for perioperative complications.

DISCLOSURE

The authors declare no potential conflicts of interest with respect to the authorship and/or publication of this article. None of the authors received financial support for this manuscript.

REFERENCES

1. Dietz HC, Cutting GR, Pyeritz RE, et al. Marfan syndrome caused by a recurrent de novo missense mutation in the fibrillin gene. Nature 1991;352(6333):337–9.

2. Loeys BL, Dietz HC, Braverman AC, et al. The revised Ghent nosology for the Marfan syndrome. J Med Genet 2010;47(7):476–85.

3. Cañadas V, Vilacosta I, Bruna I, et al. Marfan syndrome. Part 2: treatment and management of patients. Nat Rev Cardiol 2010;7(5):266–76.

4. Tan EW, Sponseller PD. Connective tissue syndromes: themes and guidelines for the Spine Deformity Surgeon. Spine Deform 2012. https://doi.org/10.1016/j.jspd.2012.04.007.

5. Byers PH, Murray ML. Heritable collagen disorders: the paradigm of the Ehlers-Danlos syndrome. J Invest Dermatol 2012;132(E1):E6–11.

6. Henderson FC, Austin C, Benzel E, et al. Neurological and spinal manifestations of the Ehlers–Danlos syndromes. Am J Med Genet C Semin Med Genet 2017. https://doi.org/10.1002/ajmg.c.31549.

7. Erkula G, Sponseller PD, Paulsen LC, et al. Musculoskeletal findings of Loeys-Dietz syndrome. J Bone Joint Surg Am 2010;92(9):1876–83.

8. Loeys BL, Chen J, Neptune ER, et al. A syndrome of altered cardiovascular, craniofacial, neurocognitive and skeletal development caused by mutations in TGFBR1 or TGFBR2. Nat Genet 2005;37(3):275–81.

9. Loeys BL, Schwarze U, Holm T, et al. Aneurysm syndromes caused by mutations in the TGF-beta receptor. N Engl J Med 2006;355(8):788–98.

10. Williams JA, Hanna JM, Shah AA, et al. Adult surgical experience with Loeys-Dietz syndrome. Ann Thorac Surg 2015;99(4):1275–81.

11. Jones TL, Papadopoulos MC. The neurosurgical manifestations of Marfan syndrome. In: Diagnosis and management of marfan syndrome. New York, NY: Lippincott Williams & Wilkens; 2016. doi:10.1007/978-1-4471-5442-6_19

12. Fishman EK, Zinreich SJ, Kumar AJ, et al. Sacral abnormalities in marfan syndrome. J Comput Assist Tomogr 1983. https://doi.org/10.1097/00004728-198310000-00019.

13. Derdabi I, Jouadi H El, Edderai M. Dural ectasia: a manifestation of type 1 neurofibromatosis. Pan Afr Med J 2018;31:226.

14. De Paepe A, Devereux RB, Dietz HC, et al. Revised diagnostic criteria for the Marfan syndrome. Am J Med Genet 1996;62(4):417–26.

15. Mesfin A, Ahn NU, Carrino JA, et al. Ten-year clinical and imaging follow-up of dural ectasia in adults with Marfan syndrome. Spine J 2013;13(1):62–7.

16. Böker T, Vanem TT, Pripp AH, et al. Dural ectasia in Marfan syndrome and other hereditary connective tissue disorders: a 10-year follow-up study. Spine J 2019. https://doi.org/10.1016/j.spinee.2019.04.010.

17. Foran JRH, Pyeritz RE, Dietz HC, et al. Characterization of the symptoms associated with dural ectasia in the Marfan patient. Am J Med Genet A 2005;134A(1):58–65.

18. Ahn NU, Sponseller PD, Ahn UM, et al. Dural ectasia is associated with back pain in marfan syndrome. Spine (Phila Pa 1976) 2000. https://doi.org/10.1097/00007632-200006150-00017.

19. Ahn NU, Sponseller PD, Ahn UM, et al. Dural ectasia in the Marfan syndrome: MR and CT findings and criteria. Genet Med 2000;2(3):173–9.

20. Oosterhof T, Groenink M, Hulsmans FJ, et al. Quantitative assessment of dural ectasia as a marker for Marfan syndrome. Radiology 2001;220(2):514–8.

21. Habermann CR, Weiss F, Schoder V, et al. MR evaluation of dural ectasia in Marfan syndrome: reassessment of the established criteria in children, adolescents, and young adults. Radiology 2005;234(2):535–41.

22. Fattori R, Nienaber CA, Descovich B, et al. Importance of dural ectasia in phenotypic assessment of Marfan's syndrome. Lancet 1999;354(9182):910–3.

23. Lundby R, Rand-Hendriksen S, Hald JK, et al. Dural ectasia in Marfan syndrome: a case control study. AJNR Am J Neuroradiol 2009;30(8):1534–40.

24. Pierro A, Cilla S, Maselli G, et al. Sagittal normal limits of lumbosacral spine in a large adult population: a quantitative magnetic resonance imaging analysis. J Clin Imaging Sci 2017;7:35.

25. Ahn NU, Nallamshetty L, Ahn UM, et al. Dural ectasia and conventional radiography in the Marfan lumbosacral spine. Skeletal Radiol 2001. https://doi.org/10.1007/s002560100323.

26. Kohns DJ. Interventional spine considerations for Dural ectasia in a patient with marfan syndrome. Am J Phys Med Rehabil 2018;97(1):e6–8.

27. Nguyen HS, Lozen A, Doan N, et al. Marsupialization and distal obliteration of a lumbosacral dural ectasia in a nonsyndromic, adult patient. J Craniovertebr Junction Spine 2015. https://doi.org/10.4103/0974-8237.167887.

28. Trapp C, Farage L, Clatterbuck RE, et al. Laparoscopic treatment of anterior sacral meningocele. Surg Neurol 2007;68(4):443–8 [discussion 448].

29. Anderson FM, Burke BL. Anterior sacral meningocele: a presentation of three cases. JAMA J Am Med Assoc 1977. https://doi.org/10.1001/jama.1977.03270280041019.

30. Gupta N, Gupta V, Kumar A, et al. Dural ectasia. Indian J Anaesth 2014;58(2):199–201.

31. Hobbs WR, Sponseller PD, Weiss A-PC, et al. The Cervical Spine in Marfan Syndrome. Spine (Phila Pa 1976) 1997;22(9):983–9.

32. Fuhrhop SK, McElroy MJ, Dietz HC 3rd, et al. High prevalence of cervical deformity and instability requires surveillance in Loeys-Dietz syndrome. J Bone Joint Surg Am 2015;97(5):411–9.

33. Lacy J, Bajaj J, Gillis CC. Atlantoaxial instability. StatPearls [Internet]. Treasure Island (FL): StatPearls Publishing; 2021.

34. Tubbs RS, Hallock JD, Radcliff V, et al. Ligaments of the craniocervical junction: a review. J Neurosurg Spine 2011. https://doi.org/10.3171/2011.1.SPINE10612.

35. Castori M, Voermans NC. Neurological manifestations of Ehlers-Danlos syndrome(s): a review. Iran J Neurol 2014;13(4):190–208.

36. Menendez JA, Wright NM. Techniques of posterior C1-C2 stabilization. Neurosurgery 2007. https://doi.org/10.1227/01.NEU.0000249220.50085.E4.

37. Herzka A, Sponseller PD, Pyeritz RE. Atlantoaxial rotatory subluxation in patients with Marfan syndrome: a report of three cases. Spine (Phila Pa 1976) 2000. https://doi.org/10.1097/00007632-200002150-00022.

38. Sponseller PD, Ahn NU, Ahn UM, et al. Osseous anatomy of the lumbosacral spine in marfan syndrome. Spine (Phila Pa 1976) 2000;25(21):2797–802.

39. Ben Amor IM, Edouard T, Glorieux FH, et al. Low bone mass and high material bone density in two patients with Loeys-Dietz syndrome caused by transforming growth factor beta receptor 2 mutations. J Bone Miner Res 2012;27(3):713–8.

40. Tan EW, Offoha RU, Oswald GL, et al. Increased fracture risk and low bone mineral density in patients with loeys-dietz syndrome. Am J Med Genet A 2013;161A(8):1910–4.

41. Eller-Vainicher C, Bassotti A, Imeraj A, et al. Bone involvement in adult patients affected with Ehlers-Danlos syndrome. Osteoporos Int 2016;27(8):2525–31.

42. Bydon M, Alvi MA, Goyal A. Degenerative lumbar spondylolisthesis: definition, natural history, conservative management, and surgical treatment. Neurosurg Clin N Am 2019. https://doi.org/10.1016/j.nec.2019.02.003.

43. Sponseller PD, Hobbs W, Riley LH, et al. The thoracolumbar spine in Marfan syndrome. J Bone Joint Surg Am 1995. https://doi.org/10.2106/00004623-199506000-00007.

44. Lavelle WF, Marawar S, Bell G. Degenerative lumbar instability. Semin Spine Surg 2013. https://doi.org/10.1053/j.semss.2013.03.003.

45. Winter RB. Severe spondylolisthesis in Marfan's syndrome: report of two cases. J Pediatr Orthop 1982. https://doi.org/10.1097/01241398-198202010-00007.

46. Taylor LJ. Severe spondylolisthesis and scoliosis in association with Marfan's syndrome. Case report and review of the literature. Clin Orthop Relat Res 1987. https://doi.org/10.1097/00003086-198708000-00024.

47. Koreckij TD, Fischgrund JS. Degenerative spondylolisthesis. J Spinal Disord Tech 2015. https://doi.org/10.1097/BSD.0000000000000298.

48. Meyerding HW. Spondylolisthesis; surgical fusion of lumbosacral portion of spinal column and interarticular facets; use of autogenous bone grafts for relief of disabling backache. J Int Coll Surg 1956;26(5 Part 1):566–91.

49. Bressner JA, MacCarrick GL, Dietz HC, et al. Management of Scoliosis in Patients With Loeys-Dietz Syndrome. J Pediatr Orthop 2017;37(8):e492–9.

50. Liu Y, Gao R, Zhou X, et al. Posterior spinal fusion for scoliosis in Ehlers-Danlos syndrome, kyphoscoliosis type. Orthopedics 2011;34(6):228.

51. Giunta C, Rohrbach M, Fauth C, et al. FKBP14 Kyphoscoliotic Ehlers-Danlos Syndrome. In: Adam MP, Ardinger HH, Pagon RA, et al., eds. GeneReviews® [Internet]. Seattle (WA): University of Washington, Seattle; 1993–2021.

52. Meester JAN, Verstraeten A, Schepers D, et al. Differences in manifestations of Marfan syndrome, Ehlers-Danlos syndrome, and Loeys-Dietz syndrome. Ann Cardiothorac Surg 2017;6(6):582–94.

53. Uehara M, Kosho T, Yamamoto N, et al. Spinal manifestations in 12 patients with musculocontractural Ehlers-Danlos syndrome caused by CHST14/D4ST1 deficiency (mcEDS-CHST14). Am J Med Genet A 2018;176(11):2331–41.

54. Lenke LG, Betz RR, Harms J, et al. Adolescent idiopathic scoliosis. A new classification to determine extent of spinal arthrodesis. J Bone Joint Surg Am 2001. https://doi.org/10.2106/00004623-200108000-00006.

55. Zenner J, Hitzl W, Meier O, et al. Surgical outcomes of scoliosis surgery in marfan syndrome. J Spinal Disord Tech 2014. https://doi.org/10.1097/BSD.0b013e31824de6f1.

56. Sponseller PD, Bhimani M, Solacoff D, et al. Results of brace treatment of scoliosis in Marfan syndrome. Spine (Phila Pa 1976) 2000. https://doi.org/10.1097/00007632-200009150-00013.

57. Gjolaj JP, Sponseller PD, Shah SA, et al. Spinal deformity correction in Marfan syndrome versus adolescent idiopathic scoliosis: learning from the differences. Spine (Phila Pa 1976) 2012;37(18):1558–65.

58. Sponseller PD, Thompson GH, Akbarnia BA, et al. Growing rods for infantile scoliosis in marfan syndrome. Spine (Phila Pa 1976) 2009. https://doi.org/10.1097/BRS.0b013e3181a9ece5.

59. Marrache M, White K, Larson AN, et al. Does the law of diminishing returns exist in early onset scoliosis with connective tissue disorders? Spine Deform 2019;7(6):1017–8.

60. Chung AS, Renfree S, Lockwood DB, et al. Syndromic scoliosis: national trends in surgical management and inpatient hospital outcomes: a 12-year analysis. Spine (Phila Pa 1976) 2019. https://doi.org/10.1097/BRS.0000000000003134.

61. Levy BJ, Schulz JF, Fornari ED, et al. Complications associated with surgical repair of syndromic scoliosis. Scoliosis 2015. https://doi.org/10.1186/s13013-015-0035-x.

Neurosurgical Evaluation and Management of Patients with Chromosomal Abnormalities

James A. Stadler III, MD

KEYWORDS

- Chromosomal abnormality • Trisomy • Atlantoaxial instability • Down syndrome
- Edwards syndrome • Patau syndrome • Klinefelter syndrome • DiGeorge syndrome

KEY POINTS

- Down syndrome (trisomy 21) is associated with atlantoaxial instability, moyamoya syndrome, and epilepsy.
- Patients with Edwards syndrome (trisomy 18) and Patau syndrome (trisomy 13) may have significant intracranial and spinal developmental concerns.
- Patients with Klinefelter syndrome (47,XXY) and velocardiofacial syndrome (22q11.2 deletion) may have spinal pathologies secondary to abnormal bone metabolism.

INTRODUCTION

Chromosomal abnormalities, as an umbrella term, have wide-ranging pathologic presentations. Inherently these disorders affect multiple genes, and by extension, numerous body systems. Patients may have an abnormal number of chromosomes, either from missing or having an extra chromosome or from structural changes following deletion, duplication, inversion, substitution, or translocation of chromosomal segments.[1] Clinical presentation may be further influenced by mosaicism and epigenetic drivers.[2]

Although there are reported cases of sporadic cranial and spinal pathologies in patients with almost all described chromosomal abnormalities, there are several syndromes with significant and relatively consistent neurosurgical concerns (**Table 1**)—Down syndrome (trisomy 21), Edwards syndrome (trisomy 18), Patau syndrome (trisomy 13), Klinefelter syndrome (47,XXY), and velocardiofacial or DiGeorge syndrome (22q11.2 deletion). Patients with these syndromes are best served by multidisciplinary teams with experience specific to their condition.

DISCUSSION

Down Syndrome

Down syndrome, or trisomy 21, is the most common survivable autosomal aneuploidy, affecting approximately 1 in 700 live births.[3,4] Down syndrome results from supernumerary representation of chromosome 21 overexpressing more than 300 genes.[5] Most patients have a complete extra copy of chromosome 21, although 2% to 4% have translocation of genetic material from chromosome 21, most often to chromosome 14, and a small percent of patients have genetic mosaicism.[6]

Patients with Down syndrome show a widely variable phenotype that often includes learning difficulties, short stature, craniofacial anomalies, and hypotonia. Systemic manifestations may include cardiac or gastrointestinal abnormalities, leukemia, and endocrine disorders.[5,7,8] Current life expectancy exceeds 60 years and continues to increase with comprehensive medical care.[9]

Cervical instability, and in particular atlantoaxial instability, is the most prominent neurosurgical concern in patients with Down syndrome.[10,11]

Department of Neurological Surgery, University of Wisconsin School of Medicine and Public Health, University of Wisconsin-Madison, 600 Highland Avenue, Madison, WI 53792, USA
E-mail address: stadler@neurosurgery.wisc.edu

Neurosurg Clin N Am 33 (2022) 61–65
https://doi.org/10.1016/j.nec.2021.09.012
1042-3680/22/© 2021 Elsevier Inc. All rights reserved.

neurosurgery.theclinics.com

Table 1
Summary of chromosomal abnormalities with neurosurgical implications

Syndrome/Eponym	Chromosomal Abnormality	Frequency	Neurosurgical Concerns	Systemic Concerns
Down	Trisomy 21	1:700	Atlantoaxial instability Moyamoya/strokes Seizures	Cardiac GI Endocrine Lymphoma
Edwards	Trisomy 18	1:6000	Myelomeningocele Encephalocele Tethered cord Cerebellar hypoplasia Callosal agenesis Polymicrogyria Seizures	Cardiac GU GI Limbs Ophthalmologic Low birth weight Arthrogryposis
Patau	Trisomy 13	1:10,000	Holoprosencephaly Myelomeningocele Tethered cord Hypotonia	Cardiac Microphthalmia Polydactyly Cleft lip/palate
Klinefelter	47,XXY	1–2:1000	Spinal fractures	Androgen deficiency Infertility Osteoporosis
Velocardiofacial (DiGeorge)	22q11.2 deletion	1:4000	Cervical abnormalities Scoliosis	Cardiac Immune deficiency GU Hypocalcemia

Abbreviations: GI, gastrointestinal; GU, genitourinary.

Atlantoaxial instability is found in 5% to 30% of patients, with rates varying likely in relation to diagnostic criteria, although only 1% to 2% become symptomatic from this.[10,12,13] Children with Down syndrome must be carefully followed with serial examinations to watch for developing myelopathy, and some investigators have advocated for routine radiographic monitoring as well.[8,12,14] Children with os odontoideum may be at particular risk for clinical progression.[12] Upright lateral images seem as effective as flexion/extension imaging, but certain organizations and activities, perhaps most notably with the Special Olympics, may request certain protocols before involvement.[14,15] Surgery is generally indicated for children with an atlantodental interval (ADI) greater than 10 mm, an ADI greater than 5 mm if myelopathic, and/or a C1-2 canal width of less than 14 mm.

Patients with Down syndrome have increased risk for moyamoya syndrome and strokes.[16] Perhaps related to underlying vasculopathy, the pathogenesis of this observation is unknown. Patients typically respond well to indirect revascularization.[17] Additional risk for strokes comes from associated cardiac abnormalities. Children with Down syndrome also have an increased risk of seizures, which affect up to 13% of patients.[10]

Edwards Syndrome

Edwards syndrome results from trisomy 18, with liveborn prevalence of approximately 1 in 6000.[3,18] Prenatally, children often have intrauterine growth restriction and may have low birth weight. Multisystem medical concerns, including significant neurodevelopmental delays and cardiac abnormalities, lead to a 5-year survival of 12%.[19]

Intracranial abnormalities classically include choroid plexus cysts, which may be appreciated prenatally and are typically benign, head shape and craniofacial abnormalities, and structural brain concerns such as holoprosencephaly or encephalocele.[18,20,21] Epilepsy is common in children with trisomy 18.[22,23] Neural tube defects and tethering of the spinal cord also seems to be relatively more common in Edwards syndrome.[21,24]

It is worth acknowledging ethical discussions regarding surgery in children with life-limiting conditions such as trisomy 18 or 13.[25–28] Although each condition has significant impact on function and survival, children should nevertheless be evaluated thoroughly by teams familiar with the condition. If this evaluation reveals opportunities to help improve the child's clinical status, surgery is often appropriate, provided truly informed parental consent with realistic understanding of surgical risks and benefits is obtained.

Patau Syndrome

Patau syndrome, or trisomy 13, is relatively less common, affecting fewer than 1 in 10,000 live births.[3,29] Complete trisomy, seen in 80% of patients, is the result of nondisjunction at meiosis; partial expression may be seen secondary to partial genetic translocation or mosaicism.[30] Significant developmental delays and physical abnormalities are common, including microcephaly, microphthalmia or proboscis, cleft lip or palate, cardiac abnormalities, and polydactyly. Mortality is greater than 90%, primarily within the first year of life.[28]

Patau syndrome is associated with significant neurologic and neurosurgical concerns. Children typically have significant intracranial malformations, including holoprosencephaly or schizencephaly. Seizures are common and should be managed by specialists familiar with the condition. Although not well studied, many children have neural tube defects including myelomeningocele or problems with secondary neurulation.[24,31] Given their neurodevelopmental status and other medical concerns, diagnosing a tethered spinal cord in children with trisomy 13 may be challenging and requires some preexistent suspicion. As discussed with Edwards syndrome, informed discussions with patients' families are critical to guide optimal care.[28]

Klinefelter Syndrome

Klinefelter syndrome is seen in men with an extra X chromosome. The most common chromosome aberration is 47,XXY, although up to 20% of patients may have higher grade aneuploidies such as 48,XXYY and 49,XXXXY.[32] At least 1 to 2 in 1000 people are diagnosed with Klinefelter syndrome, making this one of the most common chromosomal anomalies in humans. This rate is likely underestimated, given ambiguous and at times mild presentation, lack of clinician awareness, and the possibility of gonadal mosaicism.[32,33]

The syndrome is most prominently associated with androgen deficiency and infertility. Physical characteristics and symptoms vary significantly but often include decreased testicular volume, decreased libido, decreased muscle strength, and obesity.

Secondary osteoporosis may predispose this patient population to spinal fractures.[34] Atypical fracture patterns may prompt bone density analysis and investigation, as Klinefelter syndrome frequently goes undiagnosed. Patients with Klinefelter syndrome may benefit from hormone therapy for treatment of lower bone density.[35]

Velocardiofacial Syndrome

Velocardiofacial syndrome, also referred to as DiGeorge syndrome, results from a chromosomal deletion at 22q11.2.[36] Prevalence is estimated at 1:4000 live births, and the primary associations of the syndrome are with cardiac anomalies, hypoparathyroidism/hypocalcemia, immune deficiencies related to thymic aplasia, cleft lip or palate and other craniofacial abnormalities, and developmental delays. Clinical findings vary considerably due to incomplete penetrance.

Most, if not all, patients with velocardiofacial syndrome have craniocervical abnormalities, likely related to hypocalcemia and abnormal bone metabolism,[37–39] which most commonly is manifest as platybasia (although basilar invagination is relatively uncommon), dysmorphic spinal elements particularly at C2, vertebral autofusion, and absence of the posterior arch.[38] Fortunately, radiographic instability is uncommon.[40] These patients also are at significant risk for scoliosis.[41]

Although most patients with velocardiofacial syndrome do not require spinal surgery, associated medical concerns must be optimized before any operative intervention. The indications and scope of surgical intervention must be tailored to the patient's needs and medical status.[42,43]

SUMMARY

Patients with chromosomal abnormalities are at risk for numerous neurosurgical pathologies given the broad impact and multisystem involvement of these disorders. Given the heterogeneity of concerns and presentations, these patients benefit from multidisciplinary care provided by teams familiar with their specific syndrome.

CLINICS CARE POINTS

- Down syndrome carries risk of atlantoaxial instability, moyamoya syndrome, and epilepsy.
- Edwards and Patau syndromes are associated with numerous neurosurgical concerns that should be addressed in the context of their syndromes.
- Patients with Klinefelter and velocardiofacial syndromes may have spinal concerns as a

manifestation of broader pathologic processes.

- Patients with chromosomal abnormalities benefit from multidisciplinary teams experienced in caring for their syndrome.

DISCLOSURE

The author has nothing to disclose.

REFERENCES

1. National Human Genome Research Institute Home | NHGRI. Available at: https://www.genome.gov/. Accessed September 4, 2021.
2. Kurahashi H, Bolor H, Kato T, et al. Recent advance in our understanding of the molecular nature of chromosomal abnormalities. J Hum Genet 2009;54(5): 253–60.
3. Mai C, Isenburg J, Canfield M, et al. National population-based estimates for major birth defects, 2010-2014. Birth Defects Res 2019;111(18): 1420–35.
4. Sherman S, Allen E, Bean L, et al. Epidemiology of down syndrome. Ment Retard Dev Disabil Res Rev 2007;13(3):221–7.
5. Lana-Elola E, Watson-Scales SD, Fisher EMC, et al. Down syndrome: searching for the genetic culprits. Dis Model Mech 2011;4(5):586.
6. Ranweiler R. Assessment and care of the newborn with down syndrome. Adv Neonatal Care 2009; 9(1):17–24.
7. Antonarakis S, Skotko B, Rafii M, et al. Down syndrome. Nat Rev Dis Prim 2020;6(1).
8. Bull M. Health supervision for children with down syndrome. Pediatrics 2011;128(2):393–406.
9. Tsou A, Bulova P, Capone G, et al. Medical care of adults with down syndrome: a clinical guideline. JAMA 2020;324(15):1543–56.
10. Hwang S, Jea A. A review of the neurological and neurosurgical implications of down syndrome in children. Clin Pediatr (Phila) 2013;52(9):845–56.
11. Brockmeyer D. Down syndrome and craniovertebral instability. Topic review and treatment recommendations. Pediatr Neurosurg 1999;31(2):71–7.
12. Bauer J, Dhaliwal V, Browd S, et al. Repeat pediatric trisomy 21 radiographic exam: does atlantoaxial instability develop over time? J Pediatr Orthop 2021;41(8):E646–50.
13. Bertolizio G, Saint-Martin C, Ingelmo P. Cervical instability in patients with Trisomy 21: The eternal gamble. Paediatr Anaesth 2018;28(10):830–3.
14. Bouchard M, Bauer JM, Bompadre V, et al. An updated algorithm for radiographic screening of upper cervical instability in patients with down syndrome. Spine Deform 2019;7(6):950–6.
15. Myśliwiec A, Posłuszny A, Saulicz E, et al. Atlantoaxial instability in people with down's syndrome and its impact on the ability to perform sports activities – a review. J Hum Kinet 2015;48(1):17.
16. Kainth D, Chaudhry S, Kainth H, et al. Prevalence and characteristics of concurrent down syndrome in patients with moyamoya disease. Neurosurgery 2013;72(2):210–5.
17. Jea A, Smith E, Robertson R, et al. Moyamoya syndrome associated with Down syndrome: outcome after surgical revascularization. Pediatrics 2005; 116(5):e694–701.
18. Cereda A, Carey JC. The trisomy 18 syndrome. Orphanet J Rare Dis 2012;7(1):81.
19. Meyer RE, Liu G, Gilboa SM, et al. Survival of children with trisomy 13 and trisomy 18: a multi-state population-based study. Am J Med Genet A 2016; 170(4):825–37.
20. Papp C, Ban Z, Szigeti Z, et al. Role of second trimester sonography in detecting trisomy 18: a review of 70 cases. J Clin Ultrasound 2007;35(2):68–72.
21. Rosa R, Trevisan P, Rosa R, et al. Trisomy 18 and neural tube defects. Pediatr Neurol 2013;49(3): 203–4.
22. Verrotti A, Carelli A, di Genova L, et al. Epilepsy and chromosome 18 abnormalities: a review. Seizure 2015;32:78–83.
23. Grosso S, Pucci L, Di Bartolo RM, et al. Chromosome 18 aberrations and epilepsy: a review. Am J Med Genet 2005;134-A(1):88–94.
24. Bassuk A, Craig D, Jalali A, et al. The genetics of tethered cord syndrome. Am J Med Genet A 2005; 132-A(4):450–3.
25. Andrews S, Downey A, Showalter D, et al. Shared decision making and the pathways approach in the prenatal and postnatal management of the trisomy 13 and trisomy 18 syndromes. Am J Med Genet C Semin Med Genet 2016;172(3):257–63.
26. Macias G, Riley C. Trisomy 13: changing perspectives. Neonatal Netw 2016;35(1):31–6.
27. Carey JC, Kosho T. Perspectives on the care and advances in the management of children with trisomy 13 and 18. Am J Med Genet C Semin Med Genet 2016;172(3):249–50.
28. Janvier A, Farlow B, Barrington KJ. Parental hopes, interventions, and survival of neonates with trisomy 13 and trisomy 18. Am J Med Genet C Semin Med Genet 2016;172(3):279–87.
29. Levy PA, Marion R. Trisomies. Pediatr Rev 2018; 39(2):104–6.
30. Hall HE, Chan ER, Collins A, et al. The origin of trisomy 13. Am J Med Genet A 2007;143A(19):2242–8.
31. Rodríguez J, García M, Morales C, et al. Trisomy 13 syndrome and neural tube defects. Am J Med Genet 1990;36(4):513–6.

32. Lanfranco F, Kamischke A, Zitzmann M, et al. Klinefelter's syndrome. Lancet 2004;364(9430):273–83.

33. Berglund A, Stochholm K, Gravholt C. The epidemiology of sex chromosome abnormalities. Am J Med Genet C Semin Med Genet 2020;184(2):202–15.

34. Vena W, Pizzocaro A, Indirli R, et al. Prevalence and determinants of radiological vertebral fractures in patients with Klinefelter syndrome. Andrology 2020;8(6):1699–704.

35. Vogiatzi MG, Davis SM, Ross JL. Cortical bone mass is low in boys with klinefelter syndrome and improves with oxandrolone. J Endocr Soc 2021;5(4): bvab016.

36. McDonald-McGinn D, Sullivan K. Chromosome 22q11.2 deletion syndrome (DiGeorge syndrome/velocardiofacial syndrome). Medicine (Baltimore) 2011;90(1):1–18.

37. Hamidi M, Nabi S, Husein M, et al. Cervical spine abnormalities in 22q11.2 deletion syndrome. Cleft Palate Craniofac J 2014;51(2):230–3.

38. Ricchetti ET, States L, Hosalkar HS, et al. Radiographic study of the upper cervical spine in the 22Q11.2 deletion syndrome. J Bone Joint Surg Am 2004;86(8):1751–60.

39. McKay SD, Al-Omari A, Tomlinson LA, et al. Review of cervical spine anomalies in genetic syndromes. Spine (Phila Pa 1976) 2012;37(5):E269–77.

40. Kolman S, Ohara S, Bhatia A, et al. The clinical utility of flexion-extension cervical spine MRI in 22q11.2 deletion syndrome. J Pediatr Orthop 2019;39(9): E674–9.

41. Homans J, Baldew V, Brink R, et al. Scoliosis in association with the 22q11.2 deletion syndrome: an observational study. Arch Dis Child 2019;104(1): 19–24.

42. Stransky C, Basta M, McDonald-McGinn DM, et al. Perioperative risk factors in patients with 22q11.2 deletion syndrome requiring surgery for velopharyngeal dysfunction. Cleft Palate Craniofac J 2015; 52(2):183–91.

43. Campbell V, Lucas J. Beware the syndromic spine. Arch Dis Child 2019;104(1):5–6.

Syndromic Hydrocephalus

Kaamya Varagur, BA, MPhil, Sai Anusha Sanka, BA, MPH,
Jennifer M. Strahle, MD*

KEYWORDS

- Hydrocephalus • Syndromic hydrocephalus • Hydrocephalus genetics

KEY POINTS

- Hydrocephalus is a phenotypic feature associated with a diverse set of genetic syndromes in childhood
- Pathogenesis and accompanying phenotypic features, as well as inheritance patterns, vary between and within syndromes
- Next-generation sequencing studies now identify underlying genetic causes of hydrocephalus, previously categorized as "congenital hydrocephalus."

INTRODUCTION

Hydrocephalus is characterized by abnormal accumulation, and impaired circulation and clearance, of cerebrospinal fluid (CSF). CSF accumulation results in distention of the ventricular system, leading to accelerated head growth and increased intracranial pressure, and often requires surgical intervention.[1,2] Syndromic hydrocephalus encompasses a diverse group of disorders and genetic variants in which hydrocephalus is a symptom, due to congenital structural malformations, or a range of emerging pathology associated with recently described genetic variants.[3] In this review, we discuss several of the major syndromic causes of hydrocephalus, as well as emerging research on the genetic basis for congenital hydrocephalus as part of recently described genetic mutations (Table 1).

L1 SYNDROME, AND X-LINKED HYDROCEPHALUS

X-linked hydrocephalus comprises 5% of all cases of congenital hydrocephalus (Table 1)[1]. X-linked hydrocephalus, associated with hydrocephalus stenosis of the aqueduct of Sylvius (HSAS), is the most severe phenotype associated with L1 syndrome, an X-linked recessive disorder (Fig. 1).[4] Other phenotypes of L1 syndrome include MASA (mental retardation, aphasia, spastic paraplegia, adducted thumbs) and X-linked complicated corpus callosum and/or pyramidal tract agenesis.[3,5] Many of these phenotypic features commonly cooccur with X-linked hydrocephalus, especially intellectual disability.[6]

This syndrome results from mutations in *L1CAM* on chromosome region Xq28, affecting the locus of a gene coding for the neural cell adhesion molecule *L1*. Mutations in this gene are associated with disordered neuronal migration which is considered a key mechanism in the pathogenesis of this syndrome.[7] Knockout rat models of the disease have revealed early pathologic changes of periventricular white matter tracts following the development of hydrocephalus, evidenced by reductions in fractional anisotropy and axial diffusivity on DTI in the corpus callosum, external capsule, and internal capsule. Histology also revealed hypomyelination and increased extracellular fluid in the corpus callosum, yielding some insight into how mutations of *L1CAM* contribute

Department of Neurosurgery, Washington University School of Medicine, Washington University in Saint Louis, 660 South Euclid Avenue, Campus Box 8057, St Louis, MO 63110, USA
* Corresponding author.
E-mail address: strahlej@wustl.edu
Twitter: @kaamyavaragur (K.V.); @strahleMD (J.M.S.)

Neurosurg Clin N Am 33 (2022) 67–79
https://doi.org/10.1016/j.nec.2021.09.006

Table 1
Genetic basis of syndromes associated with hydrocephalus

Syndrome	Type of Disorder	Mode of Inheritance	Genetic Locus
L1 Syndrome, and X-Linked Hydrocephalus	Neuronal Adhesion	X-linked	L1CAM
Syndromic Craniosynostoses (Pfeiffer, Crouzon, Apert, Muenke)	Primary cerebral maldevelopment	Heterogeneous	FGFR1 (Pfeiffer), FGFR2 (Crouzon; Apert; Pfeiffer), FGFR3 (Muenke)
Achondroplasia	Growth Factor	Autosomal Dominant	FGFR3
NF 1	RASopathy	Autosomal Dominant	NF1 (17q11.2)
NF 2	RASopathy	Autosomal Dominant	NF2 (22q12)
Down's Syndrome	Trisomy	Nondisjunction	Chromosome 21
Tuberous Sclerosis	mTOR related	Autosomal Dominant	*DNAH5, DAIC1, CCDC151, MCIDAS, FOXJ1*
Walker–Warburg Syndrome/Brain-muscle-eye disease	Dystroglycanopathies	Autosomal Recessive	POMT1, POM*T2*, *POMGNT1, FKTN, FKRP, LARGE, ISPD*
Primary Ciliary Dyskinesia	Ciliopathy	Heterogeneous	DNAH5, MCIDAS, FOXJ1
Osteogenesis Imperfecta	Connective tissue	Autosomal Dominant	COL1A1 and COL1A2
Pettigrew Syndrome	Vesicle trafficking	X-linked	AP1S2
Costello Syndrome	RASopathy	Autosomal Dominant	HRAS
Noonon Syndrome	RASopathy	Autosomal Dominant	CBL, KRAS, NRAS, PTPN11, SOS1, SHOC2 and RAF1
Cardio-facio-cutaneous (CFC) syndrome	RASopathy	Autosomal Dominant	BRAF, MEK1, KRAS, and MEK2
Megalencephaly-polymicrogyria-polydactyly-hydrocephalus (MPPH)	PI3K-AKT-mTOR pathway	Autosomal Dominant	AKT3, CCND2 and PIK3R2
Megalencephaly-capillary-malformation (MCAP)	PI3K-AKT-mTOR pathway	N/A	PIK3CA

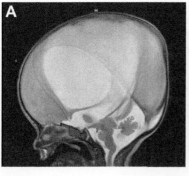
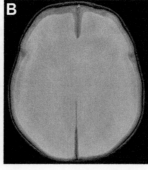

Fig. 1. 1-day-old with L1 syndrome resulting in hydrocephalus and aqueductal stenosis treated on day-of-life 1 with a VP shunt. T2-weighted MRI (*A*) sagittal and (*B*) axial views.

not only to hydrocephalus, but also to the developmental delays and intellectual deficits observed in this condition.[8]

Point mutations at branch points in introns of *L1CAM,* causing abnormal splicing, were among the first mutations implicated in the disease. Recently, duplication affecting the intracellular domain, frameshift mutations affecting translation of fibronectin type-III of *L1CAM,* and novel nonsense mutations affecting ependymal cilia have also been implicated in this syndrome.[9–13]

Beyond *L1CAM,* other X-linked mutations have recently been associated with syndromic hydrocephalus, including missense mutations in OTUD5 resulting in severe neurodevelopmental delay hydrocephalus, and early lethality.[14] Duplications of Xp22.33 also lead to an L1-like phenotype of hydrocephalus associated with stenosis of the cerebral aqueduct, and dysgenesis of the corpus callosum.[15] Modern sequencing techniques may reveal other X-linked mutations associated with L1-like syndromic hydrocephalus, though *L1CAM* remains the most common and thoroughly explored locus causing this condition.

Once an *L1CAM* pathogenic variant has been identified in a family, carrier testing, prenatal testing, and preimplantation genetic testing are available to patients and families. Treatment of individuals with X-linked hydrocephalus may vary depending on the timing of presentation; however, because many patients present with symptomatic hydrocephalus at birth, treatment often involves ventriculoperitoneal shunting (VPS), as the efficacy of endoscopic third ventriculostomy (ETV) with choroid plexus catheterization (CPC) in young infants is variable.[4]

SYNDROMIC CRANIOSYNOSTOSIS

Syndromic craniosynostosis is associated with an increased incidence of hydrocephalus.[16] Hydrocephalus is more common in syndromic compared to nonsyndromic or isolated craniosynostosis, and is seen in Crouzon's and Pfeiffer's syndromes.[17] Mechanisms underlying hydrocephalus in this group of syndromes relate to primary cerebral maldevelopment and residual structural outflow obstruction, not significantly ameliorated by posterior vault distraction strip craniectomy or cranial vault reconstruction commonly used in the treatment of craniosynostosis.[16,18] Conversely, early shunting (or overshunting) can cause iatrogenic premature fusion of the cranial sutures in patients without craniosynostosis.[19] Treatment of hydrocephalus in patients with syndromic craniosynostosis includes VP shunt and ETV +/- CPC and is usually influenced by the future need for cranial vault reconstruction; therefore, location of shunt placement may vary to accommodate future planned surgeries.

Pfeiffer Syndrome Of the syndromes associated with craniosynostosis, Pfeiffer syndrome is most frequently associated with hydrocephalus, with up to 60% to 80% of patients requiring ventriculoperitoneal shunt insertion or other treatment for hydrocephalus.[20,21] This syndrome is also associated with speech, language, hearing, and feeding issues related to mutations in FGFR2.[21,22]

Crouzon syndrome, related to mutations in *FGFR2,*[23] can be associated with a small foramen magnum and outlet obstruction associated with hydrocephalus.[24] Because of the structural predisposition to developing hydrocephalus in this form of craniosynostosis, up to 40% of patients with Crouzon's can present with or develop ventricular dilation.[25] Although ventriculomegaly is common, a smaller number will ultimately require surgical treatment of hydrocephalus.[26]

Apert Syndrome Apert syndrome, also related to mutations in *FGFR2,* is characterized by multisuture craniosynostosis, midface retrusion, syndactyly of the hands, fusion of the second through fourth nails, and nonprogressive ventriculomegaly.[27,28] Fewer patients with Apert syndrome have true or progressive hydrocephalus, and shunting is rarely required.[29] Rates of ventriculoperitoneal shunt placement in one study of a cohort of patients with Apert syndrome was 24.3%, lower than seen in Crouzon or Pfeiffer syndromes.[30]

Muenke Syndrome Muenke syndrome is an autosomal dominant syndrome associated with mutations in *FGFR3* characterized by coronal craniosynostosis and variable extracranial anomalies.[31] Though this syndrome is not regularly associated with hydrocephalus, there has been a rare familial variant of this syndrome (p.Pro250Arg) with hydrocephalus, without craniosynostosis.[32]

ACHONDROPLASIA

Achondroplasia is an autosomal dominant skeletal dysplasia caused by a gain of function G380 R mutation in *FGFR3* on chromosome 4[33,34]. This mutation alters bone growth resulting in obstruction or stenosis of the cranial skull base foramina. Increases in venous pressure secondary to stenosis of the jugular foramen can result in macrocephaly, ventriculomegaly, and hydrocephalus.[33–35] The etiology of hydrocephalus in achondroplasia is likely multifactorial, with contributions from alterations in CSF flow at the FM, venous outflow alterations, and potentially decreased CSF egress along cranial nerve sheaths due to narrowing of their respective foramina.[34,36,37]

Many patients with achondroplasia have some degree of ventriculomegaly which stabilizes overtime.[37,38] As the natural history of this ventriculomegaly and the contributions from stenosis at the FM and cervical medullary junction is better understood, there are far fewer patients who receive treatment with a VPS, which in the past was associated with significant complications.[39] Some patients are successfully treated with cervicomedullary decompression, which is associated with decreased need for shunting and stabilization of both ventriculomegaly and intracranial pressure.[37,40]

NEUROFIBROMATOSIS 1 AND NEUROFIBROMATOSIS 2

Neurofibromatosis 1 (NF1), also known as von Recklinghausen's disease, is an autosomal dominant disorder caused by mutations on chromosome 17q11.2 that affect neurofibromin production.[41,42] NF 1 has variable expression and predisposes individuals to several tumors and hamartomas in the central and peripheral nervous system, including optic pathway gliomas (OPG) and gliomas outside the optic pathway, which in some cases can lead to obstructive hydrocephalus (**Fig. 2**).[43–46] "Hydrocephalus in NF-1 can occur from alterations in CSF circulation that results from OPGs, as well as periaqueductal gliosis, aqueductal webs, nontumor hamartomatous changes, and tectal and midbrain tumors causing obstruction or narrowing of the ventricular system, particularly at the level of the cerebral aqueduct.[45,47] Treatment may involve the tumor directly, or in some cases, surgical treatment for symptomatic hydrocephalus.[42,47] Direct treatment of a tumor may involve surgical removal or treatment with chemotherapy including BRAF/MEK inhibitors.[47] Finally, treatment of NF-1 associated

hydrocephalus with ETV can be successful regardless of the type or level of obstruction.[48]

Neurofibromatosis 2 (NF2), another autosomal dominant disorder, is caused by deletions or loss of function of the tumor suppressor gene on chromosome 22q12 that encodes the protein *Merlin*.[49,50] Compared to NF1 with a prevalence of 1 in 4000 to 5000 births, NF2 is more rare with an incidence of 1 in 40,000 births.[43,51] Patients with NF2 can develop bilateral vestibular schwannomas or other intracranial tumors that can rarely cause hydrocephalus through obstruction of CSF circulation.[50,52]

DOWN SYNDROME

There have been several case reports of hydrocephalus in patients with Down syndrome. Two early reports from the 1970s describe children with Down syndrome and hydrocephalus, aqueductal stenosis, and partial agenesis of the corpus callosum.[53,54] A more recent case report describes a patient whose hydrocephalus was detected during pregnancy who required treatment with ventriculoperitoneal shunt.[55] Two additional case reports describe two patients with Down syndrome and normal pressure hydrocephalus, both of whom were treated with ventriculoperitoneal shunts.[56] The second report describes a patient with tetraventricular hydrocephalus caused by the obstruction of the foramina of Luschka and Magendie treated using ETV.[57]

Although Down syndrome is not associated with hydrocephalus, mouse models have demonstrated ventriculomegaly related to the genetic abnormalities in Down syndrome. The Ts1Rhr mouse model, with a shorter trisomic segment than previous models, exhibits PcP4-dependent ciliopathy sufficient to trigger ventricular enlargement.[58] Thus, it is possible that despite their varying presentations and treatment, some of the reported human hydrocephalus cases may be related to

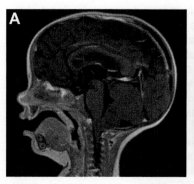
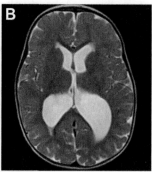

Fig. 2. 14-month-old with NF-1 presented with enlarged ventricles, transependymal CSF, and low tonsil position. Patient underwent Chiari decompression and subsequent treatment with ETV. T2-weighted MRI (*A*) sagittal and (*B*) axial views.

trisomy 21 itself rather than nonsyndromic findings. Finally, there is an increased prevalence of ventriculomegaly in very low birth weight (VLBW) infants with Down syndrome compared to other VLBW infants, suggesting that some Down Syndrome-related pathologic processes may contribute to the development of hydrocephalus or ventriculomegaly in a subset of patients with this condition.[59]

TUBEROUS SCLEROSIS

Tuberous sclerosis complex (TSC) is an autosomal dominant genetic syndrome with dysfunction of the mTOR pathway resulting in cortical and subcortical tubers, subependymal nodules along the lateral ventricles, and subependymal giant cell astrocytomas (SEGAs).[60,61] SEGAs are associated with obstructive hydrocephalus in the first 2 decades of life and are monitored for growth using frequent, serial imaging in patients with TSC.[60,61] Though they grow slowly, SEGAs can cause obstructive hydrocephalus secondary to the blockage of CSF circulation at the Foramen of Monro.[62]

Management of hydrocephalus in these cases depends on the management of the SEGAs themselves. Treatment strategies include surgical resection or mTOR inhibition. Early surgical resection was once the standard for the management of SEGAs that showed growth on serial imaging, and surgery was curative for small lesions, with low complication rates.[63] However, for larger or bilateral lesions, complication rates were higher, and in many patients with both SEGA and hydrocephalus, VPS was still necessary.[63,64] More recently, medical management using mTOR inhibitors has been used alone or in combination with surgical resection, though some concerns remain about its long-term safety considering effects on linear growth, puberty, and immunosuppression.[65–68] In patients with SEGA and asymptomatic obstructive hydrocephalus, mTOR inhibition is effective in treating hydrocephalus even in the setting of acute, symptomatic increases in intracranial pressure, though surgery is often still considered in these cases.[66,69] Endoscopic tumor removal, laser interstitial thermal therapy (LITT), and biologics targeting of the MAPK/ERK pathway, may also be used in the treatment of SEGA and associated hydrocephalus in TSC patients.[70,71]

WALKER–WARBURG SYNDROME/BRAIN–MUSCLE–EYE DISEASE

Walker–Warburg Syndrome (WWS), the most severe congenital muscular disorder, is caused by an autosomal recessive mutation that leads to type II Lissencephaly and severe hydrocephalus (**Fig. 3**)[72,73]. WWS is characterized by defective O-glycosylation of α-dystroglycan but the disease is highly heterogenous, as hypoglycosylation can occur in the protein O-mannosyltransferase 1 (POMT1) gene, present in 10% to 20% of patients, as well as in the POMT2, POMGNT1, FKTN, FKRP, LARGE, ISPD or other genes associated with dystroglycanopathy phenotypes.[73–75]

The incidence of WWS is rare, estimated at 1.2 per 100,000 births, however many cases of WWS are complicated by hydrocephalus.[76–78] Similar to the clinical and genetic variability of WWS, the nature of the concurrent hydrocephalus is also variable. Hydrocephalus can be associated with tectal enlargement resulting in aqueductal stenosis as well as cobblestone cortex.[79] One patient with WWS presented with ventriculomegaly and a bulging third ventricle along with progressive hydrocephalus, while another WWS patient presented with macrocephaly, triventricular enlargement, hypoplasia of the corpus collosum, and obstructive hydrocephalus; both were treated with VP shunts.[77] Other case studies reported prenatal findings of posterior fossa anomalies and associated hydrocephalus with a POMT2 mutation confirming WWS, and 3 affected siblings with varying levels of fetal and congenital hydrocephalus, all with fatal prognosis.[76,78] ETV-CPC was used to treat a patient with cobblestone lissencephaly, increased bulging of the anterior fontanelle and sutural separation, with a POMT1 mutation.[80]

It is important to note that the etiology of hydrocephalus in WWS is likely due to the stenosis of the aqueduct secondary to altered brain development and an enlarged tectum. This differs from an aqueductal web, for which the brain stem is otherwise normal. Given the rates of hydrocephalus and abnormal brain development in WWS, close monitoring for hydrocephalus is warranted, although many patients present at birth with symptomatic hydrocephalus requiring treatment.[76] Given the early presentation, although many patients do have aqueductal stenosis, VP shunting may be more efficacious than ETV or ETV-CPC due to the young age at presentation.

PRIMARY CILIARY DYSKINESIA/KARTAGENER'S

Primary ciliary dyskinesia (PCD) is a rare, genetically heterogeneous syndrome associated with defects in cilia and flagella motility.[81,82] Many of the mutations associated with PCD affect the dynein axonemal heavy chain 5 or dynein axonemal intermediate chain 1 genes which encode the

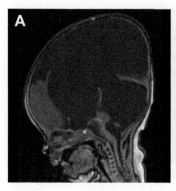
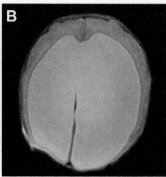

Fig. 3. 1-day-old with POMT-1 P273 L Walker–Warburg syndrome, born at 35 weeks gestation. MRI (*A*) sagittal (T1) and (*B*) axial (T2) views showing hydrocephalus with tectal dysplasia contributing to aqueductal stenosis. This patient was treated with a VP shunt on day of life 4.

outer dynein arms of cilia.[83–85] PCD has a worldwide prevalence of 1 in 16,000 children.[86] Common manifestations include Kartagener's syndrome (bronchiectasis, situs inversus, and chronic sinusitis), as well as neonatal respiratory distress, and male infertility.[86] Although hydrocephalus is infrequently seen in humans with PCD, mouse models of this disease frequently develop severe symptomatic hydrocephalus.[82] Insertional mutations in the mouse axonemal dynein heavy chain gene, *Mdnah5*, cause loss of axonemal outer arms, and reproduce most of the classic features of PCD such as recurrent respiratory infections, situs inversus, and ciliary immobility.[87] In these mice, the mutation also causes hydrocephalus and death in the perinatal period and this mouse model suggest that the degree of ciliary dysfunction caused by the mutation is causally related to the severity of PCD and the development of hydrocephalus.[87] In both human and mouse models, functional loss of the *Ccdc151* gene has also been associated with PCD, as this gene is expressed by ependymal cells and affects the ciliary axoneme. This mutation, too, is associated with hydrocephalus and perinatal death in mouse models.[88] The exact role of cilia motion in the development of hydrocephalus has yet to be determined, including whether cilia are capable of producing or maintaining bulk flow of CSF throughout the ventricular system.

Although there are case reports of hydrocephalus in Kartagener's syndrome or PCD, in humans hydrocephalus is relatively infrequent.[82,89–92] One case of PCD and hydrocephalus was associated with aqueductal stenosis and abnormal ultrastructure of the respiratory epithelium cilia.[93] Another report of autosomal recessively inherited PCD and intellectual disability in 3 generations of a Jordanian family notes that 4 of 9 affected individuals also had hydrocephalus.[94] Mutations in the multicilin gene (*MCIDAS*) are associated with choroid plexus hyperplasia and hydrocephalus in humans, possibly related to reduced generation of motile cilia.[95] Finally, mutations in *FOXJ1*, encoding a transcription factor involved in ciliogenesis, are associated with an autosomal dominant motile ciliopathy like PCD, with obstructive hydrocephalus in all reported cases. Hydrocephalus in these cases was associated with the inability to maintain patency, and resulting stenosis, of the aqueduct and/or foramina of Luschka/Magendie likely due to insufficient motile cilia function.[96] In affected individuals, pathologic specimens showed mislocalized basal bodies and incorrect localization of adhesion proteins, leading to deficits in cilia function and inadequate fluid flow.[96] Overall, whereas PCD is not consistently linked with hydrocephalus in humans, findings from mouse models and several human reports suggest that severe dysfunction of cilia motility may contribute to hydrocephalus in some cases of PCD and related ciliopathies. Possible mechanisms for symptomatic hydrocephalus include stenosis of the aqueduct due to decreased flow of fluid across this channel or from the collapse of the ependymal walls around the aqueduct due to changes in the integrity of the ependyma. Finally, as in other syndromes, concurrent altered brain development may play a role in the development of hydrocephalus.

OSTEOGENESIS IMPERFECTA

Osteogenesis imperfecta (OI) is a group of disorders of connective tissue that affects bone growth and fragility, caused by defective *COL1A1* and *COL1A2* genes and is grouped into four types—type II, type III, type IV, and type I—ordered from most to least severe.[97,98] OI can be associated with macrocephaly, hydrocephalus, basilar invagination, and cerebral atrophy.[99] Concurrent basilar invagination can lead to obstructive hydrocephalus.

Although the true incidence of hydrocephalus in OI is not well known, several studies and case reports have documented OI with associated hydrocephalus.[99,100]

In one study, OI was associated with sulcal prominence and hydrocephalus with no clear intraventricular obstruction in 22% of patients.[99] In another study of 5 neonates with OI, 4 had hydrocephalus associated with FM stenosis, cerebral parenchymal and intraventricular hemorrhage, and occipital-bone fractures.[101] All 4 infants died soon after birth.[101] One other case reported a patient that presented with a novel mutation of the COL1A2 gene and was diagnosed with type II OI with obstructive hydrocephalus; in this case, the patient was treated with ETV.[98]

EMERGING GENETIC SYNDROMES

Through the use of next-generation sequencing, novel genetic mutations associated with hydrocephalus have been identified, accounting for many cases previously classified as sporadic or as "congenital hydrocephalus."[3,102,103] It is unclear in all cases how these genetic alterations directly lead to hydrocephalus; however, mechanisms beyond disruptions to CSF dynamics or structural barriers to CSF flow such as abnormal neuronal proliferation, differentiation, and maintenance may be involved in hydrocephalus.[102]

Pettigrew Syndrome Pettigrew syndrome is an X-linked disorder, characterized by mutations in the AP1S2 gene that encodes a subunit of the AP1 adaptin protein essential in regulating lysosomal protein sorting.[104] Mutations lead to intellectual disabilities, iron and calcium deposition, and hydrocephalus.[3] The related Lethal giant larva (Lgl) protein is involved in maintaining cell polarity in mice. Loss of this protein in Lgl1−/− mice pups leads to severe hydrocephalus and neonatal death.[105]

RASopathies Various RASopathies, through mutations in the RAS-MAPK pathway, have been associated with hydrocephalus; among these disorders are NF1, discussed previously, Costello syndrome, Noonan syndrome, and cardiofaciocutaneous (CFC) syndrome, all with autosomal dominant inheritance.[3] Noonan syndrome is associated with mutations in CBL (regulators of activated TRKs), KRAS, NRAS (RAS proteins), PTPN11, SOS1, SHOC2 (modulators of RAS function), and RAF1 (downstream signal transducers); it is also associated with hydrocephalus in addition to hindbrain herniation and syringomyelia.[106,107] Costello syndrome, is caused by mutations in the HRAS proto-oncogene that lead to failure-to-thrive, along with macrocephaly,

posterior fossa crowding, low cerebellar tonsil position, and hydrocephalus.[108] CFC syndrome is most frequently caused by mutations in BRAF, but can occur due to mutations in MEK1, KRAS, and MEK2 as well. This can lead to cervical stenosis, torticollis, Chiari malformation, and hydrocephalus.[109]

RAS has a multifaceted role in CNS development. Through its involvement in the RAS-ERK pathway, it is involved in the regulation and maintenance of neural stem cells, as well as in the regulation of oligodendrocyte differentiation.[110,111] Through its regulation of the PI3K-AKT pathway, RAS is also involved in synaptic plasticity.[112,113] Despite these interactions with CNS cell growth, differentiation, and maintenance, the role of RAS in CSF clearance and flow is not well characterized, and it is possible that structural alterations due to defective neurogenesis and differentiation contribute to hydrocephalus in these cases rather than direct effects on CSF flow.

PI3K-AKT-mTOR pathway Four different mutations of genes in the PI3K-AKT-mTOR pathway, involved in cell proliferation, growth, and function, have been shown to cause megalencephaly-associated symptoms, leading to hydrocephalus.[3] Mutations in the AKT3, CCND2, and PIK3R2 genes cause different types of megalencephaly-polymicrogyria-polydactyly-hydrocephalus (MPPH), whereas mutations in the PIK3CA gene cause megalencephaly-capillary-malformations (MCAP). Both MPPH and MCAP cause megalencephaly, polymicrogyria, and ventriculomegaly that can lead to hydrocephalus.[114] PI3K pathway genes, including PIK3CA, PTEN, and MTOR contribute to neural stem cell growth, proliferation, and differentiation, especially in the developing ventricular zone, and mutations in these genes predispose patients to tumorigenesis and overgrowth syndromes.[103,115] As these syndromes have only recently been characterized, it remains to be seen whether therapeutics targeting affected molecular pathways will eventually aid in the treatment of hydrocephalus in these cases.

DISCUSSION

Hydrocephalus occurs in the setting of many well-characterized syndromes of childhood. Treatment involves a combination of treating the primary pathology (e.g. tumors that cause outflow obstruction) treatment for hydrocephalus with VPS and/or ETV +/- CPC. Next-generation sequencing has allowed for the characterization of novel genetic syndromes associated with hydrocephalus and the identification of mutations in sporadic cases of hydrocephalus. These mutations shed light on how alterations to the development and proliferation of neurons and neural stem cells contribute to sporadic hydrocephalus, and may eventually contribute to our understanding of novel syndromic causes of hydrocephalus.

Four genes regulating neural stem cell fate have recently been described in congenital hydrocephalus.[102] TRIM71 loss is associated with defective neural tube closure, and decreased proliferation of neural progenitor cells (NPCs) in mouse models.[116] SMARCC1 encodes a subunit of a chromatin remodeling complex important to the survival of NPCs and transcriptional control of telencephalon development, and knockouts develop hydrocephalus and aqueductal stenosis.[117] PTCH1 is involved in the process by which primary cilia in neuroepithelial cells sense and respond to SHH gradients, which is important in NPC differentiation and fate.[118] SHH encodes the ligand responsible for NPC migration along the dorsal-ventral axis of the neural tube.[119] TRIM71 mutations are associated with communicating hydrocephalus, while SMARCC1 and PTCH1 mutations are more likely to be associated with aqueductal stenosis. These mutations highlight that abnormal neurogenesis or brain development play a role in the development of hydrocephalus, beyond deficits in CSF accumulation or clearance.[102] In a follow-up study, mutations in the PI3K pathway genes previously discussed, as well as FOXJ1, FMN2, and FXYD2 were present in up to 22% of sporadic congenital hydrocephalus cases. Their involvement is likely related to their role in supporting embryonic neurogenesis.[103] These findings highlight that dysregulation of neurogenesis, or migration, especially in the ventricular zone, may contribute to CSF accumulation or disordered circulation in some cases of hydrocephalus.

SUMMARY

Hydrocephalus is a common phenotype in various syndromes of childhood with diverse genetic etiologies. The mechanisms behind these disorders include structural deficits, mutations affecting neuronal adhesion, vesicle trafficking, growth factors, PI3K-AKT-mTOR pathway and dystroglycanopathies, ciliopathies, and RASopathies.[3] The pathophysiology of syndromic hydrocephalus is multifactorial, and treatment is often multimodal, addressing both underlying condition and the associated hydrocephalus. Although the incidence or underlying pathogenesis of hydrocephalus in certain conditions is not known, next-generation genetic sequencing has begun to shed light on the complex underlying pathways affecting the development of the brain which result in hydrocephalus.

CLINICS CARE POINTS

- Management of syndromic hydrocephalus may require direct surgical treatment with VPS or ETV (±CPC) and/or treatment of associated pathologic condition resulting in hydrocephalus such as tumors obstructing CSF flow.
- Treatment options vary depending on a variety of patient- and syndrome-specific factors.
- In sporadic cases of congenital hydrocephalus, genetic screening for recently described variants may eventually influence treatment decisions, though at this stage few pathway-specific therapeutics are available

ACKNOWLEDGEMENTS

NIH R01 NS110793 (JMS) and Doris Duke Fund (JMS).

DISCLOSURE

The authors have nothing to disclose.

REFERENCES

1. Schrander-Stumpel C, Fryns J-P. Congenital hydrocephalus: nosology and guidelines for clinical approach and genetic counselling. Eur J Pediatr 1998;157(5):355–62.
2. Rekate HL. The definition and classification of hydrocephalus: a personal recommendation to stimulate debate. Cerebrospinal Fluid Res 2008;5:2. https://doi.org/10.1186/1743-8454-5-2.
3. Kousi M, Katsanis N. The genetic basis of hydrocephalus. Annu Rev Neurosci 2016;39(1):409–35.
4. Stumpel C, Vos YJ. L1 syndrome. In: Adam MP, Ardinger HH, Pagon RA, et al, editors. GeneReviews®. Seattle, WA: University of Washington, Seattle; 1993. Available at: http://www.ncbi.nlm.nih.gov/books/NBK1484/. Accessed January 10, 2021.
5. Adle-Biassette H, Saugier-Veber P, Fallet-Bianco C, et al. Neuropathological review of 138 cases genetically tested for X-linked hydrocephalus: evidence for closely related clinical entities of unknown

molecular bases. Acta Neuropathol 2013;126(3):427–42.

6. Willems PJ, Brouwer OF, Dijkstra I, et al. X-linked hydrocephalus. Am J Med Genet 1987;27(4):921–8.

7. Rosenthal A, Jouet M, Kenwrick S. Aberrant splicing of neural cell adhesion molecule L1 mRNA in a family with X–linked hydrocephalus. Nat Genet 1992;2(2):107–12.

8. Emmert AS, Vuong SM, Shula C, et al. Characterization of a novel rat model of X-linked hydrocephalus by CRISPR-mediated mutation in L1cam. J Neurosurg 2019;8:1–14. https://doi.org/10.3171/2018.10.JNS181015.

9. Van Camp G, Vits L, Coucke P, et al. A duplication in the L1CAM gene associated with X–linked hydrocephalus. Nat Genet 1993;4(4):421–5.

10. Kong W, Wang X, Zhao J, et al. A new frameshift mutation in L1CAM producing X-linked hydrocephalus. Mol Genet Genomic Med 2020;8(1):e1031.

11. Guo D, Shi Y, Jian W, et al. A novel nonsense mutation in the L1CAM gene responsible for X-linked congenital hydrocephalus. J Gene Med 2020;22(7):e3180.

12. Wu Q, Sun L, Xu Y, et al. Diagnosis of a fetus with X-linked hydrocephalus due to mutation of L1CAM gene. Zhonghua Yi Xue Yi Chuan Xue Za Zhi 2019;36(9):897–900.

13. Ferese R, Zampatti S, Griguoli AMP, et al. A new splicing mutation in the L1CAM gene responsible for X-Linked hydrocephalus (HSAS). J Mol Neurosci 2016;59(3):376–81.

14. Tripolszki K, Sasaki E, Hotakainen R, et al. An X-linked syndrome with severe neurodevelopmental delay, hydrocephalus, and early lethality caused by a missense variation in the OTUD5 gene. Clin Genet 2020;1. https://doi.org/10.1111/cge.13873.

15. Alhousseini A, Zeineddine S, Husseini A, et al. Familial hydrocephalus and dysgenesis of the corpus callosum associated with Xp22.33 duplication and stenosis of the aqueduct of sylvius with X-Linked recessive inheritance pattern. Gynecol Obstet Invest 2019;84(4):412–6.

16. Lin LO, Zhang RS, Hoppe IC, et al. Onset and resolution of chiari malformations and hydrocephalus in syndromic craniosynostosis following posterior vault distraction. Plast Reconstr Surg 2019;144(4):932–40.

17. Cinalli G, Sainte-Rose C, Kollar EM, et al. Hydrocephalus and craniosynostosis. J Neurosurg 1998;88(2):209–14.

18. Collmann H, Sörensen N, Krauss J, et al. Hydrocephalus in craniosynostosis. Childs Nerv Syst 1988;4(5):279–85.

19. Wang JC, Nagy L, Demke JC. Syndromic craniosynostosis. Facial Plast Surg Clin North Am 2016;24(4):531–43.

20. Fearon JA, Rhodes J. Pfeiffer syndrome: a treatment evaluation. Plast Reconstr Surg 2009;123(5):1560–9.

21. Kilcoyne S, Potter KR, Gordon Z, et al. Feeding, communication, hydrocephalus, and intracranial hypertension in patients with severe FGFR2-associated pfeiffer syndrome. J Craniofac Surg 2021;32(1):134–40.

22. Moore MH, Hanieh A. Hydrocephalus in pfeiffer syndrome. J Clin Neurosci 1994;1(3):202–4.

23. Al-Namnam NM, Hariri F, Thong MK, et al. Crouzon syndrome: genetic and intervention review. J Oral Biol Craniofac Res 2019;9(1):37–9.

24. Coll G, Arnaud E, Selek L, et al. The growth of the foramen magnum in Crouzon syndrome. Childs Nerv Syst Chns Off J Int Soc Pediatr Neurosurg 2012;28(9):1525–35.

25. Hanieh A, Sheen R, David DJ. Hydrocephalus in Crouzon's syndrome. Childs Nerv Syst Chns Off J Int Soc Pediatr Neurosurg 1989;5(3):188–9.

26. Abu-Sittah GS, Jeelani O, Dunaway D, et al. Raised intracranial pressure in Crouzon syndrome: incidence, causes, and management. J Neurosurg Pediatr 2016;17(4):469–75.

27. Wenger TL, Hing AV, Evans KN. Apert syndrome. In: Adam MP, Ardinger HH, Pagon RA, et al, editors. GeneReviews®. Seattle, WA: University of Washington, Seattle; 1993. Available at: http://www.ncbi.nlm.nih.gov/books/NBK541728/. Accessed January 10, 2021.

28. Ibrahimi OA, Chiu ES, McCarthy JG, et al. Understanding the molecular basis of Apert syndrome. Plast Reconstr Surg 2005;115(1):264–70.

29. Breik O, Mahindu A, Moore MH, et al. Apert syndrome: surgical outcomes and perspectives. J Craniomaxillofac Surg 2016;44(9):1238–45.

30. Munarriz PM, Pascual B, Castaño-Leon AM, et al. Apert syndrome: Cranial procedures and brain malformations in a series of patients. Surg Neurol Int 2020;11:361. https://doi.org/10.25259/SNI_413_2020.

31. Kruszka P, Addissie YA, Agochukwu NB, et al. Muenke syndrome. In: Adam MP, Ardinger HH, Pagon RA, et al, editors. GeneReviews®. Seattle, WA: University of Washington, Seattle; 1993. http://www.ncbi.nlm.nih.gov/books/NBK1415/. Accessed February 10, 2021.

32. González-Del Angel A, Estandía-Ortega B, Alcántara-Ortigoza MA, et al. Expansion of the variable expression of Muenke syndrome: hydrocephalus without craniosynostosis. Am J Med Genet A 2016;170(12):3189–96.

33. Baujat G, Legeai-Mallet L, Finidori G, et al. Achondroplasia. Best Pract Res Clin Rheumatol 2008; 22(1):3–18.

34. Bodensteiner JB. Neurological manifestations of achondroplasia. Curr Neurol Neurosci Rep 2019; 19(12):105.

35. Steinbok P, Hall J, Flodmark O. Hydrocephalus in achondroplasia: the possible role of intracranial venous hypertension. J Neurosurg 1989;71(1):42–8.

36. Cohen ME, Rosenthal AD, Matson DD. Neurological abnormalities in achondroplastic children. J Pediatr 1967;71(3):367–76.

37. White KK, Bompadre V, Goldberg MJ, et al. Best practices in the evaluation and treatment of foramen magnum stenosis in achondroplasia during infancy. Am J Med Genet A 2016; 170(1):42–51.

38. Pierre-Kahn A, Hirsch JF, Renier D, et al. Hydrocephalus and achondroplasia. Pediatr Neurosurg 1980;7(4):205–19.

39. King JAJ, Vachhrajani S, Drake JM, et al. Neurosurgical implications of achondroplasia. J Neurosurg Pediatr 2009;4(4):297–306.

40. Kashanian A, Chan J, Mukherjee D, et al. Improvement in ventriculomegaly following cervicomedullary decompressive surgery in children with achondroplasia and foramen magnum stenosis. Am J Med Genet A 2020;182(8):1896–905.

41. Jett K, Friedman JM. Clinical and genetic aspects of neurofibromatosis 1. Genet Med 2010; 12(1):1–11.

42. Roth J, Ber R, Constantini S. Neurofibromatosis Type 1-related hydrocephalus: treatment options and considerations. World Neurosurg 2019;128: e664–8. https://doi.org/10.1016/j.wneu.2019.04. 231.

43. Ferner RE. Neurofibromatosis 1. Eur J Hum Genet 2007;15(2):131–8.

44. Tonsgard JH. Clinical manifestations and management of neurofibromatosis type 1. Semin Pediatr Neurol 2006;13(1):2–7.

45. Glombova M, Petrak B, Lisy J, et al. Brain gliomas, hydrocephalus and idiopathic aqueduct stenosis in children with neurofibromatosis type 1. Brain Dev 2019;41(8):678–90.

46. Tanrıkulu B, Özek MM. Neurofibromatosis and hydrocephalus. In: Cinalli G, Özek MM, Sainte-Rose C, editors. Pediatric hydrocephalus. Springer International Publishing; 2019. p. 1107–18. https://doi.org/10.1007/978-3-319-27250-4_65.

47. Roth J, Constantini S, Cinalli G. Neurofibromatosis type 1-related hydrocephalus: causes and treatment considerations. Childs Nerv Syst Chns Off J Int Soc Pediatr Neurosurg 2020;36(10): 2385–90.

48. Dinçer A, Yener U, Özek MM. Hydrocephalus in patients with neurofibromatosis Type 1: MR imaging findings and the outcome of endoscopic third ventriculostomy. Am J Neuroradiol 2011; 32(4):643–6.

49. Gutmann DH, Aylsworth A, Carey JC, et al. The diagnostic evaluation and multidisciplinary management of neurofibromatosis 1 and neurofibromatosis 2. JAMA 1997;278(1):51–7.

50. Petrilli AM, Fernández-Valle C. Role of Merlin/NF2 inactivation in tumor biology. Oncogene 2016; 35(5):537–48.

51. Cinalli G, Maixner WJ, Sainte-Rose C. Pediatric hydrocephalus. New York, NY: Springer Science & Business Media; 2012.

52. Dirks PB. Genetics of Hydrocephalus. In: Cinalli G, Sainte-Rose C, Maixner WJ, editors. Pediatric hydrocephalus. Springer Milan; 2005. p. 1–17. https://doi.org/10.1007/978-88-470-2121-1_1.

53. Jayaraman A, Ballweg GP, Donnenfeld H, et al. Hydrocephalus in Down's syndrome. Childs Brain 1976;2(3):202–7.

54. Zadikoff C. Down's syndrome with hydrocephalus treated by compressive head binding. S Afr Med J 1977;51(11):353–5.

55. Forcelini CM, Mallmann AB, Crusius PS, et al. Down syndrome with congenital hydrocephalus: case report. Arq Neuropsiquatr 2006;64(3B): 869–71.

56. Marano M, Pompucci A, Motolese F, et al. Normal pressure hydrocephalus in Down Syndrome: the report of two cases. J Alzheimers Dis JAD 2020; 77(3):979–84.

57. Orlando V, Spennato P, De Liso M, et al. Fourth ventricle outlet obstruction and diverticular enlargement of luschka foramina in a child with down syndrome. Pediatr Neurosurg 2020;28:1–4. https://doi.org/10.1159/000511088.

58. Raveau M, Nakahari T, Asada S, et al. Brain ventriculomegaly in Down syndrome mice is caused by Pcp4 dose-dependent cilia dysfunction. Hum Mol Genet 2017;26(5):923–31.

59. Movsas TZ, Spitzer AR, Gewolb IH. Ventriculomegaly in very-low-birthweight infants with Down syndrome. Dev Med Child Neurol 2016;58(11): 1167–71.

60. Lu DS, Karas PJ, Krueger DA, et al. Central nervous system manifestations of tuberous sclerosis complex. Am J Med Genet C Semin Med Genet 2018;178(3):291–8.

61. Hsieh DT, Whiteway SL, Rohena LO, et al. Tuberous sclerosis complex. Neurol Clin Pract 2016;6(4): 339–47.

62. Roth J, Roach ES, Bartels U, et al. Subependymal giant cell astrocytoma: diagnosis, screening, and treatment. Recommendations from the International Tuberous Sclerosis Complex Consensus Conference 2012. Pediatr Neurol 2013;49(6): 439–44.

63. Kotulska K, Borkowska J, Roszkowski M, et al. Surgical treatment of subependymal giant cell astrocytoma in tuberous sclerosis complex patients. Pediatr Neurol 2014;50(4):307–12.

64. Fohlen M, Ferrand-Sorbets S, Delalande O, et al. Surgery for subependymal giant cell astrocytomas in children with tuberous sclerosis complex. Childs Nerv Syst Chns Off J Int Soc Pediatr Neurosurg 2018;34(8):1511–9.

65. Jóźwiak S, Nabbout R, Curatolo P. Participants of the TSC Consensus Meeting for SEGA and Epilepsy Management. Management of subependymal giant cell astrocytoma (SEGA) associated with tuberous sclerosis complex (TSC): clinical recommendations. Eur J Paediatr Neurol 2013;17(4): 348–52.

66. Ebrahimi-Fakhari D, Franz DN. Pharmacological treatment strategies for subependymal giant cell astrocytoma (SEGA). Expert Opin Pharmacother 2020;21(11):1329–36.

67. Giordano F, Moscheo C, Lenge M, et al. Neurosurgical treatment of subependymal giant cell astrocytomas in tuberous sclerosis complex: a series of 44 surgical procedures in 31 patients. Childs Nerv Syst 2020;36(5):951–60.

68. Somers MJG, Paul E. Safety considerations of mammalian target of rapamycin inhibitors in tuberous sclerosis complex and renal transplantation. J Clin Pharmacol 2015;55(4):368–76.

69. Weidman DR, Palasamudram S, Zak M, et al. The effect of mTOR inhibition on obstructive hydrocephalus in patients with tuberous sclerosis complex (TSC) related subependymal giant cell astrocytoma (SEGA). J Neurooncol 2020;147(3): 731–6.

70. Frassanito P, Noya C, Tamburrini G. Current trends in the management of subependymal giant cell astrocytomas in tuberous sclerosis. Childs Nerv Syst Chns Off J Int Soc Pediatr Neurosurg 2020;36(10): 2527–36.

71. Bongaarts A, van Scheppingen J, Korotkov A, et al. The coding and non-coding transcriptional landscape of subependymal giant cell astrocytomas. Brain J Neurol 2020;143(1):131–49.

72. Dobyns WB, Pagon RA, Armstrong D, et al. Diagnostic criteria for Walker-Warburg syndrome. Am J Med Genet 1989;32(2):195–210.

73. Vajsar J, Schachter H. Walker-Warburg syndrome. Orphanet J Rare Dis 2006;1(1):29.

74. Reeuwijk van J, Janssen M, van den Elzen C, et al. POMT2 mutations cause α-dystroglycan hypoglycosylation and Walker-Warburg syndrome. J Med Genet 2005;42(12):907–12.

75. Tully HM, Dobyns WB. Infantile hydrocephalus: a review of epidemiology, classification and causes. Eur J Med Genet 2014;57(8):359–68.

76. Rodgers BL, Vanner LV, Pai GS, Sens MA. Walker-Warburg syndrome: report of three affected sibs. Am J Med Genet 1994;49(2):198–201.

77. Preuss M, Heckmann M, Stein M, et al. Two cases of walker-warburg syndrome complicated by hydrocephalus. Pediatr Neurosurg 2010;46(1):34–8.

78. Brasseur-Daudruy M, Vivier PH, Ickowicz V, et al. Walker-Warburg syndrome diagnosed by findings of typical ocular abnormalities on prenatal ultrasound. Pediatr Radiol 2012;42(4):488–90.

79. Alharbi S, Alhashem A, Alkuraya F, et al. Neuroimaging manifestations and genetic heterogeneity of Walker-Warburg syndrome in Saudi patients. Brain Dev 2021;43(3):380–8.

80. Tanaka T, Harris CJ, Barnett SS, et al. A successful treatment of endoscopic third ventriculostomy with choroid plexus cauterization for hydrocephalus in Walker-Warburg Syndrome. Case Rep Neurol Med 2016;2016:7627289. https://doi.org/10.1155/2016/7627289.

81. Leigh MW, Pittman JE, Carson JL, et al. Clinical and genetic aspects of primary ciliary dyskinesia/Kartagener syndrome. Genet Med 2009;11(7): 473–87.

82. Lee L. Riding the wave of ependymal cilia: genetic susceptibility to hydrocephalus in primary ciliary dyskinesia. J Neurosci Res 2013;91(9):1117–32.

83. Guichard C, Harricane M-C, Lafitte J-J, et al. Axonemal Dynein Intermediate-Chain Gene (DNAI1) Mutations Result in Situs Inversus and Primary Ciliary Dyskinesia (Kartagener Syndrome). Am J Hum Genet 2001;68(4):1030–5.

84. Zariwala M, Noone PG, Sannuti A, et al. Germline mutations in an intermediate chain dynein cause primary ciliary dyskinesia. Am J Respir Cell Mol Biol 2001;25(5):577–83.

85. Omran H, Häffner K, Völkel A, et al. Homozygosity mapping of a gene locus for primary ciliary dyskinesia on chromosome 5p and identification of the heavy dynein chain DNAH5 as a candidate gene. Am J Respir Cell Mol Biol 2000;23(5):696–702.

86. Lee L. Mechanisms of mammalian ciliary motility: insights from primary ciliary dyskinesia genetics. Gene 2011;473(2):57–66.

87. Ibañez-Tallon I, Gorokhova S, Heintz N. Loss of function of axonemal dynein Mdnah5 causes primary ciliary dyskinesia and hydrocephalus. Hum Mol Genet 2002;11(6):715–21.

88. Chiani F, Orsini T, Gambadoro A, et al. Functional loss of Ccdc151 leads to hydrocephalus in a mouse model of primary ciliary dyskinesia. Dis Model Mech 2019;12(8). https://doi.org/10.1242/dmm.038489.

89. Greenstone MA, Jones RW, Dewar A, et al. Hydrocephalus and primary ciliary dyskinesia. Arch Dis Child 1984;59(5):481–2.

90. Jabourian Z, Lublin FD, Adler A, et al. Hydroceph-alus in Kartagener's syndrome. Ear Nose Throat J 1986;65(10):468–72.

91. Santi MMD, Magni A, Valletta EA, et al. Hydroceph-alus, bronchiectasis, and ciliary aplasia. Arch Dis Child 1990;65(5):543–4.

92. Picco P, Leveratto L, Cama A, et al. Immotile cilia syndrome associated with hydrocephalus and pre-cocious puberty: a case report. Eur J Pediatr Surg 1993;3(Suppl 1):20–1.

93. Vieira JP, Lopes P, Silva R. Primary ciliary dyski-nesia and hydrocephalus with aqueductal steno-sis. J Child Neurol 2012;27(7):938–41.

94. al-Shroof M, Karnik AM, Karnik AA, et al. Ciliary dyskinesia associated with hydrocephalus and mental retardation in a Jordanian family. Mayo Clin Proc 2001;76(12):1219–24.

95. Robson EA, Dixon L, Causon L, et al. Hydrocepha-lus and diffuse choroid plexus hyperplasia in pri-mary ciliary dyskinesia-related MCIDAS mutation. Neurol Genet 2020;6(4):e482.

96. Wallmeier J, Frank D, Shoemark A, et al. De Novo Mutations in FOXJ1 Result in a Motile Ciliopathy with Hydrocephalus and Randomization of Left/Right Body Asymmetry. Am J Hum Genet 2019; 105(5):1030–9.

97. Cole DE, Carpenter TO. Bone fragility, craniosynosto-sis, ocular proptosis, hydrocephalus, and distinctive facial features: a newly recognized type of osteogen-esis imperfecta. J Pediatr 1987;110(1):76–80.

98. Hachiya Y, Hayashi M, Negishi T, et al. A case of osteogenesis imperfecta type II caused by a novel COL1A2 gene mutation: endoscopic third ventricu-lostomy to prevent hydrocephalus. Neuropediatrics 2012;43(4):225–8.

99. Charnas LR, Marini JC. Communicating hydro-cephalus, basilar invagination, and other neuro-logic features in osteogenesis imperfecta. Neurology 1993;43(12):2603–8.

100. Sasaki-Adams D, Kulkarni A, Rutka J, et al. Neuro-surgical implications of osteogenesis imperfecta in children: Report of 4 cases. J Neurosurg Pediatr 2008;1(3):229–36.

101. Knisely AS, Frates RE, Ambler MW, et al. Hydro-cephalus of intrauterine onset in perinatally lethal osteogenesis imperfecta: clinical, sonographic, and pathologic correlations. Pediatr Pathol 1988; 8(4):367–76.

102. Furey CG, Choi J, Jin SC, et al. De Novo Mutation in Genes regulating neural stem cell fate in human congenital hydrocephalus. Neuron 2018;99(2): 302–14.e4.

103. Jin SC, Dong W, Kundishora AJ, et al. Exome sequencing implicates genetic disruption of prena-tal neuro-gliogenesis in sporadic congenital hydro-cephalus. Nat Med 2020;26(11):1754–65.

104. Reusch U, Bernhard O, Koszinowski U, et al. AP-1A and AP-3A Lysosomal Sorting Functions. Traffic 2002;3(10):752–61.

105. Klezovitch O, Fernandez TE, Tapscott SJ, et al. Loss of cell polarity causes severe brain dysplasia in Lgl1 knockout mice. Genes Dev 2004;18(5): 559–71.

106. Heye N, Dunne JW. Noonan's syndrome with hy-drocephalus, hindbrain herniation, and upper cer-vical intracord cyst. J Neurol Neurosurg Psychiatry 1995;59(3):338–9.

107. Roberts AE, Allanson JE, Tartaglia M, et al. Noonan syndrome. The Lancet 2013;381(9863): 333–42.

108. Gripp KW, Hopkins E, Doyle D, et al. High inci-dence of progressive postnatal cerebellar enlargement in Costello syndrome: Brain over-growth associated with HRAS mutations as the likely cause of structural brain and spinal cord ab-normalities. Am J Med Genet A 2010;152A(5): 1161–8.

109. Reinker KA, Stevenson DA, Tsung A. Orthopaedic conditions in Ras/MAPK related disorders. J Pediatr Orthop 2011;31(5):599–605.

110. Campos LS, Leone DP, Relvas JB, et al. Beta1 integrins activate a MAPK signalling pathway in neural stem cells that contributes to their maintenance. Development 2004;131(14): 3433–44.

111. Fressinaud C, Vallat JM, Labourdette G. Basic fibroblast growth factor down-regulates myelin basic protein gene expression and alters myelin compaction of mature oligodendro-cytes in vitro. J Neurosci Res 1995;40(3): 285–93.

112. Kim J-I, Lee H-R, Sim S, et al. PI3Kγ is required for NMDA receptor-dependent long-term depression and behavioral flexibility. Nat Neurosci 2011; 14(11):1447–54.

113. Choi J-H, Park P, Baek G-C, et al. Effects of PI3Kγ overexpression in the hippocampus on synaptic plasticity and spatial learning. Mol Brain 2014;7:78. https://doi.org/10.1186/s13041-014-0078-6.

114. Mirzaa GM, Conway RL, Gripp KW, et al. Megalencephaly-capillary malformation (MCAP) and megalencephaly-polydactyly-polymicrogyria-hydrocephalus (MPPH) syndromes: Two closely related disorders of brain overgrowth and abnormal brain and body morphogenesis. Am J Med Genet A 2012;158A(2):269–91.

115. Li L, Liu F, Ross AH. PTEN regulation of neural development and CNS stem cells. J Cell Biochem 2003;88(1):24–8.

116. Chen J, Lai F, Niswander L. The ubiquitin ligase mLin41 temporally promotes neural progenitor

cell maintenance through FGF signaling. Genes Dev 2012;26(8):803–15.

117. Narayanan R, Pirouz M, Kerimoglu C, et al. Loss of BAF (mSWI/SNF) Complexes Causes Global Transcriptional and Chromatin State Changes in Forebrain Development. Cell Rep 2015;13(9): 1842–54.

118. Palma V, Ruiz i Altaba A. Hedgehog-GLI signaling regulates the behavior of cells with stem cell properties in the developing neocortex. Dev Camb Engl 2004;131(2):337–45.

119. Lupo G, Harris WA, Lewis KE. Mechanisms of ventral patterning in the vertebrate nervous system. Nat Rev Neurosci 2006;7(2):103–14.

Neurosurgical Considerations of Neurocutaneous Syndromes

Rajiv R. Iyer, MD[a],*, Jennifer M. Strahle, MD[b], Mari L. Groves, MD[c]

KEYWORDS

- Neurocutaneous syndrome • Tuberous sclerosis complex • subependymal giant cell astrocytoma
- Sturge-Weber syndrome • Gorlin syndrome • Hereditary hemorrhagic telangiectasia • Epilepsy

KEY POINTS

- Phenotypic manifestations of tuberous sclerosis complex can be heterogeneous, with clinical criteria involving multiple organ systems; early detection and multidisciplinary management of these issues is important.
- Neurosurgically-relevant manifestations in TSC include SEGA formation and epilepsy. Ongoing efforts seek to elucidate the role of mTOR inhibitors in the management of these issues.
- In Sturge-Weber syndrome, there may be a causative correlation between microvascular stasis and seizures/TIAs. Ongoing studies continue to investigate the role of antiplatelet and anticonvulsive therapy in these patients.

INTRODUCTION

The phakomatoses are a group of genetic and acquired disorders characterized by neurologic, cutaneous, and often ocular manifestations, thus commonly referred to as *neurocutaneous syndromes* or *oculoneurocutaneous syndromes*. In 1932, van der Hoeve described the concept of a "phakoma," or a cutaneous birthmark such as a vascular lesion or an abnormally pigmented region seen early in life, which raises suspicion of the presence of an underlying neurocutaneous syndrome. A multitude of such conditions have since been described, and importantly, multiple organ system involvement is commonplace and requires careful multidisciplinary monitoring and management. In several neurocutaneous syndromes the underlying genetic pathophysiology has been elucidated, which will continue to play an important role in advancing therapeutic techniques. Two of the most common neurocutaneous syndromes are neurofibromatosis 1 and 2 and von-Hippel Lindau, which are discussed in another article in this issue on tumor syndromes. This article focuses on other examples of neurocutaneous syndromes, and especially on the relevant neurosurgical considerations when encountering these patients.

TUBEROUS SCLEROSIS COMPLEX
Epidemiology, Genetics, and Clinical Manifestations

Tuberous sclerosis complex (TSC) is a highly penetrant autosomal dominant disorder cause by mutation in the genes *TSC1* and *TSC2*, on chromosome 9q34 and 16p13, respectively.[1,2] TSC has a prevalence of 3.8 to 6.9 per 100,000 and an incidence of

[a] Department of Neurosurgery/Division of Pediatric Neurosurgery, University of Utah/Primary Children's Hospital, 100 N. Mario Capecchi Drive Suite 3850, Salt Lake City, UT 84113, USA; [b] Pediatric Neuro Spine Program, Pediatric Cerebrovascular Surgery, Division of Pediatric Neurosurgery, Department of Neurosurgery, Washington University School of Medicine, 1 Childrens Pl Suite 4S20, St. Louis, MO 63110, USA; [c] Department of Neurosurgery, Johns Hopkins School of Medicine, 600 N. Wolfe Street Phipps 554, Baltimore, MD 21287, USA
* Corresponding author.
E-mail address: Rajiv.Iyer@hsc.utah.edu

Neurosurg Clin N Am 33 (2022) 81–89
https://doi.org/10.1016/j.nec.2021.09.013
1042-3680/22/© 2021 Elsevier Inc. All rights reserved.

around 6.0 per 100,000 births.[3–5] In many cases TSC occurs due to de novo mutation, rather than an inherited pattern, and occurs with no gender or ethnic predilection. The proteins encoded by *TSC1* and *TSC2* are known as hamartin and tuberin, respectively, which are tumor suppressor proteins that form a heterotrimeric complex with the protein product of the *TBC1D7* gene, together known as the TSC protein complex, which is involved in the mechanistic target of rapamycin (mTOR) signaling pathway. mTOR signaling occurs through protein complexes mTORC1 and mTORC2. Depending on the timing of biallelic loss of heterozygosity in these tumor suppressor genes, phenotypic variation may also arise, including the presence of mosaicism, in which different populations of cells may or may not contain pathogenic genetic variants.[6] As a result of this multitude of factors, it is not surprising that clinical characteristics in TSC can be quite heterogeneous.

Owing to underlying overactivation of the mTOR pathway, multiple organ involvement most often results, with tumor and hamartoma formation in the central nervous system (CNS), heart, kidneys, and additional ocular and cutaneous manifestations. Although genetic testing for pathogenic mutations can yield a diagnosis of TSC, clinical diagnostic criteria also exist with 11 major and 6 minor phenotypic findings used to make the diagnosis of TSC (**Table 1**).[7] Commonly, patients with TSC are recognized due to the presence of cutaneous findings including hypopigmented "ash leaf" spots, facial angiofibromas in a butterfly pattern (also known as adenoma sebaceum), or a shagreen patch, which is a patch of excessively fibrous skin, often found on the lower back. The presence of ash leaf macules can be identified with a Wood lamp. The presence of hypopigmented macules alone is not pathognomonic for TSC, as up to 4.7% of the general population may harbor these lesions.[8]

Cardiac manifestations of TSC include cardiac rhabdomyomas, which are benign tumors typically arising in the ventricles of the heart that can be detected on echocardiography. Renal findings may include angiomyolipomas as well as renal cell carcinoma. Pulmonary issues may also arise, including lymphangioleiomyomatosis, which can lead to cystic lesions that may cause dyspnea or pneumothorax.

Neurologic Manifestations of Tuberous Sclerosis Complex

Neurologic manifestations of TSC include cortical tuber formation, neuronal migrational abnormalities, retinal hamartomas, subependymal nodules, and subependymal giant cell astrocytomas (SEGAs). These lesions can contribute to the pathogenesis of infantile spasms, refractory epilepsy, neurodevelopmental issues, tumor growth, and even hydrocephalus. Owing to the predominance and clinical significance of the neurologic sequelae associated with TSC, screening MRI is performed

Table 1
Clinical diagnostic criteria for tuberous sclerosis[a]

	Major Criteria	Minor Criteria
Dermatologic and dentistry	• Hypomelanotic macules ($\geq$3, at least 5 mm diameter) • Angiofibromas ($\geq$3) or fibrous cephalic plaque • Ungual fibromas ($\geq$2) • Shagreen patch	• "Confetti" skin lesions • Dental enamel pits ($\geq$3) • Intraoral fibromas ($\geq$2)
Ophthalmologic	• Retinal hamartoma	• Retinal achromic patch
Brain structure, tubers, and tumors	• Cortical dysplasia • Subependymal nodules • SEGA	
Cardiology	• Cardiac rhabdomyoma	
Pulmonary	• LAM	
Nephrology	• Angiomyolipomas ($\geq$2)	• Multiple renal cysts
Other (endocrine, GI)		• Nonrenal hamartomas

Definite diagnosis: 2 major features, or 1 major and 2 or more minor features.
  Possible diagnosis: 1 major feature, or 2 or more minor features.
  Abbreviations: GI, gastrointestinal; LAM, lymphangioleiomyomatosis; SEGA, subependymal giant cell astrocytoma.
  [a] *Adapted from* Northrup et al., 2013.

for identification and surveillance of these lesions in all patients suspected of having TSC and may be performed every 1 to 3 years depending on the clinical context of individual patients.[9]

The hallmark cortical dysplastic entities of TSC are cortical tubers, which are often numerous hamartomatous lesions that harbor a predilection for the frontal and parietal lobes. These lesions are typically T1 isointense or hypointense, T2 hyperintense, and diffusion restrict on MRI, and their epileptogenicity may arise either from their presence alone, or due to their surrounding effects on perituberal cortex.[10–15] Cerebellar tubers may also occur in the minority of patients and are associated with a worse neurocognitive status.[16]

Subependymal nodules are another CNS finding in patients with TSC, which are found to line the ventricle, especially around the caudothalamic groove.[17] Subependymal nodules are typically T1 hyperintense, have variable patterns of contrast enhancement, and commonly contain calcifications. These lesions may progress to SEGA in 10% to 15% of cases.[18]

SEGAs are World Health Organization grade I tumors that also line the ventricle and usually display distinct contrast enhancement with a mixed T1 and T2 appearance on MRI. The prevalence of SEGA is about 25% of the entire TSC population.[19] These lesions often occur in proximity to the foramen of Monro, and growth over time can lead to obstructive hydrocephalus. Because of their propensity to develop in patients with TSC, screening MRI is conducted to identify them, and if present, they require monitoring throughout life. Microscopically SEGAs contain balloon cells, with tumor cells often surrounding perivascular spaces, with rare mitotic figures present, consistent with their indolent nature. *BRAF* mutations have been seen in some SEGAs.[20,21]

White matter lesions and radial migration lines are also found in patients with TSC. Radial migration lines are T2 hyperintense, bandlike projections emanating from the periventricular subcortical regions, resulting from impaired neuronal migration, and may contribute to the pathogenesis of seizures or neurocognitive delays in patients with TSC.[16] In addition, patients with the *TSC2* mutation generally feature more severe neurocognitive phenotypes and seizures.[22]

Treatment

Subependymal giant cell astrocytoma
Although SEGAs are low-grade tumors, their growth around the foramen of Monro may prompt surgical resection, especially in cases of impending lateral ventricular obstruction, the current presence of hydrocephalus due to the tumor, intratumoral hemorrhage causing mass effect, and large lesions. Several case series involving surgical resection of SEGAs have demonstrated the effectiveness of this management strategy, which can be curative with gross total resection.[23,24] In patients without acute neurologic issues, medical therapy with mTOR pathway inhibitors (everolimus, sirolimus) can be considered for growing lesions, which also plays an adjuvant therapeutic role following subtotal resection, and may play a role in seizure reduction as well.[25,26] In addition to open techniques for surgical resection of SEGAs, neuroendoscopy may be used as an alternative resective strategy, as well as laser interstitial thermal therapy.[27]

Refractory epilepsy
About 80% to 90% of patients with TSC have seizures, with up to two-thirds being refractory, leading to considerable morbidity in the TSC population.[28] Baseline and routine electroencephalography (EEG) is recommended for those with seizures, and it is important to note that the neurologic phenotype present can be highly variable.

Overall, patients typically undergo standard epilepsy management as in other types of seizure disorders, bearing in mind that there is a higher likelihood for the development of medical refractoriness.[29] A multidisciplinary effort is commonly adopted to manage seizures in TSC, with comprehensive evaluation involving neurologists, neurosurgeons, neuropsychologists, and others.

Infantile spasms in patients with TSC can be treated effectively with vigabatrin, with adrenocorticotropic hormone as second-line therapy. Current, promising investigative efforts are also underway to determine the role of vigabatrin as a preventative agent in TSC seizure management.[30]

Surgical candidacy for epilepsy in the TSC population is similar to that for other causes. For example, extensive workup for medically refractory patients includes video-EEG and determination of seizure semiology, MRI, PET, magnetoencephalography, single-photon emission computed tomography (SPECT), and others in an attempt to correlate seizures with specific epileptogenic foci within the brain. For patients with focal epilepsy, concordant EEG data, including data derived from depth electrode placement, may provide sufficient correlation for surgical resection of offending dominant/secondary tubers, or perituberal cortex.[31] It has been shown that predictors of seizure freedom following seizure surgery include focal seizures rather than generalized seizures, a younger age, larger extent of resection of the epileptogenic region, and EEG/imaging concordance.[18,32] Other options for treatment of patients with severe seizure phenotypes include corpus callosotomy, vagal nerve stimulator placement, ketogenic diet, and ongoing investigative efforts into the application of cannabidiol for seizure management.[33]

Importantly, ongoing efforts are underway to help elucidate the role of preventative treatment in patients with TSC, as well as the potential disease-modifying attributes of mTOR inhibitors, which have been shown to contribute to seizure reduction, especially in younger patients and at higher doses.[34,35]

STURGE-WEBER SYNDROME
Introduction and Clinical Characteristics

Although rare, Sturge-Weber syndrome (SWS) is the third most common neurocutaneous syndrome following neurofibromatosis and TSC. SWS is a nonhereditary disorder and is also known as *encephalotrigeminal angiomatosis* or *encephalofacial angiomatosis*. Characteristic findings in this condition include the presence of a classic hemifacial port wine stain (PWS), as well as leptomeningeal angiomatosis, unilateral cerebral abnormalities, and ocular abnormalities (angiomas, glaucoma). This disorder is relevant for neurosurgeons due to the presence of seizures, possible strokelike episodes, and neurocognitive delay. The incidence of SWS is around 1 of 50,000 with no gender or ethnic predilection. Three types of SWS have been described, with type 1 involving cutaneous and neurologic manifestations (most typical), type 2 with cutaneous and ocular findings, and type 3 with neurologic manifestations alone.

The PWS in SWS is a red, sometimes salmon-colored, facial capillary malformation that is typically unilateral, present at birth, and follows trigeminal nerve distributions in a variable manner (**Fig. 1**). This facial cutaneous finding is not completely unique to SWS, and a small percentage of patients with SWS have bilateral nevi, or no PWS at all.[36] The presence of a PWS alone is not pathognomonic for SWS. Intracranial involvement in SWS is most often unilateral to the hemiface affected by the PWS, but bilateral findings, although uncommon, may be present.

Cause

Although SWS is a sporadically occurring disorder, recurrent somatic mutations in the *GNAQ* gene, which encodes for a G protein subunit involved in cellular signal transduction, have been identified as a major determining pathomechanism.[37–39] These mutations have been shown to occur in a higher rate in endothelial cells within brain lesions associated with SWS, implicating pathway impairment involving this protein in the etiopathogenesis of vascular malformations.[40] Owing to hemispheric involvement in SWS, often featuring angiomatosis, ischemic injury, and cortical dysgenesis, neurologic impairment and epilepsy can result.

Neurologic Manifestations and Imaging

Leptomeningeal angiomatosis occurs in up to 20% of patients with SWS, and although it can be present bilaterally, it most often occurs unilateral to the side of facial cutaneous involvement. The parietal and occipital lobes are typically affected. Other intracranial findings can include choroid plexus angioma formation, as well as more general resultant effects of microvascular and venous abnormalities, including gliosis, calcification, neuronal loss, and other parenchymal abnormalities (see **Fig. 1**).

Owing to the presence of these intracranial abnormalities, several neurologic issues can arise in patients with SWS. For example, headaches may occur as a result of the vascular flow dynamics. Developmentally, children may have delayed milestones and intellectual impairment, with attention-associated issues as well. Strokelike episodes, or transient ischemic attacks can also occur, which likely represent periods of vascular steal and ischemia, or Todd paralysis postseizure activity. These paroxysmal episodes often manifest in transient hemiparesis that last for a variable duration, but nearly always recover. One study evaluating transient hemiparesis in patients with SWS demonstrated that these episodes were associated with seizures or status epilepticus in more than 54% of cases, with 18% of the cases being associated with some type of head impact injury, with a median recovery time of 24 hours.[41] Importantly, the underlying cause for these episodes is still unclear, and may have a multifactorial cause involving hemispheric hypoperfusion due to abnormal SWS vasculature and chronic ischemia, postictal effects, and even traumatic effects on the underlying parenchyma.[42–44]

Epilepsy is a common neurologic manifestation of SWS, with seizures occurring in more than 75% of patients with SWS, and often early in life. Frequently, focal seizures occur, including partial motor or complex partial seizures, with occasional infantile spasms and secondary generalization.[45,46] It has been hypothesized that more extensive leptomeningeal angiomatosis or capillary malformation extent correlates with the severity of epilepsy in SWS.[47] Importantly, SPECT imaging during seizures demonstrated ischemic

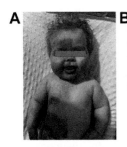 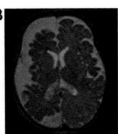 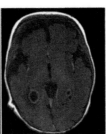

Fig. 1. (*A*) An 8-month-old female with Sturge-Weber syndrome showing cutaneous manifestations including a hemifacial port wine stain. (*B*) T2-weighted and T1 with contrast MRI images with unilateral cortical atrophy secondary to pial angiomas and reduced cortical venous drainage. Also seen is a choroid plexus cyst associated with choroid plexus hypertrophy in patients with Sturge-Weber syndrome.

vascular steal in those areas, further worsening the balance between metabolic demand and tissue oxygenation and thus creating a vicious cycle that could contribute to neurologic impairment in SWS.[48,49]

Ocular manifestations in SWS include congenital glaucoma, which may coincide with retinal vessel malformations, retinopathy of prematurity, and choroidal hemangiomas.[50,51]

MRI is the diagnostic tool of choice for evaluating the CNS manifestations of SWS. The presence of leptomeningeal angiomatosis and choroid plexus angiomas can be detected with T1 postcontrast imaging and MR angiography, with a lower sensitivity of detection in the neonatal and first 2 years of life. Therefore, if clinical suspicion of neurologic issues arises beyond these ages, repeat MRI may be warranted. Detection of other findings including venous anomalies can be augmented with susceptibility-weighted imaging, and cortical atrophy and aberrant myelination patterns found in SWS can also be identified using MRI.[52–54] Computed tomography may play a role in detecting subcortical "tram-track" calcifications, or skull hyperostosis.[55,56] Perfusion-based imaging may also play a role in evaluating patients presenting with strokelike symptoms as mentioned earlier.

Treatment

Epilepsy

Treatment of seizures in SWS begins with considerations similar to other patients with epilepsy, including appropriate medical management and multidisciplinary diagnostic workup in concert with neurology and neuropsychiatric evaluation. Owing to the high risk of intellectual disability associated with seizures in SWS, aggressive treatment has been advocated.[45] Various medications may be effective, and there are reports of sirolimus as a preventative agent in SWS epilepsy.[57,58]

Surgical options for epilepsy in SWS are often considered as up to 50% of patients with SWS develop medically refractory seizures. Multiple approaches have been undertaken, and several series exist on anatomic and functional hemispherectomy and hemispherotomy for appropriately selected patients, with good long-term seizure freedom and functional results.[59–62] Ideal candidates for hemispherectomy or hemispherotomy are those with intractable seizures with concurrent hemiparesis and visual field deficits. In some intractable cases with bilateral but asymmetric EEG findings, these surgical techniques may also play a role.[63] Other palliative surgeries such as vagus nerve stimulation (VNS) therapy insertion may also be appropriate in refractory cases.

Antiplatelet therapy

Given the possible role of microvascular stasis and thrombosis in the pathophysiology of seizures and transient ischemic events in SWS, it has been hypothesized that antiplatelet therapy with aspirin may play possible therapeutic role in these patients.[64–66] Because SWS is a progressive condition with most patients developing seizures early in life, continued studies regarding combination therapy with antiplatelet medications and anticonvulsants have shown promise in the treatment of presymptomatic patients, which may lead to improved outcomes with regard to delayed age at seizure onset and lower seizure scores.[64]

GORLIN SYNDROME
Introduction

Gorlin syndrome, also known as Gorlin-Goltz syndrome, or basal cell nevus syndrome, is a rare autosomal dominant inheritable neurocutaneous syndrome that affects approximately 1 of 30,000 individuals with no gender predilection. There is complete penetrance and variable phenotypic expression. The genetic cause of this disorder is mutation in the *PTCH1* tumor suppressor gene on chromosome 9q. Clinical features in this syndrome include basal cell carcinoma (BCC) formation, as well as jaw keratocysts, and other neurologic, ophthalmologic, and skeletal abnormalities that begin during childhood.[67] There is also a known association between Gorlin syndrome and the development of medulloblastoma, making this condition especially relevant for neurosurgeons.[68]

Pathophysiology

Mutations in the *PTCH1* gene result in abnormal signaling of the sonic hedgehog (SHH) pathway, which is involved in cellular proliferation and survival. Hedgehog proteins bind to transmembrane proteins, for example, patched (PTCH1), a regulator of SHH downstream effects. Interplay also exists between PTCH1 and Smoothened (SMO) and its downstream target proteins in the GLI family. Mutation in PTCH1 thus results in uncontrolled and constitutive activation of the SHH pathway, leading to tumorigenesis and other findings in Gorlin syndrome.[69]

Clinical Manifestations

Diagnostic criteria include the presence of 2 major criteria, or 1 major and 2 minor criteria. Major criteria include (1) multiple BCCs appearing before age 20 years, (2) histologically proven odontogenic keratocysts of the jaw, (3) palmar/plantar hyperkeratosis (3 or more pits), (4) bilamellar calcification of the falx cerebri, (5) first-degree relative with Gorlin syndrome, or (6) rib anomalies (bifid, splayed, or fused). Minor criteria include (1) macrocephaly; (2) medulloblastoma (some consider this major criteria); (3) congenital malformations such as cleft lip/palate or frontal bossing; (4) other skeletal abnormalities (sprengel, pectus, syndactyly); (5) radiological abnormalities such as hemivertebrae, bridging of the sella, or limb anomalies; or (6) ovarian or cardiac fibroma.[70]

Approximately 5% of patients with Gorlin syndrome will develop medulloblastoma, which frequently occurs within the first 2 years of life when associated with this syndrome.[71–73] These tumors frequently demonstrate mutation in PTCH1 and loss of heterozygosity on chromosome 9q.[74,75] Typical treatment of medulloblastoma in patients with Gorlin syndrome involves surgical resection and chemotherapy. Radiation therapy should be used with caution, because radiation-induced BCCs and other secondary neoplasms can arise in these exquisitely radiosensitive patients.[76]

Hereditary hemorrhagic telangiectasia

Hereditary hemorrhagic telangiectasia (HHT), also known as Osler-Weber-Rendu disease, is an autosomal dominant neurocutaneous syndrome featuring abnormal vasculogenesis that affects the lungs, liver, brain, and skin and mucous membranes. Two types, HHT1 and HHT2, are caused by mutations of the *ENG* gene on chromosome 9 and *ACVRL1* on chromosome 12, respectively. HHT1 portends a higher risk of neurologic involvement. Formation of vascular malformations such as arteriovenous malformations (AVMs) or arteriovenous fistulas (AVFs) in multiple organ systems is a key feature of this disease, which occur as a result of vascular dysplasia.

The Curacao clinical criteria for diagnosis involves epistaxis (the most common presenting symptom in HHT), multiple telangiectasias, visceral lesions, and a first-degree family relative with HHT, with a definite diagnosis present with 3 or more criteria, possible HHT diagnosis with 2 criteria, and HHT being unlikely if fewer than 2 criteria are present.[77]

Patients with HHT have an increased risk of developing an intracranial vascular malformation, such as AVM, AVF, or cavernoma, with reports suggesting that between 4% and 23% of patients with HHT will develop such a lesion.[78,79] Compared with sporadic AVMs, it has been demonstrated that AVMs in patients with HHT have a lower risk of bleeding.[80] Imaging with MR angiography or cerebral angiography is important in following these lesions when discovered, although consensus screening recommendations are controversial. Treatment of cerebral malformations associated with HHT is similar to management of sporadically occurring lesions, with surgical resection, radiotherapy and endovascular embolization being utilized. The rare presence of spinal vascular malformations is also possible.

Importantly, pulmonary AVMs or AVFs may predispose patients with HHT to neurologic manifestations such as cerebral abscesses or cerebral infarction. Paradoxic embolism may occur with right to left shunting and resultant cerebral ischemia.[81]

CLINICS CARE POINTS

- Neurological manifestations of TSC include cortical tubers, neuronal migrational abnormalities, retinal hamartomas, subependymal nodules, and SEGAs

- Treatment of SEGA may include surgical resection, mTOR pathway inhibitors, and LITT

- Infantile spasms in TSC can be effectively treated with vigabatrin, with ACTH as second-line therapy

- The presence of a port-wine stain alone is not pathognomonic for SWS

- Intracranial involvement in SWS is most frequently ipsilateral to a port-wine stain
- Treatment with antiplatelet therapy should be considered in patients with SWS, who may have microvascular stasis/thrombosis
- Paroxysmal episodes of transient hemiparesis may occur in patients with SWS
- There is a known associated of Gorlin syndrome and medulloblastoma formation
- Radiation therapy must be used with caution in patients with Gorlin syndrome due to their propensity to develop secondary neoplasms
- Patients with HHT have a propensity to develop intracranial vascular malformations, including AVM, AVF, or cavernoma
- AVMs in HHT patients have been shown to have a lower risk of bleeding than sporadic AVMs

DISCLOSURE

None.

REFERENCES

1. van Slegtenhorst M, de Hoogt R, Hermans C, et al. Identification of the tuberous sclerosis gene TSC1 on chromosome 9q34. Science 1997;277:805–8.
2. European Chromosome 16 Tuberous Sclerosis C. Identification and characterization of the tuberous sclerosis gene on chromosome 16. Cell 1993;75: 1305–15.
3. Webb DW, Fryer AE, Osborne JP. Morbidity associated with tuberous sclerosis: a population study. Dev Med Child Neurol 1996;38:146–55.
4. Shepherd CW, Beard CM, Gomez MR, et al. Tuberous sclerosis complex in Olmsted County, Minnesota, 1950-1989. Arch Neurol 1991;48:400–1.
5. Osborne JP, Fryer A, Webb D. Epidemiology of tuberous sclerosis. Ann N Y Acad Sci 1991;615:125–7.
6. Peron A, Au KS, Northrup H. Genetics, genomics, and genotype-phenotype correlations of TSC: Insights for clinical practice. Am J Med Genet C Semin Med Genet 2018;178:281–90.
7. Northrup H, Krueger DA, International Tuberous Sclerosis Complex Consensus Group. Tuberous sclerosis complex diagnostic criteria update: recommendations of the 2012 International Tuberous Sclerosis Complex Consensus Conference. Pediatr Neurol 2013;49:243–54.
8. Vanderhooft SL, Francis JS, Pagon RA, et al. Prevalence of hypopigmented macules in a healthy population. J Pediatr 1996;129:355–61.
9. Krueger DA, Northrup H, International Tuberous Sclerosis Complex Consensus G. Tuberous sclerosis complex surveillance and management: recommendations of the 2012 International Tuberous Sclerosis Complex Consensus Conference. Pediatr Neurol 2013;49:255–65.
10. Gallagher A, Grant EP, Madan N, et al. MRI findings reveal three different types of tubers in patients with tuberous sclerosis complex. J Neurol 2010;257: 1373–81.
11. Kalantari BN, Salamon N. Neuroimaging of tuberous sclerosis: spectrum of pathologic findings and frontiers in imaging. AJR Am J Roentgenol 2008;190:W304–9.
12. Mohamed AR, Bailey CA, Freeman JL, et al. Intrinsic epileptogenicity of cortical tubers revealed by intracranial EEG monitoring. Neurology 2012;79: 2249–57.
13. Kannan L, Vogrin S, Bailey C, et al. Centre of epileptogenic tubers generate and propagate seizures in tuberous sclerosis. Brain 2016;139: 2653–67.
14. Ma TS, Elliott RE, Ruppe V, et al. Electrocorticographic evidence of perituberal cortex epileptogenicity in tuberous sclerosis complex. J Neurosurg Pediatr 2012;10:376–82.
15. Major P, Rakowski S, Simon MV, et al. Are cortical tubers epileptogenic? Evidence from electrocorticography. Epilepsia 2009;50:147–54.
16. Russo C, Nastro A, Cicala D, et al. Neuroimaging in tuberous sclerosis complex. Childs Nerv Syst 2020; 36:2497–509.
17. Ridler K, Suckling J, Higgins N, et al. Standardized whole brain mapping of tubers and subependymal nodules in tuberous sclerosis complex. J Child Neurol 2004;19:658–65.
18. Lu DS, Karas PJ, Krueger DA, et al. Central nervous system manifestations of tuberous sclerosis complex. Am J Med Genet C Semin Med Genet 2018; 178:291–8.
19. Kingswood JC, d'Augeres GB, Belousova E, et al. TuberOus SClerosis registry to increase disease Awareness (TOSCA) - baseline data on 2093 patients. Orphanet J Rare Dis 2017;12:2.
20. Schindler G, Capper D, Meyer J, et al. Analysis of BRAF V600E mutation in 1,320 nervous system tumors reveals high mutation frequencies in pleomorphic xanthoastrocytoma, ganglioglioma and extra-cerebellar pilocytic astrocytoma. Acta Neuropathol 2011;121: 397–405.
21. Cotter JA. An update on the central nervous system manifestations of tuberous sclerosis complex. Acta Neuropathol 2020;139:613–24.
22. Jansen FE, Vincken KL, Algra A, et al. Cognitive impairment in tuberous sclerosis complex is a multifactorial condition. Neurology 2008;70:916–23.
23. Harter DH, Bassani L, Rodgers SD, et al. A management strategy for intraventricular subependymal giant cell astrocytomas in tuberous sclerosis complex. J Neurosurg Pediatr 2014;13:21–8.

24. Giordano F, Moscheo C, Lenge M, et al. Neurosurgical treatment of subependymal giant cell astrocytomas in tuberous sclerosis complex: a series of 44 surgical procedures in 31 patients. Childs Nerv Syst 2020;36:951–60.

25. Berhouma M. Management of subependymal giant cell tumors in tuberous sclerosis complex: the neurosurgeon's perspective. World J Pediatr 2010;6:103–10.

26. Moavero R, Pinci M, Bombardieri R, et al. The management of subependymal giant cell tumors in tuberous sclerosis: a clinician's perspective. Childs Nerv Syst 2011;27:1203–10.

27. Frassanito P, Noya C, Tamburrini G. Current trends in the management of subependymal giant cell astrocytomas in tuberous sclerosis. Childs Nerv Syst 2020;36:2527–36.

28. Nabbout R, Belousova E, Benedik MP, et al. Epilepsy in tuberous sclerosis complex: Findings from the TOSCA Study. Epilepsia Open 2019;4:73–84.

29. Curatolo P, Jozwiak S, Nabbout R, et al. Management of epilepsy associated with tuberous sclerosis complex (TSC): clinical recommendations. Eur J Paediatr Neurol 2012;16:582–6.

30. van der Poest Clement E, Jansen FE, Braun KPJ, et al. Update on drug management of refractory epilepsy in tuberous sclerosis complex. Paediatr Drugs 2020;22:73–84.

31. Neal A, Ostrowsky-Coste K, Jung J, et al. Epileptogenicity in tuberous sclerosis complex: a stereoelectroencephalographic study. Epilepsia 2020;61:81–95.

32. Fallah A, Guyatt GH, Snead OC 3rd, et al. Predictors of seizure outcomes in children with tuberous sclerosis complex and intractable epilepsy undergoing resective epilepsy surgery: an individual participant data meta-analysis. PLoS One 2013;8:e53565.

33. Hess EJ, Moody KA, Geffrey AL, et al. Cannabidiol as a new treatment for drug-resistant epilepsy in tuberous sclerosis complex. Epilepsia 2016;57:1617–24.

34. French JA, Lawson JA, Yapici Z, et al. Adjunctive everolimus therapy for treatment-resistant focal-onset seizures associated with tuberous sclerosis (EXIST-3): a phase 3, randomised, double-blind, placebo-controlled study. Lancet 2016;388:2153–63.

35. Curatolo P, Franz DN, Lawson JA, et al. Adjunctive everolimus for children and adolescents with treatment-refractory seizures associated with tuberous sclerosis complex: post-hoc analysis of the phase 3 EXIST-3 trial. Lancet Child Adolesc Health 2018;2:495–504.

36. Jagtap S, Srinivas G, Harsha KJ, et al. Sturge-Weber syndrome: clinical spectrum, disease course, and outcome of 30 patients. J Child Neurol 2013;28:725–31.

37. Shirley MD, Tang H, Gallione CJ, et al. Sturge-Weber syndrome and port-wine stains caused by somatic mutation in GNAQ. N Engl J Med 2013;368:1971–9.

38. Nakashima M, Miyajima M, Sugano H, et al. The somatic GNAQ mutation c.548G>A (p.R183Q) is consistently found in Sturge-Weber syndrome. J Hum Genet 2014;59:691–3.

39. Martins L, Giovani PA, Reboucas PD, et al. Computational analysis for GNAQ mutations: New insights on the molecular etiology of Sturge-Weber syndrome. J Mol Graph Model 2017;76:429–40.

40. Huang L, Couto JA, Pinto A, et al. Somatic GNAQ mutation is enriched in brain endothelial cells in Sturge-Weber syndrome. Pediatr Neurol 2017;67:59–63.

41. Tillmann RP, Ray K, Aylett SE. Transient episodes of hemiparesis in Sturge Weber Syndrome - causes, incidence and recovery. Eur J Paediatr Neurol 2020;25:90–6.

42. Lin DD, Barker PB, Hatfield LA, et al. Dynamic MR perfusion and proton MR spectroscopic imaging in Sturge-Weber syndrome: correlation with neurological symptoms. J Magn Reson Imaging 2006;24:274–81.

43. Jansen FE, van der Worp HB, van Huffelen A, et al. Sturge-Weber syndrome and paroxysmal hemiparesis: epilepsy or ischaemia? Dev Med Child Neurol 2004;46:783–6.

44. Zolkipli Z, Aylett S, Rankin PM, et al. Transient exacerbation of hemiplegia following minor head trauma in Sturge-Weber syndrome. Dev Med Child Neurol 2007;49:697–9.

45. Comi AM. Sturge-Weber syndrome and epilepsy: an argument for aggressive seizure management in these patients. Expert Rev Neurother 2007;7:951–6.

46. Barbagallo M, Ruggieri M, Incorpora G, et al. Infantile spasms in the setting of Sturge-Weber syndrome. Childs Nerv Syst 2009;25:111–8.

47. Sugano H, Iimura Y, Igarashi A, et al. Extent of leptomeningeal capillary malformation is associated with severity of epilepsy in Sturge-Weber Syndrome. Pediatr Neurol 2020;117:64–71.

48. Namer IJ, Battaglia F, Hirsch E, et al. Subtraction ictal SPECT co-registered to MRI (SISCOM) in Sturge-Weber syndrome. Clin Nucl Med 2005;30:39–40.

49. Aylett SE, Neville BG, Cross JH, et al. Sturge-Weber syndrome: cerebral haemodynamics during seizure activity. Dev Med Child Neurol 1999;41:480–5.

50. Hu Z, Cao J, Choi EY, et al. Progressive retinal vessel malformation in a premature infant with Sturge-Weber syndrome: a case report and a literature review of ocular manifestations in Sturge-Weber syndrome. BMC Ophthalmol 2021;21:56.

51. Ratra D, Yadav H, Dalan D, et al. Retinal vascular abnormalities in Sturge-Weber syndrome. Indian J Ophthalmol 2019;67:1223–6.

52. Andica C, Hagiwara A, Hori M, et al. Aberrant myelination in patients with Sturge-Weber syndrome

analyzed using synthetic quantitative magnetic resonance imaging. Neuroradiology 2019;61: 1055–66.

53. Hu J, Yu Y, Juhasz C, et al. MR susceptibility weighted imaging (SWI) complements conventional contrast enhanced T1 weighted MRI in characterizing brain abnormalities of Sturge-Weber Syndrome. J Magn Reson Imaging 2008;28:300–7.

54. Bar C, Pedespan JM, Boccara O, et al. Early magnetic resonance imaging to detect presymptomatic leptomeningeal angioma in children with suspected Sturge-Weber syndrome. Dev Med Child Neurol 2020;62:227–33.

55. Ragupathi S, Reddy AK, Jayamohan AE, et al. Sturge-Weber syndrome: CT and MRI illustrations. BMJ Case Rep 2014;2014. bcr2014205743.

56. Bianchi F, Auricchio AM, Battaglia DI, et al. Sturge-Weber syndrome: an update on the relevant issues for neurosurgeons. Childs Nerv Syst 2020;36: 2553–70.

57. Triana Junco PE, Sanchez-Carpintero I, Lopez-Gutierrez JC. Preventive treatment with oral sirolimus and aspirin in a newborn with severe Sturge-Weber syndrome. Pediatr Dermatol 2019;36:524–7.

58. Sun B, Han T, Wang Y, et al. Sirolimus as a potential treatment for Sturge-Weber Syndrome. J Craniofac Surg 2021;32:257–60.

59. Falconer MA, Rushworth RG. Treatment of encephalotrigeminal angiomatosis (Sturge-Weber disease) by hemispherectomy. Arch Dis Child 1960;35:433–47.

60. Kossoff EH, Buck C, Freeman JM. Outcomes of 32 hemispherectomies for Sturge-Weber syndrome worldwide. Neurology 2002;59:1735–8.

61. Bourgeois M, Crimmins DW, de Oliveira RS, et al. Surgical treatment of epilepsy in Sturge-Weber syndrome in children. J Neurosurg 2007;106:20–8.

62. Schropp C, Sorensen N, Krauss J. Early periinsular hemispherotomy in children with Sturge-Weber syndrome and intractable epilepsy–outcome in eight patients. Neuropediatrics 2006;37:26–31.

63. Tuxhorn IE, Pannek HW. Epilepsy surgery in bilateral Sturge-Weber syndrome. Pediatr Neurol 2002;26: 394–7.

64. Day AM, Hammill AM, Juhasz C, et al. Hypothesis: presymptomatic treatment of Sturge-Weber syndrome with aspirin and antiepileptic drugs may delay seizure onset. Pediatr Neurol 2019;90:8–12.

65. Lance EI, Sreenivasan AK, Zabel TA, et al. Aspirin use in Sturge-Weber syndrome: side effects and clinical outcomes. J Child Neurol 2013;28:213–8.

66. Bay MJ, Kossoff EH, Lehmann CU, et al. Survey of aspirin use in Sturge-Weber syndrome. J Child Neurol 2011;26:692–702.

67. Gorlin RJ, Goltz RW. Multiple nevoid basal-cell epithelioma, jaw cysts and bifid rib. A syndrome. N Engl J Med 1960;262:908–12.

68. Herzberg JJ, Wiskemann A. [The fifth phakomatosis. Basal cell nevus with hereditary malformation and medulloblastoma]. Dermatologica 1963;126: 106–23.

69. Pino LC, Balassiano LK, Sessim M, et al. Basal cell nevus syndrome: clinical and molecular review and case report. Int J Dermatol 2016;55:367–75.

70. Kimonis VE, Goldstein AM, Pastakia B, et al. Clinical manifestations in 105 persons with nevoid basal cell carcinoma syndrome. Am J Med Genet 1997;69: 299–308.

71. Evans DG, Ladusans EJ, Rimmer S, et al. Complications of the naevoid basal cell carcinoma syndrome: results of a population based study. J Med Genet 1993;30:460–4.

72. Evans DG, Farndon PA, Burnell LD, et al. The incidence of Gorlin syndrome in 173 consecutive cases of medulloblastoma. Br J Cancer 1991;64:959–61.

73. Foulkes WD, Kamihara J, Evans DGR, et al. Cancer surveillance in gorlin syndrome and rhabdoid tumor predisposition syndrome. Clin Cancer Res 2017;23: e62–7.

74. Ikemoto Y, Miyashita T, Nasu M, et al. Gorlin syndrome-induced pluripotent stem cells form medulloblastoma with loss of heterozygosity in PTCH1. Aging (Albany NY) 2020;12:9935–47.

75. Onodera S, Nakamura Y, Azuma T. Gorlin syndrome: recent advances in genetic testing and molecular and cellular biological research. Int J Mol Sci 2020; 21:7559.

76. Osman Ali AA, Bayoumi Y, Balbaid A, et al. Radiation induced multiple skin neoplasms following craniospinal irradiation for medulloblastoma. A case report. Am J Case Rep 2020;21:e917694.

77. Shovlin CL, Guttmacher AE, Buscarini E, et al. Diagnostic criteria for hereditary hemorrhagic telangiectasia (Rendu-Osler-Weber syndrome). Am J Med Genet 2000;91:66–7.

78. Fulbright RK, Chaloupka JC, Putman CM, et al. MR of hereditary hemorrhagic telangiectasia: prevalence and spectrum of cerebrovascular malformations. AJNR Am J Neuroradiol 1998;19:477–84.

79. Maher CO, Piepgras DG, Brown RD Jr, et al. Cerebrovascular manifestations in 321 cases of hereditary hemorrhagic telangiectasia. Stroke 2001;32: 877–82.

80. Willemse RB, Mager JJ, Westermann CJ, et al. Bleeding risk of cerebrovascular malformations in hereditary hemorrhagic telangiectasia. J Neurosurg 2000;92:779–84.

81. Labeyrie PE, Courtheoux P, Babin E, et al. Neurological involvement in hereditary hemorrhagic telangiectasia. J Neuroradiol 2016;43:236–45.

Tumor Syndromes
Neurosurgical Evaluation and Management

Aravinda Ganapathy, BS, MS[a,1], Elizabeth Juarez Diaz, BS[a,1], Justin T. Coleman[b], Kimberly A. Mackey, MD[b,c,*]

KEYWORDS

- Tumor syndrome • Neurofibromatosis • von Hippel-Lindau syndrome • Tuberous sclerosis complex
- Gorlin syndrome • Turcot syndrome • Li-Fraumeni syndrome • Cowden syndrome

KEY POINTS

- In a patient with a central nervous system malignancy, it is critical for the clinician to be aware of associated tumor syndromes to guide management and therapy.
- Neurofibromatosis-1 is the most common syndromic disorder of the central nervous system.
- First-line therapy for the most common tumor associated with tuberous sclerosis complex, subependymal giant cell astrocytoma, now primarily consists of mammalian target of rapamycin inhibition.
- Treatment of tumor syndromes involving the central nervous system requires a multidisciplinary approach.

INTRODUCTION

Historically, clinicians made observations in their clinical practice regarding certain associations of specific central nervous system (CNS) tumors and other clinical findings, which led to the description of several CNS tumor syndromes. Advances in the fields of genetics and molecular biology have brought forth a deeper understanding of various syndromic conditions associated with CNS tumors. Some of the most common tumor syndromes the neurosurgeon will encounter are also neurocutaneous disorders, namely, neurofibromatosis-1 (NF-1) and tuberous sclerosis complex (TSC). Tumor syndromes can also be associated with multiple extra-CNS findings. Herein, the authors discuss the most clinically relevant CNS tumor syndromes, including a brief discussion of their genetics, diagnosis, and treatment.

NEUROFIBROMATOSIS 1

NF-1, previously known as von Recklinghausen disease, is the most common autosomal dominant (AD) syndromic disorder of the CNS and neurocutaneous disorder.[1,2] It has an estimated incidence of 1 in 2500, and a prevalence of 1 in 2000 to 1 in 3000 individuals, regardless of ethnic background, race, or sex.[3–6] The NF-1 mutation is located on locus 17q.11.2 that encodes neurofibromin, a 2818-amino-acid protein that accelerates the inactivation of Ras; when impaired, this leads to an increase in cell growth.[1,3,7] Approximately half of the patients with NF-1 have sporadic de novo mutations in the absence of known family history.[8] Although NF-1 has complete penetrance, it has variable expression. Patients with NF-1 have a lifetime cancer risk of 59.6%.[8] It is necessary to approach patient care

[a] Washington University School of Medicine, 660 S Euclid Avenue, St Louis, MO 63110, USA; [b] South Georgia Medical Center, 2409 North Patterson Street, Suite 210, Valdosta, GA 31605, USA; [c] Department of Neurosurgery, Children's Hospital of the King's Daughters, 601 Children's Ln, Norfolk, VA 23507, USA
[1] These authors contributed equally.
* Corresponding author. South Georgia Medical Center, 2409 North Patterson Street, Suite 210, Valdosta, GA 31605.
E-mail address: Kimberly.mackey@sgmc.org

Neurosurg Clin N Am 33 (2022) 91–104
https://doi.org/10.1016/j.nec.2021.09.007

with a multidisciplinary team, including malignancy surveillance and genetic counseling.

Diagnosis of NF-1 is established by fulfilling 2 or more of the 7 National Institutes of Health (NIH) criteria as shown in **Table 1**. Approximately 97% of all patients with NF-1 meet criteria by their eighth birthday.[3,4] Those with sporadic NF-1 mutations may reach that threshold later than the first decade of life.[3]

During childhood and early adolescence, plexiform neurofibromas (pNFs), benign tumors of peripheral nerve sheath, can be seen in 30% to 50% of patients.[4] pNFs grow along multiple nerve fascicles along the length of the nerve and can cause pain, local compression, loss of function of nerves, aneurysms, vascular dysplasia, and disfigurement. On MRI scan, pNFs are generally gadolinium-enhancing masses.[5,9] After adolescence, the growth of pNFs slows or arrests completely. The risk that pNFs may transform into malignant peripheral nerve sheath tumors (MPNSTs) highlights the importance of early detection.[3,8] Patients with new neurologic symptoms, such as limb weakness, sensory changes, or pain, should undergo evaluation by MRI and PET scans to evaluate degree of malignancy.[3,4,8,10]

MPNSTs occur in 8% to 16% of patients and are the leading cause of death in the NF-1 population.[11] The 5-year survival rate among MPNSTs is 5% to 50%. Gross total resection (GTR) with wide negative margins is the best current treatment for MPNSTs; chemotherapy doxorubicin and ifosfamide may be recommended for incomplete surgical resection.[4,11,12] There remains controversy over the use of radiotherapy (RT) because of the potential for radiation-induced higher-grade secondary malignancies.[12,13]

Optic pathway glioma (OPG), most commonly low-grade glioma (LGG), affects 15% to 20% of patients and can arise anywhere along the optic pathway.[1,3,4,6] Nearly half of OPGs are asymptomatic; however, when they manifest, patients present with impaired visual acuity, visual field defect, and precocious puberty because of hypothalamic involvement.[6,14] Annual examinations are recommended for all NF-1 patients under the age of 10 to 12 years and are more sensitive than imaging.[3,11] Yearly height and weight monitoring is used to screen for precocious puberty. First-line therapy for optic gliomas consists of chemotherapy (carboplatin and vincristine).[4,13] Surgery is indicated in large orbital tumors with complete

---

Table 1
Diagnostic criteria for neurofibromatosis-1, neurofibromatosis-2, and Li-Fraumeni syndrome

NF-1	NF-2	Li-Fraumeni
If 2 or more of the following are found: • 6 or more cafe-au-lait macules over 5 mm in maximum diameter in prepubertal individuals, and over 15 mm in longest diameter in postpuberty • 2 or more neurofibromas of any type or one plexiform neurofibroma • Freckling in axillary or inguinal region • Optic glioma • 2 or more Lisch nodules (iris hamartomas) • Distinctive osseous lesion, such as sphenoid dysplasia or thinning of long bone cortex with or without pseudoarthrosis • A first-degree relative (parent, sibling, or offspring) with NF-1 by the above criteria	1. Bilateral 8 nerve masses seen with appropriate imaging (CT or MRI) or 2. First-degree relative with NF-2 and either: Unilateral 8 nerve mass, or Two of the following • Neurofibroma • Meningioma • Glioma • Schwannoma • Juvenile posterior subcapsular lenticular opacity	1. Sarcoma diagnosed before age 45 2. First-degree relative, meaning a parent, sibling, or child, with any cancer before age 45 3. First-degree relative or second-degree relative, meaning grandparent, aunt/uncle, niece/nephew, or grandchild, with any cancer before age 45 or a sarcoma at any age

loss of vision, and/or in the setting of obstructive hydrocephalus.[1] RT is avoided in the treatment of OPG because of secondary malignancy risk.

LGG can also be found in the brainstem, make up approximately 4% of NF-1-associated lesions, and tend to be indolent.[8,9,11,14] In a patient known to have NF-1, biopsy is generally not indicated, particularly in the midbrain area, and can be followed with radiographic surveillance. Treatment of obstructive hydrocephalus from expansion of brainstem or exophytic component can often be achieved by ventricular shunting but may often be amenable to endoscopic third ventriculostomy.

Importantly, NF-1 patients have at least a 5-fold increase for developing World Health Organization (WHO) grade IV astrocytoma (glioblastoma). Therapy for this population is similar to sporadic glioblastomas, with maximal safe resection followed by adjuvant chemotherapy (temozolomide) and fractionated RT.[10]

NEUROFIBROMATOSIS 2

Neurofibromatosis-2 (NF-2) is an AD disorder with an incidence of one in every 25,000, with complete penetrance by age 60 and no difference in sex.[6,15–17] Approximately half of NF-2 cases are de novo mutations of patients without family history of NF-2.[18] In NF-2, a mutation on a region of chromosome 22q12 that encodes for a tumor suppressor gene *merlin* is defective, most commonly expressed in Schwann and meningeal cells.[7] NF-2 is rarely a pediatric disease, as it tends to present in young adulthood around 20 to 30 years of age. NF-2 often clinically presents with dermatologic findings (plaquelike cutaneous schwannomas), ophthalmologic findings, peripheral neuropathies, and/or hearing loss.[1,6,16,17,19,20] Diagnostic criteria used in clinical practice, based on the NIH consensus criteria, are delineated in **Table 1**; ongoing research is working to refine diagnostic criteria. The pathognomonic finding in NF-2 is bilateral vestibular schwannoma (VS), with meningiomas and spinal cord ependymomas, ocular manifestations, and peripheral neuropathies also typical findings.

Bilateral VS are found in 90% to 95% of individuals and arise from the superior and inferior vestibular branches of the eighth cranial nerve.[1,16,17] Hearing loss from VS associated with morbidity affects 30% of children and 60% of adults. Less common clinical symptoms include balance difficulty, facial nerve weakness, and potential neurologic deficit from hydrocephalus and/or brainstem compression from large tumors.[14,16] These schwannomas are best visualized as enhancing masses at the cerebellopontine angle (CPA) on contrasted T1-weighted MRI scan.[17] Hearing loss is not directly correlated to tumor size or growth rate, but the presence of hearing loss can be used to determine appropriate timing for intervention.[1,16]

Controversy over the exact timing of surgery along with associated risks in this population has historically led to poor preservation of hearing and facial function. Management of smaller VS, often asymptomatic, remains controversial. Although early surgical management of VS less than 3 cm has been shown to preserve hearing in 30% to 65%, and facial nerve function in 75% to 92% of NF-2 patients, there is no consensus on the management of VS less than 3 cm.[16] Stereotactic radiosurgery (SRS) has shown local control in 74% to 100% of VS, but there is evidence of potential increased risk of malignant progression complicating treatment.[16] Recent level 3 recommendations suggest SRS as an option for treatment in patients with NF-2 with VS that is enlarging or causing hearing loss.[6,21–23] Once the tumor is greater than 3 cm, there is brainstem compression or hydrocephalus, or in patients not interested in SRS, surgical resection is often recommended. Surgical approaches include the middle cranial fossa approach, often used in patients with small, mostly intracanalicular tumors with good hearing status but with greater risk of facial dysfunction; posterior suboccipital (retrosigmoid) approach for larger tumors with components in the CPA and the option to preserve hearing; and translabyrinthine approach, which always sacrifices hearing but has the lowest recurrence rate. Patients with mosaic NF-2 have better prognosis.[14]

Meningioma can be found in NF-2 patients, but of course, most patients with meningiomas are not associated with NF-2. Intracranial meningiomas are seen in 45% to 58% of NF-2 patients, and spinal meningiomas are diagnosed in 20% of patients.[1,15,17,22] The presence of intracranial meningiomas is associated with a 2 to 5 times increase in relative risk for mortality. NF-2 meningiomas are associated with greater anaplastic grades than sporadic meningiomas. Most meningiomas can be safely resected if in the cerebral hemispheres and spinal canal; however, optic nerve sheath and skull-base pose greater surgical risk. For those appropriate for SRS, a 5-year progression-free survival rate of 86% has been shown but has not been followed long term.[24] Again, RT and/or SRS could be associated with malignant transformation and future tumor development, and the treatment modality remains somewhat controversial.

Ependymoma is the most common intramedullary spinal cord tumor (IMSCT) associated with NF-2 (75% of IMSCT are ependymoma in this population).[15] Ependymomas are diagnosed in up to half of all NF-2 patients.[17] Most often in WHO grade II tumors, patients with IMSCT present with weakness, often unilateral, sensory change, bladder dysfunction, scoliosis, and/or back pain. Ependymoma is truly a surgical disease, and GTR has been shown to be successful without regrowth.[16,17] For patients with NF-2, treatment at a specialty medical center has been associated with decreased risk of mortality, highlighting yet again the importance of a comprehensive medical team when treating patients with tumor syndromes.[16,25]

COWDEN SYNDROME

Cowden syndrome is a rare AD disease that affect approximately one in 250,000 live births.[26–28] This rare syndrome is caused by a germline mutation of the PTEN gene located on chromosome 10q23, that acts as a negative regulator of cell proliferation and cell-cycle progression through Akt and mammalian target of rapamycin (mTOR) inhibition.[9,28] Patients with this mutation are at higher risk of developing thyroid, breast, and uterine cancers, as well as hamartomas, meningiomas, and skin tumors.[29] Macrocephaly has been reported in 80% to 100% of CS patients.[27]

Cowden syndrome is associated with Lhermitte-Duclos disease (LDD), occurring in 9% to 15% of patients.[28] LDD occurs during the third or fourth decade of life and usually presents with headache, ataxia, cranial nerve palsies, obstructive hydrocephalus, gastrointestinal polys, and penile freckling.[6,9,30] A characteristic finding of LDD is diffuse enlargement of cerebellar folia owing to slow growth of benign neoplastic cells.[26] On MRI scan, a characteristic finding on T2-weighted imaging is a striated pattern called "tiger-striping," and diffusion-weighted imaging can help delineate surgical resection margins.[30]

Surgical resection of LDD is the mainstay of treatment, aimed at reduction in intracranial pressure associated with mass effect. Resection may relieve obstructive hydrocephalus in LDD, but will not improve cerebellar symptoms.[26] A suboccipital approach is performed, and ventricular shunting may be required.[31] Given that abnormal tissue may blend into normal cerebellar hemisphere, GTR is not always achieved.[9,31] Adjuvant therapy is not required postoperatively. Follow-up long term for recurrence and other malignancy is important.

TURCOT SYNDROME

Turcot syndrome is a rare AD disease characterized by the presence of primary CNS malignancy in conjunction with colorectal neoplasms.[6,32] Type 1 Turcot syndrome is known as hereditary nonpolyposis related colorectal cancer (HNPCC, or Lynch syndrome). HNPCC is caused by a germline mutation in DNA mismatch repair genes: PMS2 located on Ch 7p22, MLH1 located on Ch 3p22, and MSH2 located on chromosome 2p21.[33,34] Type 2 Turcot syndrome (familial adenomatous polyposis or FAP) arises from a mutation on the APC (Ch 5q21).[7,9,18] APC protein is part of the wingless-related integration site signaling pathway that controls cell proliferation and differentiation.[9]

FAP-diagnosed individuals with APC gene mutations have a 3-fold risk of brain tumors, specifically, a 13-fold risk of medulloblastoma (MB) with the highest incidence before 10 to 20 years of age.[9,18] Astrocytoma, ependymoma, and pituitary adenomas have also been found in patients with FAP.[18,32-] Treatment for FAP-associated Turcot syndrome tumors is identical to sporadic forms of tumors, including maximal safe surgical resection, chemotherapy, and RT, depending on age of the child.[9]

HNPCC or Lynch syndrome presents in the CNS with gliomas, commonly glioblastoma, before the age of 30 years.[9] HNPCC glioblastomas are treated similar to the sporadic counterparts with standard regimen of resection, chemotherapy, and radiation.[9,35] Surveillance with neuroaxis MRI scan is critical for individuals with Turcot syndrome from 2 years of age onward, in 1- to 3-year intervals.[9,18] For family members of patients with known Turcot syndrome–related CNS tumors, neurologic evaluation is recommended.[32]

LI-FRAUMENI SYNDROME

Li-Fraumeni syndrome (LFS) is caused by a mutation in the TP53 gene located on chromosome 17p13.[6,7,26,36] P53 is a tumor suppressor tetrameric protein that acts as a gatekeeper in regulation of cell-cycle arrest, apoptosis, senescence, and DNA repair. The prevalence of this disorder is one in 5000, and these individuals have a life-long risk of multiple tumors in various organ systems.[9] Diagnostic criteria for LFS are shown in **Table 1**. Germline TP53 mutations are found in 50% of pediatric adrenocortical tumors, 2% to 10% of childhood brain tumors, 9% of rhabdomyosarcoma, and 2% to 3% of osteosarcomas. Approximately half of LFS patients will develop a cancer by age 30.[9,28,37] Some common brain tumors in LFS include choroid plexus carcinoma (CPC), MB, astrocytoma, and, with less frequency, ependymoma.[1]

CPC are less than 0.8% of primary brain tumors,[36] arising in the ventricle as a lobulated "cauliflower-like" mass; in LFS, they are associated with an increased severity when compared with sporadic counterparts.[9,36] Treatment usually consists of GTR with adjuvant chemotherapy. RT in known LFS patients is avoided because of potential secondary tumor effect.[38]

Astrocytomas (grade II to IV) are the most common brain tumors associated with LFS.[36] In adults, infiltrating astrocytoma is predominately supratentorial; however, in children, infratentorial tumors are more common.[9] MRI scans of grade II diffuse astrocytoma have infiltrative homogenous T1 hypointensity and fluid-attenuated inversion recovery (FLAIR) hyperintensity with no contrast enhancement,[9] whereas grade III and, nearly universally, grade IV are associated with enhancement. Whether astrocytoma associated with LFS with a concomitant IDH mutation carries a better prognosis, much like the sporadic counterpart (non-LFS but with IDH mutation) is still undetermined.[36] Annual dedicated brain MRI scan is recommended on all tumors associated with LFS.[28] Therapy consists of maximal safe resection with or without adjuvant chemotherapy. RT may not be used in lower-grade lesions because of observed risk of secondary malignancy and worse outcomes.[36]

MB may present in children with LFS during their first 5 years, as well as in early adulthood in the third decade.[9,36] MB with germline TP53 mutations has worse overall survival when compared with sporadic TP53 MB. These tumors arise in the posterior fossa, most commonly the fourth ventricle but can invade or involve cerebellar parenchyma.[36] Therapy consists of GTR (<1.5 cm^3) with chemotherapy.[9,39] Genetic counseling for LFS families is vital because of the high prevalence of tumors in this population.[6,26]

GORLIN SYNDROME

Gorlin syndrome (GS), also known as nevoid basal cell carcinoma syndrome or Gorlin-Goltz syndrome, is a rare AD cancer syndrome inherited with high penetrance but variable expression.[40] The prevalence varies between 1/31,000 and 1/235,800, with no predilection between men and women.[41] The disorder is characterized primarily by mutations in the patched 1 (PTCH1) gene, a tumor suppressor located on chromosome 9q: the gene encodes a 12-transmembrane domain receptor that acts as a receptor for the hedgehog protein (SHH).[40] In addition, heterozygous loss-of-function mutations in the SUFU gene on chromosome 10 have been found in individuals meeting the diagnostic criteria for GS.[42] Affected

patients characteristically acquire multiple developmental abnormalities, such as multiple basal cell carcinomas (BCCs) and odontogenic keratocysts of the jaw, at an early age, as well as an increased risk of MB development in early childhood.[42] Clinical presentation appears to vary by ethnicity: up to 90% of white patients with GS develop BCCs, compared with only about 40% of black patients. Patients with GS develop MB (mostly the desmoplastic type) at an early age; although sporadic MBs typically present between ages 6 and 10 years, MBs often present in patients with GS by age 3.[43] The prevalence of MBs is significantly higher in patients with the SUFU gene mutation than in patients with the PTCH1 mutation[41,42,44] and likely more prevalent in women than men by 3:1.[45,46] Because of the presence of MB at such an early age, children under the age of 5 years with MB should be carefully screened for other syndromic signs.[46,47] Other tumors have been reported less frequently in GS, including meningioma, oligodendroglioma, and craniopharyngioma.[45] Other intracranial and facial findings include ectopic calcifications of the falx cerebri, cleft lip or palate, bridging of the sella turcica, and ocular manifestations (hypertelorism, congenital cataracts).[48,49] Imaging modalities are primarily used to confirm diagnoses: skull radiograph or head computed tomographic (CT) scan can be used to identify calcified falx cerebri or sella turcica bridging, whereas panoramic films are recommended for odontogenic keratocysts.[50] Molecular genetic testing can be done as well to identify PTCH1 or SUFU variants in suspected individuals. Treatment typically involves surveillance for development of cancers and specific treatment for syndrome-related complications.[51] Importantly, RT is contraindicated in patients with GS who develop MBs because of the propensity to develop secondary malignancies.[52] Surgical resection and chemotherapy should be considered the mainstay of treatment in these cases.

ATAXIA-TELANGIECTASIA

Ataxia-telangiectasia (AT) is a rare autosomal recessive (AR) primary immunodeficiency disorder with an estimated incidence of 1 in 20,000 to 100,000 live births.[53,54] The disorder is characterized by a mutation in the ATM gene localized to chromosome 11.[55] Clinically, the disorder is marked by several neurologic abnormalities, the earliest of which is ataxia, manifesting between 6 and 18 months of age, along with spinocerebellar neurodegeneration in homozygotes.[56] Because of the ataxia at a young age, the most common misdiagnoses include Friedreich ataxia and cerebral palsy.[57,58] Beyond 10 years of age, patients are typically confined to a wheelchair.[59]

Although the most prevalent malignancies for patients with AT are leukemia and lymphoma,[60–62] patients also show higher incidence of brain malignancies, especially MBs, gliomas, and pilocytic astrocytomas.[9,63] Regarding relevant variants, the D1853N polymorphism is considered the most fundamental variant in genotyping the *ATM* gene in patients with brain tumors: studies have begun to elucidate a role for the variant in not only disease susceptibility but also metastatic progression as well.[63–65] Importantly, because of the role *ATM* plays in DNA repair, patients are particularly sensitive to cell damage from chemotherapy and RT, making this disorder difficult to treat. Diagnostic testing using radiographs and ionizing radiation should also be limited to mitigate risk of subsequent complications; surveillance MRI scan is the primary imaging modality. With such limited treatment options, gene therapy is being investigated, such as the lentiviral vector to rescue defects in the *ATM* cells.[9,66]

MULTIPLE ENDOCRINE NEOPLASIA TYPE 1

Multiple endocrine neoplasia type 1 (MEN1) is a rare AD genetic syndrome with an estimated prevalence of 1 in 30,000 individuals.[67] The disorder is characterized by the cooccurrence of multiple endocrine (parathyroid glands, pituitary, pancreas) and nonendocrine tumors in the same or related individuals.[67,68] Clinically, the disorder has a nearly 100% penetrance by age 50 years.[68] MEN1 is caused by an inactivating mutation of the tumor suppressor gene *MEN1* located on chromosome 11.[69] CNS neoplasms, such as meningiomas, ependymomas, and schwannomas, are among the nonendocrine tumors of MEN1 syndrome.[70–72] Pituitary tumors are a more common occurrence however, with prevalence reports ranging between 10% and 60% in patients with MEN1.[73] Up to 3% of patients who develop a pituitary tumor will have MEN1, with the most common subset of secreting tumor being a prolactinoma.[69] The clinical diagnosis is based on the presence of 2 or more primary MEN1 endocrine tumors (parathyroid, pancreas, pituitary) or by identifying a germline-inactivating mutation in the MEN1 gene.[68] MEN1 typically presents during or after the second decade of life, with reports demonstrating primary hyperparathyroidism and pituitary tumors as the most common first clinical manifestations.[74] Patients and at-risk family members should be carefully screened (either genetically or biochemically) and monitored for development of MEN1-associated tumors. Treatment for MEN1 tumors is generally similar to that for sporadic disease.

VON HIPPEL-LINDAU SYNDROME

Von Hippel-Lindau syndrome (vHL) is an AD disorder with an approximate prevalence of 1/36,000 individuals.[75,76] Clinically, the disorder is characterized by multiple benign and malignant tumors: primary CNS manifestations include hemangioblastoma of the brain (cerebellum and brainstem), spine, and retina. Other tumorigenic manifestations include clear cell renal cell carcinoma (RCC), pheochromocytomas and paragangliomas, pancreatic neuroendocrine tumors, endolymphatic sac tumors of the middle ear, and papillary cystadenomas of the epididymis and broad ligament.[77,78]

Molecularly, vHL syndrome is characterized by loss of function of the tumor suppressor gene *vHL* on chromosome 3.[79] Classification of vHL syndrome primarily depends on the risk for pheochromocytoma development: type 1 patients have a low risk, whereas type 2 patients have an increased risk of developing pheochromocytoma (with subdivisions for type 2 depending on risk of developing RCC).[80] CNS hemangioblastomas affect 60% to 80% of all vHL syndrome patients, making them the most common lesions.[81] Patients with vHL, with a mean age of presentation around 30 years, affected by hemangioblastomas are typically younger than those with sporadic hemangioblastoma, who normally present within the fifth and sixth decades of life.[75,78,82] Lesions appear to predominantly present in the cerebellum and spinal cord, with other lesions presenting in the brainstem, cauda equina, and supratentorial region.[83,84] Although sporadic hemangioblastoma lesions typically present solitarily, vHL is associated with multiple lesions and cerebellar presentations.[85]

Current recommendations include genetic screening patients with CNS hemangioblastomas for vHL mutations, especially patients presenting under the age of 50 years, as well as at-risk relatives.[86] Furthermore, genetic counseling should be provided for at-risk families and surveillance by routine MRI scan for brain and spine hemangioblastomas, as well as for other benign and malignant lesions.

TUBEROUS SCLEROSIS COMPLEX

TSC is an AD disorder with an incidence of approximately 1/6000 to 10,000 live births.[87] It results from a mutation in either the *TSC1* or the *TSC2* tumor suppressor genes. *TSC1* is found on chromosome 9 and encodes the protein hamartin, whereas *TSC2* is found on chromosome 16 and encodes the protein tuberin.[88] Heterodimerization of hamartin and tuberin results in inhibition of the mTOR pathway, a pathway that plays critical roles in regulation of cell growth and proliferation.[89] De novo mutations account for around 80% of all TSC cases, with *TSC2* mutations being approximately 4 times as common as mutations in *TSC1*. Familial TSC cases show no predilection toward either gene.[90] A high rate of mosaicism has been detected in families with TSC, which is thought to play a role in the disease's de novo propagation.[91] The disorder displays nearly complete penetrance but highly variable expressivity: the severity varies significantly among affected members, even individuals of the same family.[92,93]

Clinically, TSC is characterized by the development of benign tumors in multiple organs, including the brain, retina, heart, kidneys, skin, liver, and lungs.[87] Neurologic manifestations are among the most common in patients with TSC: up to 90% of children with TSC have demonstrated neuropsychiatric disorders, such as attention-deficit/hyperactivity disorder (ADHD), intellectual disability, and autism spectrum disorders,[94] whereas epileptic spasms are seen in nearly 50% of children with TSC.[95] In one study, seizures were found to occur in 78% of patients, with most occurring before 1 year of age.[96] Structural brain malformations in patients with TSC include glioneuronal hamartomas (also called cortical tubers) in at least 80% of patients, subependymal nodules in around 90% of patients, and subependymal giant cell tumors (also known as subependymal giant cell astrocytomas, or SEGAs) in 5% to 20% of patients with TSC.[97–99] Glioneuronal hamartomas are composed of abnormally disorganized neurons and glia with astrocytosis, whereas subependymal nodules are small, usually calcified asymptomatic intraventricular protrusions typically located in the lateral ventricle adjacent to the caudate nucleus.[97,100,101] SEGAs are considered the characteristic brain tumor in patients with TSC: a benign, slow-growing tumor that typically arises from the periventricular area adjacent to the foramen of Monro and comprises mixed glioneuronal cells.[102] Immunohistochemistry studies in mouse models have suggested both SEGAs and glioneuronal hamartomas share a related neuroglial progenitor cell of origin.[103] The main difference between subependymal nodules and SEGAs is their size (SEGAs are typically >1 cm) and location, as discussed previously.[97,104] Furthermore, although SEGAs will continue to grow over time, subependymal nodules will typically remain stable in size.[97]

SEGA tumors may become symptomatic between the ages of 10 and 30 years, but symptomatic tumors only occur in approximately 6% to 9% of patients with TSC.[9,102,105] Affected children typically present with neurologic cues, such as

---

Table 2
Diagnostic criteria for tuberous sclerosis complex

***Confirmed* Diagnosis: 2 Major Features[a] OR 1 Major and ≥2 Minor Features**
***Possible* Diagnosis: With 1 Major OR ≥2 Minor Features**

Major Features	Minor Features
• Hypomelanotic macules (≥3, at least 5 mm diameter) • Angiofibromas (≥3) • Ungual fibromas (≥2) • Shagreen patch • Multiple retinal hamartomas • Subependymal nodules • Cortical dysplasias (includes tubers and cerebral white matter radial migration lines) • Subependymal giant cell astrocytoma (SEGA) • Cardiac rhabdomyoma • Angiomyolipomas (≥2) • Lymphangioleiomyomatosis	• "Confetti" skin lesions • Dental enamel pits (≥3) • Intraoral fibromas (≥2) • Retinal achromatic patch • Multiple renal cysts • Nonrenal hamartomas

[a] Two major features of lymphangioleiomyomatosis and angiomyolipomas do NOT meet criteria for diagnosis.

Table 3
Tumor syndrome characteristics

Syndrome	Inheritance	Gene	Molecular Mechanism	Associated CNS Tumors	Other Neurologic Manifestations
Ataxia-telangiectasia	AR	*ATM* (11q22)	DNA double-stranded break repair impairment, cell-cycle dysregulation	Medulloblastoma, glioma, pilocytic astrocytoma Lymphoma/leukemia	Ataxia, spinocerebellar neurodegeneration
Cowden	AD	*PTEN* (10q23)	Dysregulation of cell cycle, proliferation	Cerebellar tumor	Cranial nerve palsies, obstructive hydrocephalus, ataxia, headache
Gorlin	AD	*PTCH1* (9q22) *SUFU* (10q24)	SHH pathway dysregulation	Medulloblastoma, meningioma, oligodendroglioma, craniopharyngioma	Ectopic calcifications of falx cerebri, cleft lip or palate, bridging of sella turcica, odontogenic keratocysts, hypertelorism, congenital cataracts
Li-Fraumeni		*TP53* (17p13)	Tumor suppressor	Choroid plexus carcinoma, astrocytoma, medulloblastoma	Tumors in various organ systems
Multiple endocrine neoplasia type I	AD	*MEN1* (11q13)	Not well established	Meningioma, ependymoma, schwannoma	Pituitary tumors
NF-1	AD	*Neurofibromin* (17q11)	Dysregulation of tumor suppressor, Ras activity	Neurofibromas, peripheral nerve sheath tumors, optic gliomas, astrocytoma	Cognitive impairment, epilepsy
NF-2	AD	*Merlin* (22q12)	Dysregulation cell proliferation	Bilateral vestibular schwannomas, meningiomas, intramedullary spinal cord tumors	Optic nerve sheath meningiomas, retinal hamartomas, cataracts

Tuberous sclerosis complex	AD	TSC1 (9q34) TSC2 (16q13)	Dysregulation of mTOR pathway	Glioneuronal hamartomas, subependymal nodules, subependymal giant cell tumors	Neuropsychiatric disorders: ADHD, intellectual disability, autism spectrum, epileptic spasms, seizures
Turcot	AD	MLH1 (3p22), MSH2 (2p21), PMS2 (7p22), APC (5q21)	DNA mismatch repair dysregulation, proliferation, and differentiation	Glioblastoma, astrocytoma, ependymoma, pituitary adenomas, medulloblastoma	Colorectal neoplasms in conjunction with CNS malignancies
Von Hippel-Lindau syndrome	AD	VHL (3p25)	Dysregulation of hypoxia inducible factors HIF-1α and HIF-2α	Hemangioblastomas of cerebellum, spinal cord, brainstem, cauda equina, and supratentorial region	Retinal hemangioblastoma

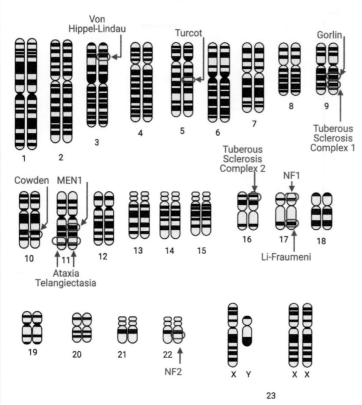

Fig. 1. CNS tumor syndrome.

headaches, vomiting, visual deficits, or seizures, or they may present with other nonspecific symptoms, such as loss of appetite, fatigue, depression, and epilepsy.[96,102,106] Treatment is aimed at the management of seizures and obstructive hydrocephalus, should it occur. Resection can be undertaken open or endoscopically; electrocorticography can be used as a surgical adjunct when intervention is aimed at seizure control. Recently, mTOR inhibitors, such as rapamycin, everolimus, and others, have largely replaced surgery as the primary treatment for SEGA.[107]

Finally, white matter abnormalities are relatively common in TSC and include superficial abnormalities associated with glioneuronal hamartomas, radial migration lines, and cystlike white matter lesions.[108–110] These abnormalities appear to be suggestive of lesions of demyelination, dysmyelination, hypomyelination, or lines of migration disorder.[111]

Diagnosis of TSC is either based on genetic testing or meeting multiple clinical criteria.[112] **Tables 2** and **3** provide the full criteria. Contrasted MRI scan remains the primary means of identifying TSC-associated cortical malformations.[9] In patients diagnosed with TSC, routine electroencephalographic monitoring is suggested, as well as

long-term surveillance by MRI scan. Seizure control remains one of the most difficult aspects of managing patients with TSC, and these children therefore require multidisciplinary management, including an epileptologist; vigabatrin has demonstrated effectiveness and is considered a first-line therapeutic, along with corticotropin as an alternative.[113]

SUMMARY

Although most tumors in the CNS occur sporadically, it is important to identify when a CNS malignancy is related to a genetic syndrome. This become critical for guiding screening modalities and timing, treatment options, and familial counseling. The pediatric neurosurgeon may serve as the first clinician involved in the care of CNS tumor, and so it is necessary that she or he be able to identify when a syndrome may be underlying the patient's disease. The authors reviewed the most common genetic tumor syndromes, including genetics, molecular mechanism, associated CNS tumors, and other neurologic manifestations. There are certainly other CNS tumor syndromes, including but not limited to, Rubinstein-Taybi syndrome, melanoma-astrocytoma syndrome, and

Carney complex. Importantly, the care of patients with CNS tumor syndromes must involve a multi-disciplinary approach (**Fig. 1**).

CLINICS CARE POINTS

- In a patient with a central nervous system malignancy, it is critical for the clinician to be aware of associated tumor syndromes to guide management and therapy.
- Neurofibromatosis-1 is the most common syndromic disorder of the central nervous system, and the pediatric neurosurgeon should be well versed in the diagnostic criteria.
- Management of the most common tumor associated with tuberous sclerosis complex, called subependymal giant cell astrocytoma, now primarily consists of mammalian target of rapamycin inhibition as first-line therapy.
- Tumor syndromes in the pediatric neurosurgery patient population are best approached with a multispecialty team, including, but not limited to, the neurosurgeon, neurologist, and/or epileptologist, geneticist, radiologist, pathologist, hematologist/oncologist, radiation oncologist, and the pediatrician.

DISCLOSURE

The authors have nothing to disclose.

REFERENCES

1. Ranger AM, Patel YK, Chaudhary N, et al. Familial syndromes associated with intracranial tumours: a review. Childs Nerv Syst 2014;30(1):47–64.
2. Stefanaki K, Alexiou GA, Stefanaki C, et al. Tumors of central and peripheral nervous system associated with inherited genetic syndromes. Pediatr Neurosurg 2012;48(5):271–85.
3. Ferner RE, Gutmann DH. Neurofibromatosis type 1 (NF1): diagnosis and management. Handbook Clin Neurol 2013;115:939–55.
4. Cimino PJ, Gutmann DH. Neurofibromatosis type 1. Handb Clin Neurol 2018;148:799–811.
5. Hastings B, Mortele K, Lee EY. Genetic syndromes affecting both children and adults: a practical guide to imaging-based diagnosis, management, and screening recommendations for general radiologists. Radiol Clin North Am 2020;58(3):619–38.
6. Farrell CJ, Plotkin SR. Genetic causes of brain tumors: neurofibromatosis, tuberous sclerosis, von Hippel-Lindau, and other syndromes. Neurol Clin 2007;25(4):925–46, viii.
7. Melean G, Sestini R, Ammannati F, et al. Genetic insights into familial tumors of the nervous system. Am J Med Genet C Semin Med Genet 2004; 129C(1):74–84.
8. Ly KI, Blakeley JO. The diagnosis and management of neurofibromatosis type 1. Med Clin 2019; 103(6):1035–54.
9. Vijapura C, Saad Aldin E, Capizzano AA, et al. Genetic syndromes associated with central nervous system tumors. Radiographics 2017;37(1):258–80.
10. Hirbe AC, Gutmann DH. Neurofibromatosis type 1: a multidisciplinary approach to care. Lancet Neurol 2014;13(8):834–43.
11. Anderson JL, Gutmann DH. Neurofibromatosis type 1. Handbook Clin Neurol 2015;132:75–86.
12. Dunn GP, Spiliopoulos K, Plotkin SR, et al. Role of resection of malignant peripheral nerve sheath tumors in patients with neurofibromatosis type 1. J Neurosurg 2013;118(1):142–8.
13. Campen CJ, Gutmann DH. Optic pathway gliomas in neurofibromatosis type 1. J Child Neurol 2018; 33(1):73–81.
14. Blakeley JO, Plotkin SR. Therapeutic advances for the tumors associated with neurofibromatosis type 1, type 2, and schwannomatosis. Neuro-oncology 2016;18(5):624–38.
15. Asthagiri AR, Parry DM, Butman JA, et al. Neurofibromatosis type 2. Lancet 2009;373(9679):1974–86.
16. Ruggieri M, Pratico AD, Serra A, et al. Childhood neurofibromatosis type 2 (NF2) and related disorders: from bench to bedside and biologically targeted therapies. Acta Otorhinolaryngol Ital 2016; 36(5):345–67.
17. Coy S, Rashid R, Stemmer-Rachamimov A, et al. Correction to: an update on the CNS manifestations of neurofibromatosis type 2. Acta Neuropathol 2020;139(4):667.
18. Dinarvand P, Davaro EP, Doan JV, et al. Familial adenomatous polyposis syndrome: an update and review of extraintestinal manifestations. Arch Pathol Lab Med 2019;143(11):1382–98.
19. Evans D. Neurofibromatosis type 2. Handbook Clin Neurol 2015;132:87–96.
20. Aboukais R, Bonne NX, Baroncini M, et al. Management of multiple tumors in neurofibromatosis type 2 patients. Neurochirurgie 2018;64(5):364–9.
21. Germano IM, Sheehan J, Parish J, et al. Congress of Neurological Surgeons systematic review and evidence-based guidelines on the role of radiosurgery and radiation therapy in the management of patients with vestibular schwannomas. Neurosurgery 2018;82(2):E49–51.
22. Nguyen T, Chung LK, Sheppard JP, et al. Surgery versus stereotactic radiosurgery for the treatment of multiple meningiomas in neurofibromatosis type 2: illustrative case and systematic review. Neurosurg Rev 2019;42(1):85–96.

23. Chung LK, Nguyen TP, Sheppard JP, et al. A systematic review of radiosurgery versus surgery for neurofibromatosis type 2 vestibular Schwannomas. World Neurosurg 2018;109:47–58.

24. Farschtschi S, Mautner VF, McLean ACL, et al. The neurofibromatoses. Dtsch Arztebl Int 2020;117(20): 354–60.

25. Evans DGR, Salvador H, Chang VY, et al. Cancer and central nervous system tumor surveillance in pediatric neurofibromatosis 2 and related disorders. Clin Cancer Res 2017;23(12):e54–61.

26. Hottinger AF, Khakoo Y. Update on the management of familial central nervous system tumor syndromes. Curr Neurol Neurosci Rep 2007;7(3):200.

27. Dhamija R, Hoxworth JM. Imaging of PTEN-related abnormalities in the central nervous system. Clin Imaging 2020;60(2):180–5.

28. Kim B, Tabori U, Hawkins C. An update on the CNS manifestations of brain tumor polyposis syndromes. Acta Neuropathol 2020;139(4):703–15.

29. Pilarski R, Burt R, Kohlman W, et al. Cowden syndrome and the PTEN hamartoma tumor syndrome: systematic review and revised diagnostic criteria. J Natl Cancer Inst 2013;105(21):1607–16.

30. Chen Y-S, Chong YB, Lin C-H, et al. Cowden syndrome diagnosed by Lhermitte–Duclos disease. Formos J Surg 2019;52(5):197.

31. Nowak D, Trost H. Lhermitte–Duclos disease (dysplastic cerebellar gangliocytoma): a malformation, hamartoma or neoplasm? Acta Neurol Scand 2002;105(3):137–45.

32. Galiatsatos P, Foulkes WD. Familial adenomatous polyposis. Am J Gastroenterol 2006;101(2): 385–98.

33. Hottinger AF, Khakoo Y. Neurooncology of familial cancer syndromes. J child Neurol 2009;24(12): 1526–35.

34. Gorovoy IR, de Alba Campomanes A. A potential life-saving diagnosis–recognizing Turcot syndrome. J AAPOS 2014;18(2):186–8.

35. Lusis EA, Travers S, Jost SC, et al. Glioblastomas with giant cell and sarcomatous features in patients with Turcot syndrome type 1: a clinicopathological study of 3 cases. Neurosurgery 2010;67(3):811–7 [discussion 817].

36. Orr BA, Clay MR, Pinto EM, et al. An update on the central nervous system manifestations of Li–Fraumeni syndrome. Acta Neuropathol 2020; 139(4):669–87.

37. Johansson G, Andersson U, Melin B. Recent developments in brain tumor predisposing syndromes. Acta Oncol 2016;55(4):401–11.

38. McBride KA, Ballinger ML, Killick E, et al. Li-Fraumeni syndrome: cancer risk assessment and clinical management. Nat Rev Clin Oncol 2014;11(5):260.

39. Thompson EM, Hielscher T, Bouffet E, et al. Prognostic value of medulloblastoma extent of resection after accounting for molecular subgroup: a retrospective integrated clinical and molecular analysis. Lancet Oncol 2016;17(4):484–95.

40. Okamoto N, Naruto T, Kohmoto T, et al. A novel PTCH1 mutation in a patient with Gorlin syndrome. Hum Genome Var 2014;1(1):1–3.

41. Onodera S, Nakamura Y, Azuma T. Gorlin syndrome: recent advances in genetic testing and molecular and cellular biological research. Int J Mol Sci 2020;21(20):7559.

42. Smith MJ, Beetz C, Williams SG, et al. Germline mutations in SUFU cause Gorlin syndrome-associated childhood medulloblastoma and redefine the risk associated with PTCH1 mutations. J Clin Oncol 2014;4155–61.

43. Amlashi SF, Riffaud L, Brassier G, et al. Nevoid basal cell carcinoma syndrome: relation with desmoplastic medulloblastoma in infancy: a population-based study and review of the literature. Cancer 2003;98(3):618–24.

44. Anupindi SA, Bedoya MA, Lindell RB, et al. Diagnostic performance of whole-body MRI as a tool for cancer screening in children with genetic cancer-predisposing conditions. Am J Roentgenol 2015;205(2):400–8.

45. Thalakoti S, Geller T. Basal cell nevus syndrome or Gorlin syndrome. Handbook Clin Neurol 2015;132: 119–28.

46. Lacombe D, Chateil J, Fontan D, et al. Medulloblastoma in the nevoid basal-cell carcinoma syndrome: case reports and review of the literature. Genet Couns 1990;1(3–4):273–7.

47. Evans DGR, Farndon P, Burnell L, et al. The incidence of Gorlin syndrome in 173 consecutive cases of medulloblastoma. Br J Cancer 1991; 64(5):959–61.

48. Moramarco A, Himmelblau E, Miraglia E, et al. Ocular manifestations in Gorlin-Goltz syndrome. Orphanet J rare Dis 2019;14(1):1–7.

49. Pandeshwar, P., K. Jayanthi, and D. Mahesh, Gorlin-Goltz syndrome. Case reports in dentistry, 2012. 2012;4.

50. Kimonis VE, Mehta SG, Digiovanna JJ, et al. Radiological features in 82 patients with nevoid basal cell carcinoma (NBCC or Gorlin) syndrome. Genet Med 2004;6(6):495–502.

51. Barankin B, Goldenberg G, Robinson JK. Nevoid basal cell carcinoma syndrome (Gorlin syndrome). UpToDate; 2021. Available at: https://www.uptodate.com/contents/nevoid-basal-cell-carcinoma-syndrome-gorlin-syndrome?search=nevoid-basal-cell-carcinomasyndrome&source=search_result&selectedTitle=1~41&usage_type=default&display_rank=1. Accessed February 11, 2021.

52. O'Malley S, Weitman D, Olding M, et al. Multiple neoplasms following craniospinal irradiation for medulloblastoma in a patient with nevoid basal

cell carcinoma syndrome: case report. J Neurosurg 1997;86(2):286–8.

53. Swift M, Reitnauer PJ, Morrell D, et al. Breast and other cancers in families with ataxia-telangiectasia. N Engl J Med 1987;316(21):1289–94.

54. Swift M, Morrell D, Cromartie E, et al. The incidence and gene frequency of ataxia-telangiectasia in the United States. Am J Hum Genet 1986;39(5):573.

55. Lavin MF. Ataxia-telangiectasia: from a rare disorder to a paradigm for cell signalling and cancer. Nat Rev Mol Cel Biol 2008;9(10):759–69.

56. Amirifar P, Ranjouri MR, Yazdani R, et al. Ataxia-telangiectasia: a review of clinical features and molecular pathology. Pediatr Allergy Immunol 2019; 30(3):277–88.

57. Cabana MD, Crawford TO, Winkelstein JA, et al. Consequences of the delayed diagnosis of ataxia-telangiectasia. Pediatrics 1998;102(1):98–100.

58. Rothblum-Oviatt C, Wright J, Lefton-Greif MA, et al. Ataxia telangiectasia: a review. Orphanet J rare Dis 2016;11(1):1–21.

59. Crawford TO. Ataxia telangiectasia. In: Seminars in Pediatric Neurology. Elsevier; 1998;5(4):287–94.

60. Olsen JH, Hahnemann JM, Børresen-Dale A-L, et al. Cancer in patients with ataxia-telangiectasia and in their relatives in the Nordic countries. J Natl Cancer Inst 2001;93(2):121–7.

61. Morrell D, Cromartie E, Swift M. Mortality and cancer incidence in 263 patients with ataxia-telangiectasia. J Natl Cancer Inst 1986;77(1):89–92.

62. Reiman A, Srinivasan V, Barone G, et al. Lymphoid tumours and breast cancer in ataxia telangiectasia; substantial protective effect of residual ATM kinase activity against childhood tumours. Br J Cancer 2011;105(4):586–91.

63. Estiar MA, Mehdipour P. ATM in breast and brain tumors: a comprehensive review. Cancer Biol Med 2018;15(3):210.

64. Mehdipour P, Habibi L, Mohammadi-Asl J, et al. Three-hit hypothesis in astrocytoma: tracing the polymorphism D1853N in ATM gene through a pedigree of the proband affected with primary brain tumor. J Cancer Res Clin Oncol 2008; 134(11):1173–80.

65. Mehdipour P, Mahdavi M, Mohammadi-Asl J, et al. Importance of ATM gene as a susceptible trait: predisposition role of D1853N polymorphism in breast cancer. Med Oncol 2011;28(3):733–7.

66. Carranza D, Torres-Rusillo S, Ceballos-Pérez G, et al. Reconstitution of the ataxia-telangiectasia cellular phenotype with lentiviral vectors. Front Immunol 2018;9:2703.

67. Al-Salameh A, Baudry C, Cohen R. Update on multiple endocrine neoplasia type 1 and 2. La Presse Médicale 2018;47(9):722–31.

68. Thakker RV, Newey PJ, Walls GV, et al. Clinical practice guidelines for multiple endocrine

neoplasia type 1 (MEN1). J Clin Endocrinol Metab 2012;97(9):2990–3011.

69. Kamilaris CD, Stratakis CA. Multiple endocrine neoplasia type 1 (MEN1): an update and the significance of early genetic and clinical diagnosis. Front Endocrinol 2019;10:339.

70. Asgharian B, Chen Y-J, Patronas NJ, et al. Meningiomas may be a component tumor of multiple endocrine neoplasia type 1. Clin Cancer Res 2004; 10(3):869–80.

71. Cuevas-Ocampo AK, Bollen AW, Goode B, et al. Genetic confirmation that ependymoma can arise as part of multiple endocrine neoplasia type 1 (MEN1) syndrome. Acta Neuropathol 2017;133(4): 661–3.

72. Almeida MQ, Stratakis CA. Solid tumors associated with multiple endocrine neoplasias. Cancer Genet Cytogenet 2010;203(1):30–6.

73. Syro LV, Scheithauer BW, Kovacs K, et al. Pituitary tumors in patients with MEN1 syndrome. Clinics 2012;67:43–8.

74. Marini F, Falchetti A, Del Monte F, et al. Multiple endocrine neoplasia type 1. Orphanet J rare Dis 2006;1(1):1–9.

75. Maher E, Yates J, Harries R, et al. Clinical features and natural history of von Hippel-Lindau disease. QJM 1990;77(2):1151–63.

76. Neumann HH, Wiestler O. Clustering of features and genetics of von Hippel-Lindau syndrome. Lancet 1991;338(8761):258.

77. Aronow ME, Wiley HE, Gaudric A, et al. von Hippel–Lindau disease: update on pathogenesis and systemic aspects. Retina 2019;39(12):2243–53.

78. Varshney N, Kebede AA, Owusu-Dapaah H, et al. A review of von Hippel-Lindau syndrome. J Kidney Cancer VHL 2017;4(3):20.

79. Latif F, Tory K, Gnarra J, et al. Identification of the von Hippel Lindau disease tumor suppressor gene. Science 1993;260(5112):1317–20.

80. Zbar B, Kishida T, Chen F, et al. Germline mutations in the von Hippel-Lindau disease (VHL) gene in families from North America, Europe, and Japan. Hum Mutat 1996;8(4):348–57.

81. Wind JJ, Lonser RR. Management of von Hippel–Lindau disease-associated CNS lesions. Expert Rev Neurother 2011;11(10):1433–41.

82. Noujaim DL, Therrien JA. 16 - Hemangioblastoma. In: Neuroradiology JE Small, et al, editors. Philadelphia: Elsevier; 2019. p. 153–7.

83. Chittiboina P, Lonser RR. von Hippel–Lindau disease. Handbook Clin Neurol 2015;132:139–56.

84. Wanebo JE, Lonser RR, Glenn GM, et al. The natural history of hemangioblastomas of the central nervous system in patients with von Hippel—Lindau disease. J Neurosurg 2003;98(1):82–94.

85. Conway JE, Chou D, Clatterbuck RE, et al. Hemangioblastomas of the central nervous system in von

Hippel-Lindau syndrome and sporadic disease. Neurosurgery 2001;48(1):55–63.

86. Binderup M, Bisgaard ML, Harbud V, et al. Von Hippel-Lindau disease (vHL). National clinical guideline for diagnosis and surveillance in Denmark. 3rd edition. Dan Med J 2013;60(12): B4763.

87. Curatolo P, Bombardieri R. Tuberous sclerosis. Handbook Clin Neurol 2007;87:129–51.

88. Randle SC. Tuberous sclerosis complex: a review. Pediatr Ann 2017;46(4):e166–71.

89. Tee AR, Manning BD, Roux PP, et al. Tuberous sclerosis complex gene products, Tuberin and Hamartin, control mTOR signaling by acting as a GTPase-activating protein complex toward Rheb. Curr Biol 2003;13(15):1259–68.

90. Au KS, Williams AT, Roach ES, et al. Genotype/ phenotype correlation in 325 individuals referred for a diagnosis of tuberous sclerosis complex in the United States. Genet Med 2007;9(2):88–100.

91. Verhoef S, Bakker L, Tempelaars AM, et al. High rate of mosaicism in tuberous sclerosis complex. Am J Hum Genet 1999;64(6):1632–7.

92. Smalley SL, Burger F, Smith M. Phenotypic variation of tuberous sclerosis in a single extended kindred. J Med Genet 1994;31(10):761–5.

93. Leung AK, Robson WLM. Tuberous sclerosis complex: a review. J Pediatr Health Care 2007;21(2): 108–14.

94. De Vries PJ, Whittemore VH, Leclezio L, et al. Tuberous sclerosis associated neuropsychiatric disorders (TAND) and the TAND checklist. Pediatr Neurol 2015;52(1):25–35.

95. Hsieh DT, Jennesson MM, Thiele EA. Epileptic spasms in tuberous sclerosis complex. Epilepsy Res 2013;106(1–2):200–10.

96. Webb DW, Fryer AE, Osborne JP. Morbidity associated with tuberous sclerosis: a population study. Dev Med Child Neurol 1996;38(2):146–55.

97. Roth J, Roach ES, Bartels U, et al. Subependymal giant cell astrocytoma: diagnosis, screening, and treatment. Recommendations from the International Tuberous Sclerosis Complex Consensus Conference 2012. Pediatr Neurol 2013;49(6): 439–44.

98. Yates JR, MacLean C, Higgins JNP, et al. The Tuberous Sclerosis 2000 study: presentation, initial assessments and implications for diagnosis and management. Arch Dis Child 2011;96(11):1020–5.

99. Hallett L, Foster T, Liu Z, et al. Burden of disease and unmet needs in tuberous sclerosis complex with neurological manifestations: systematic review. Curr Med Res Opin 2011;27(8):1571–83.

100. Józwiak S, Schwartz RA, Janniger CK, et al. Usefulness of diagnostic criteria of tuberous sclerosis complex in pediatric patients. J Child Neurol 2000;15(10):652–9.

101. Altman N, Purser R, Post MJ. Tuberous sclerosis: characteristics at CT and MR imaging. Radiology 1988;167(2):527–32.

102. Goh S, Butler W, Thiele EA. Subependymal giant cell tumors in tuberous sclerosis complex. Neurology 2004;63(8):1457–61.

103. Ess KC, Kamp CA, Tu BP, et al. Developmental origin of subependymal giant cell astrocytoma in tuberous sclerosis complex. Neurology 2005; 64(8):1446–9.

104. Michelozzi C, Di Leo G, Galli F, et al. Subependymal nodules and giant cell tumours in tuberous sclerosis complex patients: prevalence on MRI in relation to gene mutation. Child's Nervous Syst 2013;29(2):249–54.

105. O'Callaghan FJ, Martyn CN, Renowden S, et al. Subependymal nodules, giant cell astrocytomas and the tuberous sclerosis complex: a population-based study. Arch Dis Child 2008; 93(9):751–4.

106. Torres OA, Roach E, Delgado MR, et al. Early diagnosis of subependymal giant cell astrocytoma in patients with tuberous sclerosis. J Child Neurol 1998;13(4):173–7.

107. Ebrahimi-Fakhari D, Franz DN. Pharmacological treatment strategies for subependymal giant cell astrocytoma (SEGA). Expert Opin Pharmacother 2020;21(11):1329–36.

108. Griffiths P, Bolton P, Verity C. White matter abnormalities in tuberous sclerosis complex. Acta Radiologica 1998;39(5):482–6.

109. Van Tassel P, Curé JK, Holden KR. Cystlike white matter lesions in tuberous sclerosis. Am J Neuroradiol 1997;18(7):1367–73.

110. Von Ranke FM, Faria IM, Zanetti G, et al. Imaging of tuberous sclerosis complex: a pictorial review. Radiol Bras 2017;50(1):48–54.

111. Iwasaki S, Nakagawa H, Kichikawa K, et al. MR and CT of tuberous sclerosis: linear abnormalities in the cerebral white matter. Am J Neuroradiol 1990;11(5):1029–34.

112. Northrup H, Krueger DA, Roberds S, et al. Tuberous sclerosis complex diagnostic criteria update: recommendations of the 2012 International Tuberous Sclerosis Complex Consensus Conference. Pediatr Neurol 2013;49(4):243–54.

113. Krueger DA, Northrup H, Roberds S, et al. Tuberous sclerosis complex surveillance and management: recommendations of the 2012 International Tuberous Sclerosis Complex Consensus Conference. Pediatr Neurol 2013;49(4):255–65.

Syndromic Craniosynostosis
Unique Management Considerations

David S. Hersh, MD[a,b,*], Christopher D. Hughes, MD MPH[b,c]

KEYWORDS

- Craniosynostosis • Syndromic • Apert • Crouzon • Muenke • Pfeiffer • Saethre–Chotzen

KEY POINTS

- Syndromic craniosynostosis is characterized by the premature closure of multiple cranial sutures, as well as congenital anomalies of the facial skeleton, limbs, and/or cardiac system.
- Management by a multidisciplinary "craniofacial team" is necessary to coordinate the care of this complex patient population.
- Team members may include neurosurgery, plastic surgery, ophthalmology, otolaryngology, audiology, speech language pathology, oral/maxillofacial surgery, orthodontics, dentistry, nutrition, psychology, neurodevelopmental pediatrics, social work, and a coordinator.
- Intracranial hypertension is common among patients with syndromic craniosynostosis, and may result from craniocerebral disproportion, obstructive sleep apnea, venous outflow obstruction, and/or hydrocephalus.
- Surgical options include fronto-orbital advancement with cranial vault remodeling, posterior vault expansion, endoscopic-assisted suturectomy with postoperative orthotic therapy, and midface advancement. Surgical intervention and its timing should be considered carefully for each individual patient.

INTRODUCTION

Craniosynostosis refers to the premature fusion of one or more of the cranial sutures. In patients with craniosynostosis, calvarial growth is restricted in the direction that is perpendicular to the affected suture, and compensatory growth occurs parallel to the suture, resulting in abnormal skull development. Craniosynostosis occurs in approximately 1 per 2500 births, and most commonly presents as isolated, single-suture craniosynostosis.[1–3] Approximately 10% to 20% of patients present with syndromic craniosynostosis, which is typically characterized by multisuture involvement and additional congenital anomalies.[4]

COMMON CRANIOSYNOSTOSIS SYNDROMES

Technological advances have facilitated the molecular characterization of more than 180 syndromes associated with craniosynostosis.[5] The 5 most common syndromes associated with craniosynostosis include Crouzon syndrome, Apert syndrome, Pfeiffer syndrome, Muenke syndrome, and Saethre–Chotzen syndrome. The genetic and clinical features associated with each of these syndromes are summarized in **Table 1**. Genetic mutations involving members of the transmembrane fibroblast growth factor receptor (FGFR) family have been implicated in a number of syndromes, which may be inherited in an autosomal

a Division of Neurosurgery, Connecticut Children's, 282 Washington Street, Hartford, CT 06106, USA;
b Department of Surgery, UConn School of Medicine, 200 Academic Way, Farmington, CT 06032, USA;
c Divisions of Plastic Surgery and Craniofacial Surgery, Connecticut Children's, 282 Washington Street, Hartford, CT 06106, USA
* Corresponding author.
E-mail address: dhersh@connecticutchildrens.org

Neurosurg Clin N Am 33 (2022) 105–112
https://doi.org/10.1016/j.nec.2021.09.008

Table 1
Features of most common craniosynostosis syndromes

Syndrome	Gene	Phenotype	Associated Findings
Apert	FGFR2	Turribrachycephaly, ocular proptosis, downslanting palpebral fissures, midfacial retrusion, high palatal arch, occasional cleft palate	Variable syndactyly of hands and feet
Crouzon	FGFR2	Brachycephaly, midfacial retrusion, ocular proptosis, high palatal arch	
Pfeiffer	FGFR2	Type I: turribrachycephaly, ocular proptosis, downslanting palpebral fissures, midfacial retrusion	Broad thumbs and toes
	FGFR1	Type II: Kleeblattschädel (cloverleaf skull)	Intracranial anomalies, hydrocephalus
		Type III: Severe proptosis, shortened anterior cranial base	
Muenke	FGFR3	Coronal craniosynostosis	Hearing loss
Saethre Chotzen	TWIST1	Low frontal hairline, biparietal foraminae	Hearing loss, variable syndactyly, ear anomalies

dominant fashion but which most often arise sporadically owing to de novo mutations.[1,6,7] Epigenetic phenomena are known to play a critical role as well, and cases are often characterized by variable expressivity.

MULTIDISCIPLINARY MANAGEMENT

The involvement of structures beyond the cranium itself is a hallmark feature of syndromic craniosynostosis, and abnormal development of the facial skeleton, limbs, and/or cardiac system is often present. As a result, management by a multidisciplinary "craniofacial team" has become the core model for the coordination of care in this complex patient population. Key members of the craniofacial team are listed in **Box 1**. Unique aspects of the management of patients with syndromic craniosynostosis are addressed by the following specialists.

Ophthalmology

Proptosis and exophthalmos are often present in patients with syndromic craniosynostosis owing to orbital and midface hypoplasia. This condition can result in exposure of the sclera, dryness, and corneal injury unless intervention is performed. Temporary tarsorraphies may be required, and careful attention to the eyes is needed to prevent long-term damage. One of the goals of a frontoorbital advancement (and later, a midface advancement) is to protect the globes.[1]

Otolaryngology, Audiology, and Speech Language Pathology

Hearing loss occurs frequently in patients with syndromic craniosynostosis. Pure sensorineural hearing loss occurs in Muenke syndrome owing to abnormal development of the organ of Corti, whereas in Crouzon, Apert, and Pfeiffer syndrome conductive hearing loss predominates owing to otitis media with effusions as well as abnormal middle ear anatomy. A thorough evaluation by otolaryngology and audiology is therefore mandated, and when hearing loss is identified, management ranges from sound field amplification and preferential seating in school to tympanostomy tube insertion to hearing aids or cochlear implants.[8]

Airway obstruction is also a common feature of patients with syndromic craniosynostosis. Midface hypoplasia may constrict the upper airway, and

Box 1
Members of the craniofacial team

- Neurosurgery
- Plastic surgery
- Ophthalmology
- Otolaryngology
- Audiology
- Speech language pathology
- Oral/maxillofacial surgery
- Orthodontics
- Dentistry
- Nutrition
- Psychology
- Neurodevelopmental pediatrics
- Social work
- Coordinator

primary airway pathologies such as laryngomalacia, tracheomalacia, and tracheal–cartilaginous sleeves contribute to obstruction and sleep-disordered breathing.[1,9] A number of treatment approaches have been described and include adenotonsillectomy, nasopharyngeal airways, continuous positive airway pressure therapy, tracheostomy, and midface advancement.[1]

Oral and Maxillofacial Surgery, Orthodontics, Dentistry, and Nutrition

Midface hypoplasia is one of the core features of many craniosynostosis syndromes and can result in significantly abnormal dentofacial anatomy. Midface advancement can be performed early in life in cases of severe airway compromise, but this is often delayed until after 5 to 7 years of age. Particularly as skeletal maturity is reached, oral/maxillofacial surgeons, orthodontists, and dentists become integral parts of the team, because orthognathic surgery is often needed to correct any residual dentofacial deformities.[1,10] Owing to the potential impact of these deformities on oral intake, involvement by a nutritionist is recommended as well.

Psychology and Neurodevelopmental Pediatrics

The association between nonsyndromic, single-suture craniosynostosis and developmental delay remains highly controversial. Some craniosynostosis syndromes, however, are known to have a higher incidence of intellectual disability. Screening by a neuropsychologist and/or developmental pediatrician is therefore typically recommended at 1 to 2 years of age and again when entering elementary school, so that early intervention can be instituted and modified learning plans can be formulated when appropriate.[7,11] Regardless of the patient's neurodevelopmental status, the craniofacial phenotype associated with many forms of syndromic craniosynostosis can result in social stigma, and counseling by a psychologist can be helpful.

INTRACRANIAL HYPERTENSION

Although a minority of patients with nonsyndromic, single-suture craniosynostosis may develop elevated intracranial pressure, the incidence of intracranial hypertension is significantly higher among patients with syndromic craniosynostosis, particularly those with Crouzon syndrome (61%) and Apert syndrome (45%–83%).[4,12–15] A number of potential etiologies have been implicated in the pathogenesis of intracranial hypertension in this unique patient population, including craniocerebral disproportion, obstructive sleep apnea, venous outflow obstruction, and hydrocephalus.[4]

Craniocerebral Disproportion

Early theories attributed intracranial hypertension in syndromic craniosynostosis patients to craniocerebral disproportion. Brain growth within a rigid cranium with inadequate volume (owing to premature closure of multiple sutures) can result in elevated intracranial pressure.[16,17] Surgical intervention was, therefore, designed to increase the intracranial volume through various forms of cranial vault expansion techniques. Although other factors are now known to contribute to the development of intracranial hypertension, cranial vault expansion may still be effective in decreasing the intracranial pressure through indirect mechanisms.

Obstructive Sleep Apnea

Obstructive sleep apnea during REM sleep results in hypercapnia, which in turn stimulates vasodilation and increased cerebral perfusion. The increase in cerebral blood flow ultimately produces an increased intracranial pressure.[4,18–20] Moderate to severe obstructive sleep apnea has been associated with a significantly increased risk of intracranial hypertension among patients with syndromic craniosynostosis.[4]

Venous Outflow Obstruction

Syndromic craniosynostosis is associated not only with dysmorphism of the calvarial vault, but also skull base changes that can result in narrowing of the venous sinuses. Similar to patients with achondroplasia, venous sinus narrowing may produce venous hypertension, which can impact cerebrospinal fluid absorption and contribute to hydrocephalus and/or intracranial hypertension.[21–25]

Hydrocephalus

Ventriculomegaly, which is present in up to 40% of patients with syndromic craniosynostosis, may contribute to intracranial hypertension as well. Communicating hydrocephalus may result from venous sinus stenosis and subsequent venous hypertension, although obstructive hydrocephalus may occur in the setting of aqueductal stenosis or a fourth ventricular outlet obstruction. Close monitoring is necessary to differentiate static ventriculomegaly from progressive hydrocephalus, for whom ventriculoperitoneal shunting should be considered.[26]

SURGICAL MANAGEMENT

A number of surgical techniques have been developed to address the craniofacial dysmorphism associated with syndromic craniosynostosis. These techniques can be categorized into several core strategies: fronto-orbital advancement with cranial vault remodeling, posterior vault expansion, endoscopic-assisted suturectomy with postoperative orthotic therapy, and midface advancement.

Fronto-orbital Advancement and Cranial Vault Remodeling

The traditional approach to the treatment of patients with syndromic craniosynostosis has been an open procedure to achieve anterior skull expansion with a fronto-orbital advancement. Many syndromic patients with craniosynostosis exhibit significant frontal and orbital retrusion, forehead dysmorphology, and turricephaly, prompting the need for fronto-orbital advancement and cranial vault remodeling. The procedure is designed to normalize the forehead shape, provide globe protection by advancing the orbital bandeau, and increase the intracranial volume.

The frontal bone comprising the forehead is often removed and recontoured as 1 bone flap, while the orbital bandeau is removed separately. The bandeau typically measures between 10 to 15 mm in height above the orbital rims, and extends in a mortise and tenon fashion from the lateral temporal fossa, through the sphenoid wing, through the lateral orbital wall near the fronto-zygomatic suture, across the superior orbit, into the medial orbit, and across the region of the nasofrontal suture. The frontal bone and orbital bandeau are reshaped and customized to form a neocranio-orbital construct that is then repositioned and secured using a combination of sutures and resorbable plates and screws.

The ultimate degree of advancement that is required can be estimated from the baseline level of orbital retrusion by measuring the distance from the orbitale superioris to the anterior projection of the cornea.[27] Practically, the advancement may be limited by the ability to close the scalp over the expanded cranium after remodeling. Periosteal or galeal scoring can be used to facilitate a tension-free closure. Some surgeons advocate modifications to the fronto-orbital advancement; for example, some investigators suggest abandoning the orbital bandeau in favor of a 1-piece reconstruction.[28] Individual patient morphology dictates the nuances of each procedure, but the fronto-orbital advancement and its modifications represent the traditional approach to intracranial

expansion for patients with syndromic craniosynostosis.

Centers vary with respect to the age at which fronto-orbital advancement is typically undertaken; some data suggest that delaying the operation until an older age minimizes retrusion and the need for reoperation.[3] When increased intracranial pressure is suspected, however, early intervention becomes necessary. To decrease the risk of developing intracranial hypertension, many centers advocate an initial, early posterior vault distraction to prophylactically increase the intracranial volume, often followed by a fronto-orbital advancement later in life.

Posterior Vault Expansion via Distraction Osteogenesis

Since its first description in 2009, posterior vault distraction osteogenesis has become the initial treatment of choice for syndromic craniosynostosis in many centers.[29] Citing evidence of greater intracranial volume gains per unit of sagittal advancement,[30] proponents of posterior vault distraction osteogenesis highlight the procedure's ability to more efficiently address intracranial hypertension in patients with syndromic craniosynostosis.[31,32] In addition to improved intracranial volume expansion, posterior vault distraction osteogenesis tends to be a comparatively less morbid procedure compared with a fronto-orbital advancement, with less time in the operating room, less blood loss, and a shorter hospital stay.

The procedure involves a posterior incision in the coronal plane. Dissection typically proceeds in the subgaleal plane until the nuchal region, where a subperiosteal plane is entered for an additional few centimeters. Craniotomies are made in the biparietal and occipital regions, and vertically oriented barrel staves are made in the occipital region to allow for a more gradual posterior contour as the distraction progresses. Internal distractors are placed in a parallel fashion to create a straight posterior or a slight posteroinferior distraction vector.

As with all distraction procedures, posterior vault distraction osteogenesis does require an additional procedure for hardware removal after the consolidation phase of distraction. Proponents of posterior vault distraction osteogenesis as an initial operation for patients with syndromic craniosynostosis, however, suggest that the early volume expansion provided by the procedure provides significant patient benefit. Subsequent fronto-orbital advancement can even be avoided in some patients after successful posterior vault distraction osteogenesis[33]; in others, a fronto-orbital advancement may still be required, but can be performed in a delayed fashion.

Endoscopic-Assisted Suturectomy with Adjuvant Helmeting

Endoscopic-assisted suturectomy with adjuvant orthotic therapy has arisen as an alternative to both fronto-orbital advancement and posterior vault distraction osteogenesis as an initial treatment for some patients. Advocates of this approach favor the procedure's shorter operative time and favorable morbidity profile. The procedure is typically undertaken early in life, ideally before 4 months of age. In the most common form of multisutural craniosynostosis—bilateral coronal craniosynostosis—small bilateral incisions are made overlying the fused sutures. Burr holes are created and enlarged, and a roughly 1 cm wide craniectomy is performed along the fused suture and carried down to the inferior aspect of the squamosal temporal bone. Patients are typically fitted for a helmet 1 week postoperatively and are instructed to wear it 23 hours per day. The duration of helmet use varies; some centers discontinue the orthosis once the head shape has normalized, whereas others continue its use until the patient reaches 1 year of age.

One series from Boston demonstrated significant improvements in head shape, head circumference, and the cephalic index after an endoscopic-assisted suturectomy with helmeting, even among a subset analysis of syndromic patients.[34] The authors found that close to 50% of syndromic patients ultimately required a subsequent fronto-orbital advancement, and long-term follow-up data for syndromic patients are forthcoming. A subsequent series of 6 patients from Johns Hopkins also demonstrated that, although some patients will require a subsequent fronto-orbital advancement, an early endoscopic suturectomy may delay the need for an open procedure.[35] Notably, endoscopic surgery seems to have been sufficient for patients who were less than 2 months of age at the time of the index procedure, and those patients were classified as Whitaker category I at their most recent follow-up. Head-to-head comparisons of volume expansion and head shape normalization between endoscopic-assisted suturectomy with helmeting and posterior vault distraction osteogenesis have not yet been performed; although both procedures have been advocated as early options with the potential to delay or even avoid a fronto-orbital advancement, future analyses will be needed to determine which procedure produces optimal results.

Midface Treatment: Le Fort III and Monobloc Advancement

Patients with syndromic craniosynostosis often exhibit characteristic midface deformities, which can be severely functionally limiting. In particular, midfacial hypoplasia and sagittal maxillary deficiency can narrow the diameter of the pharyngeal airway and can lead to life threatening obstructive sleep apnea. All patients with syndromic craniosynostosis should be regularly evaluated by an ENT specialist and undergo polysomnography. Severe sleep apnea with elevated apnea–hypopnea indices may indicate the need for midface advancement sooner rather than later in a subset of patients.

In general, delaying midfacial operations until the patient has reached a more advanced skeletal age (between 7 and 12 years of age) is preferable to limit the impact on subsequent skeletal growth and minimize the odds of needing a revision. There are several choices when considering the surgical correction of midfacial hypoplasia in this patient population, and each patient will have a unique set of considerations. The spectrum of deformities, including intracranial volume, brow position and degree of globe protection, exorbitism, degree of midfacial hypoplasia, and the presence of an open bite, should be considered on a case-by-case basis to select the appropriate approach for the midface.

The subcranial Le Fort III osteotomy is designed to advance the midface (maxilla, nasal bones, and central zygoma) as a single unit. It has a long history and is generally well-tolerated with a lower morbidity profile compared with other techniques. Many centers advocate for the Le Fort III osteotomy with halo distraction, in contrast with the traditional Le Fort III osteotomy, to achieve greater degrees of advancement, greater soft tissue accommodation, and more control over the vector of midfacial movement.[36] Patients with adequate globe protection and minimal occlusal anomalies are likely best served through either of the Le Fort III osteotomy techniques, depending on the degree of desired advancement.

Some investigators have challenged the notion of an en bloc midfacial advancement for certain patients with syndromic craniosynostosis. In patients with Apert syndrome, the characteristic maxillary hypoplasia may not be uniformly distributed throughout the midface. Therefore, the central midface and the lateral orbitozygomatic complex may require separate and different vectors of advancement and expansion. In such patients, a Le Fort II osteotomy with zygomatic repositioning has been advocated by some, and this has been demonstrated to achieve "normalized" facial ratios compared with Le Fort III osteotomy alone.[37]

When the patient's residual deformity comprises both the midface and the orbital bandeau, however, midface advancement alone, whether with a Le Fort III osteotomy or a Le Fort II osteotomy with zygomatic repositioning, fails to address the full spectrum of the functional and phenotypic challenges. In cases where both the bandeau and the midface need to be corrected, surgical options typically include a revision fronto-orbital advancement followed by a subcranial Le Fort III osteotomy, or a monobloc advancement (with or without facial bipartition).

Monobloc advancement attempts to address the frontofacial disproportion by advancing and normalizing both components in a single unit, or bloc. This goal may be achieved with or without distraction. Monobloc advancement tends to be associated with a greater risk of surgical morbidity, and in particular cerebrospinal fluid leak. However, many centers have a robust experience with monobloc advancement and they have demonstrated beneficial functional outcomes with respect to vision and breathing with acceptable complication profiles.[38,39] Proponents cite the ability to address both frontal retrusion and midfacial hypoplasia in 1 step; those who favor a subcranial Le Fort III osteotomy approach cite evidence of the increased morbidity associated with a monobloc advancement.[40] Ultimately, the patients and their unique considerations should dictate the surgical approach.

FUTURE DIRECTIONS

The use of virtual surgical planning has been established in adult craniofacial surgery for some time, especially in oncologic, orthognathic, and complex craniomaxillofacial reconstruction. The adoption of virtual surgical planning within the pediatric craniofacial community has been more recent and uneven. Several centers have documented benefits in specific clinical situations, including orthognathic operations and customized reconstruction of secondary craniofacial defects with alloplastic implants.[41] The use of virtual surgical planning for craniosynostosis, however, has seen a slower universal adoption, with mixed data regarding clinical benefits and cost effectiveness.[42,43] Future developments and improvements in virtual surgical planning design and implementation may result in increased applicability within craniosynostosis surgery.

In addition, our understanding of syndromic craniosynostosis has evolved rapidly in recent years.

Molecular and genomic advances have facilitated the classification of craniosynostosis syndromes based on the underlying genotype, rather than the currently used eponymous nomenclature.[15,44,45] Genomic subtyping may allow for better prognostication and guide individualized treatment in the future.

A better understanding of the underlying molecular pathways that are involved in craniosynostosis may also ultimately yield molecular targets that can be pharmacologically inhibited. Murine models of syndromic craniosynostosis have been used to analyze a variety of pharmaceutical agents, including a soluble form of *FGFR2* with the Ser252Trp mutation, a small hairpin RNA targeting the dominant mutant form of *FGFR2*, and inhibitors of the mitogen-activated protein kinase 1 and 2 (MEK1/2)/ERK pathway.[6,46–50] Unfortunately, given the usual onset of craniosynostosis as a prenatal event and the challenges of in utero diagnosis and treatment, pharmaceutical strategies such as these currently remain confined to the laboratory.[51]

SUMMARY

Craniosynostosis involves the premature fusion of 1 or more cranial sutures, and most commonly presents as an isolated, nonsyndromic diagnosis. However, a subset of patients have syndromic craniosynostosis, which typically involves multiple sutures and extracranial structures such as the facial skeleton, limbs, and/or cardiac system. A number of unique considerations must be taken into account when managing patients with syndromic craniosynostosis. A multidisciplinary craniofacial team with a central coordinator is particularly useful for the coordination of care among various specialists, and close monitoring is mandatory owing to the increased risk of intracranial hypertension. Surgical management varies widely among centers, but core options include fronto-orbital advancement with cranial vault remodeling, posterior vault expansion, endoscopic-assisted suturectomy with postoperative orthotic therapy, and midface advancement. Surgical intervention and its timing should be considered carefully for each individual patient.

CLINICS CARE POINTS

- Patients with suspected syndromic craniosynostosis should be referred to a multidisciplinary craniofacial team for further evaluation.

- Maintain a high index of suspicion for intracranial hypertension.
- A variety of surgical approaches are available; tailor surgical interventions to individual patients.

DISCLOSURE

The authors have nothing to disclose.

REFERENCES

1. Buchanan EP, Xue Y, Xue AS, et al. Multidisciplinary care of craniosynostosis. J Multidiscip Healthc 2017; 10:263–70.
2. French LR, Jackson IT, Melton LJ 3rd. A population-based study of craniosynostosis. J Clin Epidemiol 1990;43(1):69–73.
3. Fearon JA. Evidence-based medicine: craniosynostosis. Plast Reconstr Surg 2014;133(5):1261–75.
4. Spruijt B, Joosten KFM, Driessen C, et al. Algorithm for the management of intracranial hypertension in children with syndromic craniosynostosis. Plast Reconstr Surg 2015;136(2):331–40.
5. Sawh-Martinez R, Steinbacher DM. Syndromic craniosynostosis. Clin Plast Surg 2019;46(2):141–55.
6. Azoury SC, Reddy S, Shukla V, et al. Fibroblast growth factor receptor 2 (FGFR2) mutation related syndromic craniosynostosis. Int J Biol Sci 2017; 13(12):1479–88.
7. Taylor JA, Bartlett SP. What's new in syndromic craniosynostosis surgery? Plast Reconstr Surg 2017; 140(1):82e–93e.
8. Agochukwu NB, Solomon BD, Muenke M. Hearing loss in syndromic craniosynostoses: otologic manifestations and clinical findings. Int J Pediatr Otorhinolaryngol 2014;78(12):2037–47.
9. Nash R, Possamai V, Manjaly J, et al. The management of obstructive sleep apnea in syndromic craniosynostosis. J Craniofac Surg 2015;26(6):1914–6.
10. Azoulay-Avinoam S, Bruun R, MacLaine J, et al. An overview of craniosynostosis craniofacial syndromes for combined orthodontic and surgical management. Oral Maxillofac Surg Clin North Am 2020; 32(2):233–47.
11. Mathijssen IM. Guideline for care of patients with the diagnoses of craniosynostosis: working group on craniosynostosis. J Craniofac Surg 2015;26(6): 1735–807.
12. Abu-Sittah GS, Jeelani O, Dunaway D, et al. Raised intracranial pressure in Crouzon syndrome: incidence, causes, and management. J Neurosurg Pediatr 2016;17(4):469–75.
13. Marucci DD, Dunaway DJ, Jones BM, et al. Raised intracranial pressure in Apert syndrome. Plast Reconstr Surg 2008;122(4):1162–8.
14. Taylor WJ, Hayward RD, Lasjaunias P, et al. Enigma of raised intracranial pressure in patients with complex craniosynostosis: the role of abnormal intracranial venous drainage. J Neurosurg 2001;94(3):377–85.
15. O'Hara J, Ruggiero F, Wilson L, et al. Syndromic craniosynostosis: complexities of clinical care. Mol Syndromol 2019;10(1–2):83–97.
16. Renier D, Sainte-Rose C, Marchac D, et al. Intracranial pressure in craniostenosis. J Neurosurg 1982; 57(3):370–7.
17. Gault DT, Renier D, Marchac D, et al. Intracranial pressure and intracranial volume in children with craniosynostosis. Plast Reconstr Surg 1992;90(3): 377–81.
18. Gonsalez S, Hayward R, Jones B, et al. Upper airway obstruction and raised intracranial pressure in children with craniosynostosis. Eur Respir J 1997;10(2):367–75.
19. Hayward R, Gonsalez S. How low can you go? Intracranial pressure, cerebral perfusion pressure, and respiratory obstruction in children with complex craniosynostosis. J Neurosurg 2005;102(1 Suppl): 16–22.
20. Driessen C, Joosten KF, Bannink N, et al. How does obstructive sleep apnoea evolve in syndromic craniosynostosis? A prospective cohort study. Arch Dis Child 2013;98(7):538–43.
21. Hayward R. Venous hypertension and craniosynostosis. Childs Nerv Syst 2005;21(10):880–8.
22. Ghali GZ, Zaki Ghali MG, Ghali EZ, et al. Intracranial venous hypertension in craniosynostosis: mechanistic underpinnings and therapeutic implications. World Neurosurg 2019;127:549–58.
23. Sainte-Rose C, LaCombe J, Pierre-Kahn A, et al. Intracranial venous sinus hypertension: cause or consequence of hydrocephalus in infants? J Neurosurg 1984;60(4):727–36.
24. de Goederen R, Cuperus IE, Tasker RC, et al. Dural sinus volume in children with syndromic craniosynostosis and intracranial hypertension. J Neurosurg Pediatr 2020;1–8.
25. Florisson JM, Barmpalios G, Lequin M, et al. Venous hypertension in syndromic and complex craniosynostosis: the abnormal anatomy of the jugular foramen and collaterals. J Craniomaxillofac Surg 2015; 43(3):312–8.
26. Collmann H, Sorensen N, Krauss J. Hydrocephalus in craniosynostosis: a review. Childs Nerv Syst 2005;21(10):902–12.
27. Mulliken JB, Godwin SL, Pracharktam N, et al. The concept of the sagittal orbital-globe relationship in craniofacial surgery. Plast Reconstr Surg 1996; 97(4):700–6.
28. Fearon JA, Ditthakasem K, Garcia JC, et al. Abandoning the supraorbital bandeau in anterior craniosynostosis repairs, for a single-segment reconstruction. Plast Reconstr Surg 2018;142(3):334e–41e.

29. White N, Evans M, Dover MS, et al. Posterior calvarial vault expansion using distraction osteogenesis. Childs Nerv Syst 2009;25(2):231–6.

30. Choi M, Flores RL, Havlik RJ. Volumetric analysis of anterior versus posterior cranial vault expansion in patients with syndromic craniosynostosis. J Craniofac Surg 2012;23(2):455–8.

31. Derderian CA, Wink JD, McGrath JL, et al. Volumetric changes in cranial vault expansion: comparison of fronto-orbital advancement and posterior cranial vault distraction osteogenesis. Plast Reconstr Surg 2015;135(6):1665–72.

32. Steinbacher DM, Skirpan J, Puchala J, et al. Expansion of the posterior cranial vault using distraction osteogenesis. Plast Reconstr Surg 2011;127(2):792–801.

33. Swanson JW, Samra F, Bauder A, et al. An algorithm for managing syndromic craniosynostosis using posterior vault distraction osteogenesis. Plast Reconstr Surg 2016;137(5):829e–41e.

34. Rottgers SA, Lohani S, Proctor MR. Outcomes of endoscopic suturectomy with postoperative helmet therapy in bilateral coronal craniosynostosis. J Neurosurg Pediatr 2016;18(3):281–6.

35. Hersh DS, Hoover-Fong JE, Beck N, et al. Endoscopic surgery for patients with syndromic craniosynostosis and the requirement for additional open surgery. J Neurosurg Pediatr 2017;20(1):91–8.

36. Fearon JA. Halo distraction of the Le Fort III in syndromic craniosynostosis: a long-term assessment. Plast Reconstr Surg 2005;115(6):1524–36.

37. Hopper RA, Kapadia H, Morton T. Normalizing facial ratios in Apert syndrome patients with Le Fort II midface distraction and simultaneous zygomatic repositioning. Plast Reconstr Surg 2013;132(1):129–40.

38. Khonsari RH, Haber S, Paternoster G, et al. The influence of fronto-facial monobloc advancement on obstructive sleep apnea: an assessment of 109 syndromic craniosynostoses cases. J Craniomaxillofac Surg 2020;48(6):536–47.

39. Raposo-Amaral CE, Denadai R, Zanco GL, et al. Long-term follow-up on bone stability and complication rate after monobloc advancement in syndromic craniosynostosis. Plast Reconstr Surg 2020;145(4):1025–34.

40. Zhang RS, Lin LO, Hoppe IC, et al. Retrospective review of the complication profile associated with 71 subcranial and transcranial midface distraction procedures at a single institution. Plast Reconstr Surg 2019;143(2):521–30.

41. Kalmar CL, Xu W, Zimmerman CE, et al. Trends in utilization of virtual surgical planning in pediatric craniofacial surgery. J Craniofac Surg 2020;31(7):1900–5.

42. Shah A, Patel A, Steinbacher DM. Simulated frontoorbital advancement and intraoperative templates enhance reproducibility in craniosynostosis. Plast Reconstr Surg 2012;129(6):1011e–2e.

43. Cho RS, Lopez J, Musavi L, et al. Computer-assisted design and manufacturing assists less experienced surgeons in achieving equivalent outcomes in cranial vault reconstruction. J Craniofac Surg 2019;30(7):2034–8.

44. Forrest CR, Hopper RA. Craniofacial syndromes and surgery. Plast Reconstr Surg 2013;131(1):86e–109e.

45. Agochukwu NB, Solomon BD, Muenke M. Impact of genetics on the diagnosis and clinical management of syndromic craniosynostoses. Childs Nerv Syst 2012;28(9):1447–63.

46. Tanimoto Y, Yokozeki M, Hiura K, et al. A soluble form of fibroblast growth factor receptor 2 (FGFR2) with S252W mutation acts as an efficient inhibitor for the enhanced osteoblastic differentiation caused by FGFR2 activation in Apert syndrome. J Biol Chem 2004;279(44):45926–34.

47. Morita J, Nakamura M, Kobayashi Y, et al. Soluble form of FGFR2 with S252W partially prevents craniosynostosis of the apert mouse model. Dev Dyn 2014;243(4):560–7.

48. Eswarakumar VP, Ozcan F, Lew ED, et al. Attenuation of signaling pathways stimulated by pathologically activated FGF-receptor 2 mutants prevents craniosynostosis. Proc Natl Acad Sci U S A 2006;103(49):18603–8.

49. Shukla V, Coumoul X, Wang RH, et al. RNA interference and inhibition of MEK-ERK signaling prevent abnormal skeletal phenotypes in a mouse model of craniosynostosis. Nat Genet 2007;39(9):1145–50.

50. Shukla V, Coumoul X, Deng CX. RNAi-based conditional gene knockdown in mice using a U6 promoter driven vector. Int J Biol Sci 2007;3(2):91–9.

51. Rachwalski M, Khonsari RH, Paternoster G. Current approaches in the development of molecular and pharmacological therapies in craniosynostosis utilizing animal models. Mol Syndromol 2019;10(1–2):115–23.

Epilepsy Syndromes: Current Classifications and Future Directions

Laura C. Swanson, MD, PhD[a], Raheel Ahmed, MD, PhD[b],*

KEYWORDS

- Epilepsy syndromes • Structural epilepsy • Epilepsy surgery • Precision medicine

KEY POINTS

- Summary of the current ILAE classifications of epilepsy syndromes
- Describe common structural etiologies of epilepsy and surgical interventions
- Discuss technological advancements and future directions for the classification and treatment of epilepsy syndromes

INTRODUCTION

Epilepsy is one of the most common neurologic diseases with an estimated lifetime prevalence of 7.6 per 1000 people.[1] It is a heterogeneous disorder with significant variability in etiology, clinical presentation, treatment, and prognosis across the human lifespan. Individual epilepsies were, therefore, initially categorized in syndromes, with shared clinicopathological features, to facilitate a uniform approach for diagnosis and treatment.[2,3] However, ongoing diagnostic advancements and delineation of epilepsy subtypes challenge the concept and utility of syndromic classifications in clinical practice.[4] Classification of epilepsy syndromes is, therefore, expected to evolve from shared clinical features toward the molecular underpinnings of the disease process that may facilitate tailored therapeutic approaches.[5–7]

Although the most recent report from the International League Against Epilepsy (ILAE) in 2017 classifies seizure types based on initial clinical manifestation (focal, generalized, mixed, and unknown), this review will discuss major pediatric epilepsy syndromes categorized by the age of onset.[8] This rationale highlights the age of onset as a defining characteristic of epilepsy and illustrates the age-specific spectrum of clinical presentations in pediatric epilepsy. The review will provide summarized clinical descriptions of current syndromic epilepsies (**Table 1**) and will characterize epilepsies of structural etiology that may be amenable to surgical intervention (**Table 2**). Lastly, emerging technologies are highlighted that will facilitate future syndromic classifications through an improved understanding of the underlying pathophysiological basis of epilepsy.

COMMON EPILEPSY SYNDROMES
Neonatal and infantile epilepsies

Of the 4 recognized epilepsy syndromes that present during the neonatal period, 2 are medication-responsive with a relatively benign course and spontaneously resolve by 1 to 2 years of age: self-limited neonatal seizures and self-limited familial neonatal epilepsy[9] (see **Table 1**). The remaining 2 syndromes, early myoclonic encephalopathy (EME) and Ohtahara Syndrome (OS), are notable for a severe clinical presentation often with intractable seizures.[10] These 2 syndromes are distinguished mainly by the predominant seizure type. Neonates with EME will experience frequent myoclonic seizures, focal seizures, and

[a] Department of Pediatrics, Ann & Robert H. Lurie Children's Hospital of Chicago, 225 E. Chicago Ave. #18, Chicago, IL 60611, USA; [b] Department of Neurosurgery, University of Wisconsin-Madison School of Medicine and Public Health, 1675 Highland Avenue #0002, Madison, WI 53705, USA
* Corresponding author.
E-mail address: raheel.ahmed@neurosurgery.wisc.edu

Neurosurg Clin N Am 33 (2022) 113–134
https://doi.org/10.1016/j.nec.2021.09.009
1042-3680/22/© 2021 Elsevier Inc. All rights reserved.

Table 1
Summary of epilepsy syndromes

Syndrome	Seizure Semiology	Clinical Features	Background EEG	Initial MRI	Genetic Factors	Treatment Options
Neonatal						
Benign Neonatal Seizures	Focal Unifocal clonic seizures	Typical onset at 4–7 d of life Spontaneous remission around 6 mo	May be discontinuous or normal	Normal	KCNQ2, KCNQ3	AEDs: phenobarbital, fosphenytoin, levetiracetam
Benign Familial Neonatal Epilepsy	Focal Focal or multifocal clonic or tonic seizures	Typical onset at 4–7 d of life Spontaneous remission around 6 mo	May be discontinuous or normal	Normal	Family history of neonatal seizures KCNQ2, KCNQ3, SCN2A	AEDs: phenobarbital, fosphenytoin, levetiracetam
Early Myoclonic Encephalopathy	Focal and Generalized Frequent myoclonus; mixed focal seizures and GTCS	Early mortality Developmental and psychomotor delays Often develop DRE	Interictal burst-suppression pattern	Variable; some structural causes	ERBB4, SLC25A22, SIK1, GABRB2	AEDs: phenobarbital, fosphenytoin, levetiracetam
Ohtahara Syndrome	Focal and Generalized Tonic flexion; single or in series	Early mortality Developmental and psychomotor delays Often develop DRE	Interictal burst-suppression pattern	Variable; some structural causes	STXBP1, SLC25A22, CDKL5, ARX, KCNT1, KCNQ2,[10,13,137]	AEDs: vigabatrin, zonisamide, Other: ACTH, steroids, ketogenic diet
Infantile						
West Syndrome	Focal and Generalized Epileptic spasms; focal seizures may develop	Global developmental impairment	Hypsarrhythmia Disorganized with high voltage irregular slow waves and polyspikes	Variable; some structural causes	ARX, CDKL5, SPTAN1, STXBP1	1st line: ACTH, vigabatrin AEDs: valproate, zonisamide, Other: pyridoxine, ketogenic diet

Syndrome	Seizure types	Clinical features	EEG	Genes	Treatment
Dravet Syndrome	Focal and generalized Tonic-clonic, hemiclonic, myoclonic, atonic, atypical absence	Cognitive and behavioral impairments May develop ataxia or pyramidal signs	Post-ictal slowing that develops into diffuse slowing over time	Majority of cases: SCN1A Other genes: PCDH19, SCN1B, GABRA1, STXBP1, CHD2, SCN2A, HCN1, KCNA2, GABRG2[138]	1st line: valproate, clobazam AEDs: topiramate, stiripentol, levetiracetam, cannabidiol Other: fenfluramine, bromides, ketogenic diet
Myoclonic Epilepsy In Infancy	Generalized Myoclonic	Cognitive and behavioral impairments may occur Spontaneous remission at 6 mo – 5 y	Normal	None known	AEDs: valproate, clobazam, clonazepam
Epilepsy in Infancy with Migrating Focal Seizures	Focal Focal motor, focal tonic	Reduced life expectancy Severe neurologic disabilities Often develop DRE	Normal at onset, diffuse slowing occurs with time	KCNT1, SCN1A, SCN2A, PLCB1, TBC1D24, CHD2	AEDs: oxcarbazepine, phenytoin, bromides, topiramate, levetiracetam, vigabatrin, stiripentol, lacosamide.
Genetic Epilepsy with Febrile Seizures Plus (GEFS+)	Generalized Generalized tonic-clonic, atonic, myoclonic, absence	Febrile seizures that occur beyond 6 y of age Often remits at adolescence	Normal	SCN1A, SCN1B, GABRG2, SCN2A, SCN9A, GABRD	Treatment often unnecessary AEDs: valproate, clobazam, ethosuximide, levetiracetam, topiramate

(continued on next page)

Table 1
(continued)

Syndrome	Seizure Semiology	Clinical Features	Background EEG	Initial MRI	Genetic Factors	Treatment Options
Self-limited Infantile Epilepsy	Focal Behavioral arrest, impaired awareness, automatisms, clonic movements	Typical onset at 3–20 mo Seizures often intractable, but spontaneously resolve within 1 y	Normal	Normal	Majority of cases: PRRT2 SCN2A, KCNQ2, KCNQ3	AEDs: phenobarbital, fosphenytoin, levetiracetam
Myoclonic Encephalopathy in Nonprogressive Disorders	Generalized Myoclonic status epilepticus lasting days-weeks	Poor prognosis Severe developmental and neurologic impairments	Abnormal background with slow (theta-delta) activity, mainly in the central or parieto-occipital regions. Interictal multifocal continuous spikes and sharp waves	Variable; some structural causes	Chromosomal abnormalities including: Angelman syndrome, Wolf Hirschhorn syndrome	AEDs: benzodiazepines
Hemiconvulsion-Hemiplegia Epilepsy	Focal Unilateral convulsive status epilepticus, focal seizures	Extended convulsions lead to unilateral cerebral atrophy and hemiplegia	Ipsilateral slowing and low voltage activity on background EEG	Edema in the affected hemisphere	Not known	Often intractable AEDs: phenobarbital, carbamazepine, valproate Surgery: hemisphereotomy
Childhood Absence	Generalized Frequent and brief absence seizures; may develop GTCS	Normal development and cognition Seizures tend to disappear in adolescence	Normal background May see 2.5-4 Hz occipital intermittent rhythmic delta activity (OIRDA) Generalized 3 Hz spike-and-wave on interictal EEG	Normal	SLC2A1, GABRA1, GABRB3, GABRG2, CACNA1H[20]	1st line: ethosuximide AEDs: valproate, lamotrigine

Syndrome	Seizure Type	Development / Outcome	EEG	Genetics	Treatment
Childhood Epilepsy with Centrotemporal Spikes (BECTS)	Focal and Generalized Brief hemifacial seizures; may evolve to nocturnal GTCS	Normal development and cognition Seizures generally resolve by age 13 Many do not require AED therapy	Normal background Interictal high amplitude centrotemporal spikes or sharp-and-slow wave complexes in drowsiness and sleep	Normal	GRIN2A, RBFOX1, RBFOX2, DEPDC5[20]	AEDs: valproate, gabapentin
Atypical Childhood Epilepsy with Centrotemporal Spikes	Focal Focal frontoparietal seizures; may develop focal motor seizures with negative myoclonus	Normal development and cognition Neurologic and motor impairments in the active phase of epilepsy. Spontaneous remission by age 15	Background may be normal or demonstrate diffuse slowing Interictal high amplitude centrotemporal spikes or sharp-and-slow wave complexes in drowsiness and sleep	Normal	GRIN2A	AEDs: ethosuximide Other: ACTH, steroids
Lennox–Gastaut	Generalized Primarily tonic seizures; can also develop GTCS, atypical absence, atonic, or myoclonic seizures	Developmental and cognitive delays with regression after seizure onset Often develop DRE	Abnormal background with generalized or focal slowing Multifocal spike-and-wave with anterior predominance, slow spike-and-wave in slow sleep on interictal EEG	Variable; some structural causes	GABRB3, CHD2, FOXG1, DNM1, STXBP1, SCN8A, ALG13[29,139]	AEDs: felbamate, lamotrigine, topiramate, levetiracetam, cannabidiol Surgery: VNS corpus callosotomy Other: ketogenic diet
Panayiotopoulos Syndrome	Focal Focal autonomic seizure; often prolonged	Normal development and cognition 25% of cases experience only one seizure Spontaneous remission by adolescence	Normal background Multifocal high voltage repetitive spikes or sharp and slow-waves on interictal EEG	Normal	Not known	Treatment often not necessary AEDs: valproate, carbamazepine

(continued on next page)

Table 1
(continued)

Syndrome	Seizure Semiology	Clinical Features	Background EEG	Initial MRI	Genetic Factors	Treatment Options
Late-Onset Childhood Occipital Epilepsy	Focal and Generalized Primarily brief focal sensory visual seizures; can develop other occipital lobe seizures, impaired awareness, hemiclonic seizures, or focal to bilateral GTCS	Normal development and cognition Spontaneous remission within 2–4 y of onset	Normal background Occipital spike-and-wave on interictal EEG	Normal	Not known	AEDs: Very responsive to carbamazepine
Epilepsy with Myoclonic/Atonic Seizures (Doose Syndrome)	Focal and Generalized Primarily myoclonic-atonic seizures; can develop febrile seizures, absence, tonic seizures, GTCS	Normal development and cognition; may develop impairments after seizure onset	Normal or generalized slowing in background Generalized spike-and-wave on interictal EEG	Normal	SCN1A, SLC2A1	AEDs: valproate, lamotrigine, levetiracetam, topiramate, zonisamide, clobazam, felbamate Other: VNS ketogenic diet
Epilepsy with Myoclonic Absences (Tassinari Syndrome)	Generalized Primarily frequent myoclonic absences; can develop GTCS, absence seizures	Normal development and cognition initially; 70% will develop a learning disability 50% last into adulthood	Normal background Generalized spike-and-wave on interictal EEG	Normal	Not known	Often intractable AEDs: valproate, ethosuximide, lamotrigine, clobazam

Syndrome	Seizure Type	Development/Cognition	EEG	Imaging	Genetics	Treatment
Epilepsy with Eyelid Myoclonia (Jeavons Syndrome)	Focal and Generalized Primarily frequent and brief eyelid myoclonias; may develop febrile seizures, GTCS	Normal development and cognition	Normal background Fast generalized polyspike-and-wave (3–6 Hz) on interictal EEG	Normal	Not known	Often intractable AEDs: levetiracetam, valproate, ethosuximide, lamotrigine, topiramate, clobazam Other: ketogenic diet
Photosensitive Occipital Lobe Epilepsy	Focal and Generalized Primarily brief focal sensory visual seizures; may evolve to GTCS, myoclonic seizures, absences	May have impaired development and cognition	Normal background Occipital spike-and-wave may be present on interictal EEG	Normal	GRIN2A	Treatment often not necessary AEDs: valproate, levetiracetam, lamotrigine, carbamazepine, clobazam
Epileptic Encephalopathy During Sleep	Focal If seizures occur, they are infrequent, nocturnal, focal motor seizures; frequency increases with time	Progressive decline in development, cognition, and behavior with residual deficits following seizure resolution Spontaneous remission at 1mo–7 y	Normal or diffuse slowing on background EEG Continuous slow (1.5-2 Hz) spike-and-wave in slow sleep on interictal EEG	Variable; some structural causes	GRIN2A	AEDs: diazepam, clobazam, ethosuximide, valproate, acetazolamide, levetiracetam Surgery: subpial transections resection of structural lesions
Landau–Kleffner Syndrome	Focal and Generalized Seizures occur in 70% of cases and are infrequent and nocturnal. May demonstrate focal, atonic, or atypical absence seizures	Presents with subacute onset of progressive aphasia Cognitive and behavioral abnormalities often observed Residual language impairment Spontaneous remission	Normal background High amplitude epileptiform activity in the temporal-parietal region on interictal EEG	Normal	GRIN2A	*Often intractable* AEDs: diazepam, clobazam, ethosuximide, valproate, acetazolamide, levetiracetam

(continued on next page)

Table 1
(continued)

Syndrome	Seizure Semiology	Clinical Features	Background EEG	Initial MRI	Genetic Factors	Treatment Options
Sleep-related Hyper-motor Epilepsy	Focal Brief, nocturnal frontal lobe seizures with tonic or dystonic motor features, often with preserved awareness	Normal development and cognition Some cases of cognitive disturbance or decline	Normal background Rare frontal sharp waves or spikes on interictal EEG	Normal	CHRNA4, CHRNB2, CHRNA2, DEPDC5	AEDs: low-dose carbamazepine
Adolescence						
Juvenile Absence Epilepsy	Generalized Absence; often develop GTCs	Onset at 9–13 y of age Normal development Good response to AEDs	Normal background May see occipital intermittent rhythmic delta activity (OIRDA)	Normal	CACNAB4, GABRA1, GABRG2	AEDs: valproate, lamotrigine, ethosuximide
Juvenile Myoclonic Epilepsy	Generalized Myoclonic; can develop GTCs	Normal development and cognition	Normal background Spike-and-wave (3.5-6 Hz) on interictal EEG	Normal	CACNB4, GABRA1, CLCN2, GABRD, EFHC1[37,38]	*1st line:* valproate, lamotrigine AEDs: topiramate, levetiracetam
Epilepsy with Generalized Tonic-Clonic Seizures	Generalized GTCs; generally upon awakening	Normal development and cognition Seizures precipitated by sleep deprivation, fatigue, and excessive alcohol consumption	Normal background Spike-and-wave on interictal EEG	Normal	CLCN2	AEDs: valproate, lamotrigine, levetiracetam, phenobarbital, topiramate
Autosomal Dominant Epilepsy with Auditory Features (ADEAF)	Focal Focal sensory auditory or focal cognitive seizures; mainly nocturnal	Normal development and cognition Good response to AEDs	Normal	Normal	LGI1[20]	AEDs: carbamazepine, phenytoin, valproate, levetiracetam

Variable						
Family Focal Epilepsy with Variable Foci (FFEVF)	Focal Has a single focal seizure type, varies per individual	Normal development and cognition Good response to AEDs	Normal background Interictal focal epileptiform abnormalities corresponding to seizure onset zone	Normal	DEPDC5	AEDs: carbamazepine, lacosamide, lamotrigine, oxcarbazepine, topiramate
Reflex Epilepsies	Focal or Generalized Myoclonic jerks, focal atonic or tonic seizures, can progress to GTC	Normal development and cognition Seizures either induced exclusively by reading, or by startle. Startle seizures often secondary to a structural cause	Normal background Interictal EEG may reflect structural cause if present	Variable; some structural causes	Not known	Depends on seizure type AEDs: valproate, levetiracetam, clonazepam, lamotrigine, carbamazepine
Progressive Myoclonus Epilepsies	Generalized Myoclonic; sometimes develop GTCs	Progressive cognitive decline and motor impairment Cerebellar signs Often becomes DRE	Progressive background slowing	Variable	EPM2A, EPM2B[140]	1st line: valproate AEDs: levetiracetam, topiramate, clonazepam, zonisamide, clobazam, brivaracetam

Data from Refs.[16,141,142].

Table 2
Summary of structural epilepsies

Structural Etiology	Seizure Semiology	Percent with Seizures	Percent with DRE	Surgical Options	Seizure Outcomes
Neurocutaneous Syndromes					
Neurofibromatosis-1 (NF-1)	Focal and Generalized GTCs, absence, myoclonic, focal seizures	6%–10%[51]	Uncommon, generally well controlled with AEDs	Lesionectomy Lobectomy	66% seizure free in single case series[65]
Sturge–Weber Syndrome (SWS)	Focal and Generalized Focal seizures in location of leptomeningeal angioma, GTCs, epileptic spasms	72%[51]	46%[143]	Gold Standard: hemispherectomy or hemispherectomy Alternatives: Lesionectomy	80% seizure free with hemispherectomy/ hemisphereotomy[60]
Tuberous Sclerosis Complex (TSC)	Focal and Generalized Focal seizures, GTCs, epileptic spasms	90%[51]	70%	Preferred: Tuberectomy Lobectomy	59% seizure free[55]
Malformation of Cortical Development (MCD)					
Polymicrogyria (PMG)	Focal and Generalized Presents with focal seizures, may transition to focal or bilateral GTCS.	78%[88]	65%[91]	Often not feasible due to multifocal lesions Some success with lesionectomy or hemispherectomy in selected cases	50% seizure free[144]
Focal Cortical Dysplasia (FCD)	Focal and Generalized Presents with focal seizures, may transition to focal or bilateral GTCS, epileptic spasms	~100%	80%[79]	Preferred: Lesionectomy For extensive lesions: lobectomy or hemispherectomy	60%–80% seizure free[80,81]
Lissencephaly (LIS)	Focal and Generalized Primarily epileptic spasms; atypical absence, atonic, tonic seizures also seen	>90%	~100%[145]	Not feasible	N/A

Subcortical Band Heterotopia	Focal and Generalized Presents with focal seizures; may develop focal to bilateral GTCS	~80%[146]	~50%	Inadequate results[147]	N/A
Periventricular Nodular Heterotopia (PVNH)	Focal and Generalized Focal seizures originating from the site of the lesion; GTCS, epileptic spasms	90%	Most known cases	Often not feasible due to overlap with eloquent cortex Some success with laser interstitial thermal therapy (LITT)	50% seizure free with LITT[76]
Hypothalamic Hamartoma	Focal and Generalized Presents with brief gelastic seizures; focal impaired awareness seizures, bilateral GTCS may develop	Unknown	100%[148]	Lesionectomy of hamartoma	50% seizure free[149]
Hemimegalencephaly	Focal and Generalized Focal seizures originating from hemimegalencephalic hemisphere; Focal to bilateral GTCS, epileptic spasms	100%	100%[86]	Anatomic or functional hemispherectomy	Individual case reports of 100% seizure freedom[150]
Vascular Malformations					
Cerebral Angioma (CA)	Focal Focal seizures originating from the site of the CA	50%	40%	Surgical lesionectomy of angioma	70%–90% seizure free[105]
Arteriovenous Malformation (AVM)	Focal and Generalized Focal seizures originating from the site of the AVM; Focal to bilateral GTCS	22%–47%	22%–58%	In cases of DRE or high risk of rupture, options include: radiosurgery, endovascular embolization, microsurgical resection	42.5%–77% seizure free[97]

(continued on next page)

Table 2
(continued)

Structural Etiology	Seizure Semiology	Percent with Seizures	Percent with DRE	Surgical Options	Seizure Outcomes
Other Causes					
Aicardi Syndrome	Focal and Generalized Infantile/spasms that often asymmetric or unilateral; may develop focal seizures[110]	95%–100%	>73%[113]	Palliative corpus callosotomy	Seizure reduction possible, seizure freedom unlikely[114]
Hypoxic-Ischemic Brain Injury (HIE)	Focal and Generalized Focal seizures originating from the site of injury; may develop focal to bilateral GTCS, epileptic spasms	9%–33%[151]	Unknown	Not feasible	N/A

Data from Refs. [141,142]

tonic spasms, whereas those afflicted with OS will mainly develop tonic spasms.[11] The etiologies of EME and OS are similar, with errors of inborn metabolism more often resulting in EME, and structural abnormalities favoring OS.[11] EME and OS share a characteristic electrographic pattern of "burst-suppression" on interictal EEG, consisting of periods of high-voltage electrical activity followed by periods of minimal brain activity.[10–12] Individuals with either diagnosis have a poor prognosis with high mortality in infancy, and severe psychomotor delays and neurologic disability in survivors. Few antiepileptic drugs (AEDs), ACTH, pyridoxine, and corticosteroids are effective in reducing seizure frequency or developmental delay.[11] Recent incorporation of improved genetic sequencing in clinical practice has helped delineate genetic causes for both OS and EME.[10,13,14]

Individuals with OS may develop another severe epilepsy syndrome that presents slightly later in infancy: West syndrome (WS).[12,15] WS has an estimated incidence of approximately 0.43 in 1000 live births and presents between 3 and 12 months of age. In cases arising from OS, the presentation onset is typically earlier at 3 to 4 months of age.[16] Similar to OS, the etiologies of WS can include structural brain abnormalities, genetic mutations, or chromosomal disruptions, and in certain cases, inborn errors of metabolism. WS is defined by the classical triad of: (1) infantile spasms, (2) hypsarrhythmia on EEG, and (3) developmental arrest or regression.[15] Standard therapy for infants with WS includes adrenocorticotrophic hormone (ACTH), vigabatrin, and corticosteroids, although recent studies have suggested prednisolone may be as effective as ACTH.[17] Alternatively, the ketogenic diet has been found effective at seizure reduction in roughly 45% of affected infants.[18] Long-term outcomes are highly variable and dependent on etiology—structural and genetic causes are associated with globally delayed development or developmental regression.[19]

In addition to WS, there are additional epilepsy syndromes that present during infancy, with a wide range of clinical severity. The incidence of syndromes with spontaneous remission including genetic epilepsy with febrile seizures plus (GEFS+) and myoclonic epilepsy of infancy,[20] has not been well described, potentially due to their transient nature or overlap with neonatal syndromes. More severe infantile syndromes often associated with developmental and cognitive delays include: Dravet syndrome, which has an estimated incidence of 1/20,000 to 1/40,000, as well as rarer syndromes such as epilepsy in infancy with migrating focal seizures (0.11/100,000), myoclonic encephalopathy in nonprogressive disorders, and hemiconvulsion-hemiplegia epilepsy.[20–22] These syndromes, as well as those with later onset in childhood and adolescence, have been summarized in **Table 1**.

Childhood epilepsies

The most common epilepsy syndrome of childhood, accounting for 25% of childhood epilepsy diagnoses, is benign epilepsy with centrotemporal spikes (BECTS), or benign rolandic epilepsy.[20] This syndrome presents between ages 4 and 11 years, with a peak at age 7 to 8 and a male predominance. Typically, short focal-onset seizures present nocturnally and consist of ipsilateral facial paresthesias, followed by dysarthria, facial jerking, and drooling.[20,23] Given that seizures occur infrequently and nearly all cases of BECTS spontaneously remit by adolescence (14–16 years), pharmacotherapy is not universally prescribed, although AEDs are effective in individuals who do experience frequent events.[20,24] Although children will experience universal resolution of seizures, they are at risk for developing neurocognitive deficits.[25]

Another common epilepsy syndrome in childhood absence epilepsy (pyknolepsy), idiopathic generalized epilepsy (IGE) that accounts for ~15% of childhood epilepsy diagnoses.[20,26] Clinical observations suggest that it is likely inherited; however, unlike many recognized inherited epilepsy syndromes, few genes have been found to be directly associated with this syndrome.[27] Onset typically begins between ages 4 and 10 with a peak incidence between years 5 and 7, and unlike BECTS, has a female predominance. Clinically, this syndrome presents with frequent absence seizures consisting of the impairment of consciousness that can often be accompanied by automatisms, eyelid fluttering, staring, and/or behavioral arrest. EEG consistently demonstrates generalized 3 to 4 Hz spike-and-wave discharges during the ictal period.[20] Generally, absence seizures can be well controlled with ethosuximide or valproic acid, and in most cases, seizures will spontaneously resolve as the child enters adolescence.[28]

A more severe, but less prevalent (1%–10% of cases) childhood epilepsy syndrome is Lennox–Gastaut syndrome (LGS).[29,30] Similar to OS and EME presenting in infancy, LGS is defined as an epileptic encephalopathy, because patients suffer cognitive and behavioral deficits as a direct result of epileptic activity.[29] Diagnosis requires the following criteria: (1) multiple seizure types (tonic seizures are the most common), (2) a distinctive diffuse, slow spike-and-wave pattern on EEG (2.5 Hz) with slow background activity, and (3) neurocognitive decrement. Around 75% of cases have an identifiable cause including structural abnormalities, perinatal trauma, CNS infections, or metabolic disorders. For the remaining 25%, recent studies have identified genetic predispositions including copy number variants or mutations in SCN1A, CHD2, FOXG1, or DNM1.[29] Seizures are generally refractory to medication; however, AEDs such as valproate, clobazam, felbamate, lamotrigine, and topiramate may help limit injurious seizures such as drop attacks and generalized tonic-clonic seizures (GTCS).[31] Ketogenic diet may help reduce seizure burden.[32] Surgical treatment includes the resection of seizure focus in selected focal cases,[33,34] whereas corpus callosotomy and vagal nerve stimulation may be effective as palliative interventions to reduce drop attacks and overall seizure burden, respectively.[35,36]

Adolescent epilepsies

Juvenile myoclonic epilepsy (JME) is the most prevalent genetic generalized epilepsy syndrome, accounting for roughly 5% to 10% of all epilepsies in this age group. Although its mechanism is not yet understood, JME is associated with mutations in CACNB4, EFHC1, and GABRA1.[37,38] The age of onset ranges from 12 to 18 years of age, with a slight female predominance.[9] All individuals diagnosed with JME have myoclonic seizures, the vast majority (~90%) will have GCTS, and 20% to 40% will have absence seizures. Seizures most often present after awakening.[37] JME seizures can be triggered by sleep deprivation, stress, anxiety, or alcohol intake, and many individuals are photosensitive.[37] EEG findings in JME may include diffuse 4 to 6 Hz polyspike and wave discharges, primarily in the fronto-central region, and all patients will demonstrate abnormal EEGs during sleep.[39,40] Most JME cases are responsive to AEDs, especially valproic acid, with many individuals achieving seizure freedom on monotherapy.[37,41–43]

The second common generalized epilepsy syndrome of adolescent onset is juvenile absence epilepsy (JAE), with a prevalence of 2% to 3% out of all epilepsy syndromes in adults, and 10% to 15% of all patients diagnosed with IGE.[44] The age of onset for most cases is ages 9 to 13, but a range as wide as 5 to 20 years has been reported.[44–46] Most JAE patients experience 1 to 10 absence seizures per day, whereas 80% will additionally have GTCS. A smaller subset (20%) will also suffer from mild myoclonic jerks. Absence seizures are triggered by mental arousal stimuli, whereas GTCS are more often triggered by sleep deprivation,

stress, and alcohol consumption. Background interictal EEG is generally normal, but ictal EEG will show 3–4 Hz generalized polyspike and wave discharges.[45,47] Treatment for JAE is similar to that for other IGEs, with valproic acid as the first-line treatment. However, there is disagreement on the efficacy of treatment in JAE, with seizure-free outcomes ranging from 15% to 70%.[44,45,48,49]

STRUCTURAL EPILEPSIES

Epilepsy syndromes associated with epileptogenic lesions identifiable on radiographic evaluation encompass a broad group of epilepsies that are predisposed to evolve into a medication refractory state but are conversely amenable to surgical resection for seizure relief (see **Table 2**). Identification of a structural etiology is of prognostic significance in surgical treatment and odds of achieving seizure freedom.[50] The following section will provide an overview of the prevalent syndromic epilepsies associated with identifiable epileptogenic lesions.

Neurocutaneous syndromes

Neurocutaneous syndromes are a group of heritable diseases that present with skin lesions and peripheral or central nervous system involvement and include tuberous sclerosis (TSC), neurofibromatosis (NF), and Sturge–Weber syndrome (SWS). Although the specific pathologic mechanisms differ, all 3 are linked to disruptions in the Ras and mTOR pathways.[51] TSC is caused by autosomal dominant mutations in the tumor repressor genes TSC1 or TSC2 resulting in tubers: growths of dysplastic and immature neurons and glia in the cerebral cortex.[51,52] Seizures occur in up to 90% of patients with TSC and include combinations of focal and multifocal seizures, and infantile spasms.[51] TSC-associated seizures invariably evolve into drug-resistant epilepsy (DRE).[51,53] Alternative therapies include the ketogenic diet, vagal nerve stimulation, and the mTOR inhibitor rapamycin.[54] In cases whereby a dominant epileptogenic tuber is identified, early surgical resection is encouraged. A meta-analysis of 229 patients with TSC who underwent epilepsy surgery indicated that the rate of postoperative seizure freedom was 59%, with favorable seizure outcomes more likely with a unilateral seizure focus on EEG, and seizure onset after 1 year of age. Lobectomy was also associated with better outcomes than localized tuberectomy.[55]

SWS is caused by a somatic mosaic mutation in GNAQ, and is characterized by malformations in the vasculature of the brain, skin, and eyes.[51,56] Clinical manifestations include facial angiomas (port-wine stain), leptomeningeal blood vessel malformations, and ocular angiomas. SWS typically has a unilateral presentation, but in certain cases occurs bilaterally and has a worse prognosis.[57] Seizures present with a focal onset followed by secondary generalization and tend to occur in clusters.[58] The seizure mechanism in SWS is hypothesized to be a result of abnormal cerebral blood vessel development leading to perfusion deficits and hypoxic-ischemic brain injury.[59] Surgical treatment is recommended in cases of unilateral SWS with DRE.[60] Surgical disconnection through hemispherectomy remains the gold standard for surgical intervention in unilateral SWS, with seizure-free outcomes in ~80% of cases.[60–63]

The incidence of epilepsy is relatively less common (4%–13%) in NF-1, an autosomal dominant condition caused by a mutation in the NF1 gene. Seizures are associated with intracranial tumors, hippocampal sclerosis, or polymicrogyria.[64,65] Compared with TSC and SWS, these seizures are generally responsive to medication. In DRE cases, positive outcomes following surgery have been reported; specifically for cases with a single epileptogenic zone.[65,66]

Malformations of cortical development

Malformations of cortical development (MCD) are structural anomalies in the cerebral cortex that can be categorized into 3 groups associated with abnormalities in neuronal migration, neuronal or glial proliferation/differentiation, and cortical organization. The secondary alterations in neural circuitry result in the development of epilepsy, affecting an estimated 75% of individuals with MCD.[67] Due to their underlying structural anomalies, MCD-associated epilepsy Is typically medication refractory and MCDs account for approximately 25% to 40% of all DRE diagnosed in childhood.[68,69]

Common neurodevelopmental diseases of abnormal neuronal migration include lissencephaly (LIS) and gray matter heterotopia. In LIS, the mature brain lacks gyration, and the cerebral cortex is thickened with a poorly organized cytoarchitecture. Given the extensive involvement of the cortex, surgical intervention to improve seizures is generally not feasible, and seizure response to AED therapy is limited.[70,71] Gray matter heterotopias result when neurons fail to migrate to their appropriate location in the cortical mantle.[72] The most common subtype is periventricular nodular heterotopia (PVNH) associated with rests of ectopic gray matter tissue within the lateral ventricle walls.[73] 90% of individuals with PVNH will have seizures due to intrinsic

epileptogenic properties of the nodules.[70,74,75] Surgical resection is effective in cases with focal seizure networks associated with limited nodules.[74] Recent advances in laser interstitial thermal therapy (LITT) have demonstrated seizure improvement in selected individuals.[76]

Focal cortical dysplasia (FCD) and hemimegalencephaly (HMEG) are the 2 most common structural disorders that arise from the abnormal proliferation of neurons and glia in-utero. FCDs are a heterogenous group of lesions that consist of abnormalities in cortical architecture accompanied by hypertrophic, dysmorphic, or immature neurons.[77] Based on the presence and extent of these features, which corresponds to overall disease severity, FCDs are classified into types I, II, and III.[78] FCDs most commonly present as DRE, which can develop at any age but most commonly presents in childhood.[79] Surgical resection in FCD DRE is associated with good seizure outcomes, with 60% to 80% of patients achieving near-complete seizure freedom.[77,80,81] In patients with more extensive lesions, lobectomies, or hemispherectomies have demonstrated good efficacy.[82] Individuals with HMEG present with a grossly dysplastic, single enlarged hemisphere with cortical dysgenesis, hypertrophy of white matter, and dilated ventricles.[73,83] The clinical presentation of HMEG typically includes intractable partial seizures, hemiparesis, and developmental delay.[84] Hemispherectomy approaches can yield excellent seizure control.[85,86]

Polymicrogyria (PMG) is one of the most common structural abnormalities, making up ~20% of all cases of MCDs.[87] It is a heterogenous condition characterized by abnormally dense microgyria resulting in the disruption of the normal cortex.[73] PMG can present either unilaterally or bilaterally, as an isolated lesion or in conjunction with additional MCDs. It most commonly occurs in a bilateral perisylvian pattern.[88] Though its etiology is largely unknown, it is often associated with cerebral artery ischemia, hypoxia, congenital infections, as well as certain genetic factors.[88,89] The most common symptoms of PMG are epilepsy and global developmental delay which occur in 78% and 70% of cases, respectively.[88,90] 65% of PMG cases develop DRE. Despite the presence of multiple cortical malformations, invasive monitoring in select individuals often demonstrates predominant epileptogenic foci that are amenable to ablative or resective interventions with good seizure relief.[91–93]

Vascular malformations

Common epileptogenic vascular malformations associated with epilepsy include arteriovenous malformations (AVMs) and cerebral angiomas. Focal epilepsy has been reported in 22% to 47% of patients with an AVM, and is the second most common clinical presentation for AVMs, preceded only by hemorrhage.[94–97] AVMs can precipitate an epileptic event either as a result of hemorrhage from a ruptured AVM, or from vascular steal and peri-nidal edema surrounding the AVM. Although the precise means of epileptogenicity has not been determined, posited mechanisms include the degeneration of neurons and glia, reactive oxygen species, and alterations in cellular signaling in the tissue surrounding the malformation.[95,98] Across studies, AVM location has been one of the strongest predictors of seizure incidence, with cortical location associated with a higher seizure incidence.[95,97] Larger AVM size, venous dilation, and male sex have also been identified as positive predictors of seizures.[94,95,97] Although AED therapy is effective (45%–78% chance of seizure improvement[99,100]), there is a high incidence of developing DRE that can be addressed through surgical options including radiosurgery, endovascular embolization, and/or microsurgical resection.[97,101–103]

Cerebral angiomas (CA), otherwise known as cerebral cavernous malformations (CCM), may present as sporadic single malformations, or as multiple clustered lesions associated with a developmental venous anomaly.[104] Although most CAs arise sporadically, inherited autosomal dominant forms of CA arise as a result of a loss-of-function mutation in the genes CCM1, CCM2, or CCM3. CCMs consist of abnormally dilated blood vessels with immature vessel walls that are prone to sporadic and chronic hemorrhage. They can be associated with secondary development of seizures that can occur in approximately 50% of patients.[104–106] CA lesions are not intrinsically epileptogenic. Rather, seizures arise from the peri-nidal cortical region as a result of the hemosiderin deposits and secondary gliosis.[98,105] Patients with CAs can develop DRE in 35% to 40% of cases.[107] Early surgical resection is associated with seizure freedom and can effectively eliminating seizure burden in patients with cavernoma-related epilepsy and its secondary disability.[108,109]

Aicardi syndrome

Aicardi syndrome (AS) is a rare *de novo* neurodevelopmental disorder defined by a triad of infantile spasms, corpus callosum agenesis, and central chorioretinal lacunae.[110] In addition, many individuals with AS will exhibit symptoms of neuronal migration defects. Although the mechanism for AS is largely unknown, its strong female predominance suggests an X-linked genetic

mechanism.[110] Patients with AS present with infantile spasms at 3 to 4 months of age, which may evolve into focal seizures with age.[111] Seizure activity is frequently asymmetric or unilateral, with EEG demonstrating multifocal epileptiform discharges and burst suppression with dissociation between the cerebral hemispheres.[112] Seizures are generally medically refractory, but some of the later developed focal seizures may respond to AED therapy.[113] Evidence is limited regarding the efficacy of resective epilepsy surgery in AS; however, palliative corpus callosotomy has recently been implemented in cases of severe medically refractory AS.[114]

FUTURE DIRECTIONS
Modern classification of epilepsy syndromes

The first standardized classification systems for epilepsy were established by the ILAE in 1969 and 1989, respectively.[4,115,116] The purpose of these classifications has been to establish objective criteria to assist clinicians in formulating diagnosis, prognosis, and treatment plans for an individual patient based on uniform criteria. Originally, this system focused on a shared "cluster of signs & symptoms" that primarily used the site of origin for the seizure (focal vs generalized), and seizure etiology, if known, to classify the known syndromes.[116] However, with technological advancements in neuroimaging, electrophysiology, and genetic testing, these classification systems have proven insufficient.[5,117–119] The newest ILAE classification, released in 2017, has incorporated additional information into clinical descriptions of epilepsy syndromes with emphasis on seizure etiology.[8] Description of epilepsy syndromes was updated as "a cluster of features incorporating seizure types, EEG, and imaging features that tend to occur together."[8,120] Although individual seizure presentations or syndromes may be influenced by genetic and environmental factors unique to each patient, these classifications continue to provide a common standardized terminology for clear communication and assessment of epilepsy among clinicians, patients, and researchers. The following section highlights ongoing advances in diagnostic modalities that can potentially impact future syndromic classifications for epilepsy.

Advances in genetic sequencing and its role in precision medicine

The rapid development in genetic technology over the last decade has helped uncover a genetic association or direct monogenic cause in over half of the known epilepsies.[5,121] This discovery, and accessibility of genetic sequencing, has dramatically impacted epilepsy on multiple levels: (1) as investigative tools for establishing and confirming the diagnosis, (2) improved understanding of the underlying molecular mechanisms of epilepsy pathogenesis, and (3) identifying genetic targets for precision medicine and potential gene therapy. Current diagnostic techniques to assess genetic linkages for epilepsy include clinical exome and genome sequencing, microarrays, and cytogenetic studies.[122–125] More recent diagnostic approaches assessing microRNA expression may help identify diagnostic and prognostic biomarkers of disease, as potentially therapeutic targets.[126]

Although genetic testing can help identify potential disease-causing mutations, implementing this information in an effective treatment approach remains challenging, especially for rare or previously uncharacterized mutations. To address this problem, the NIH established the Undiagnosed Disease Network (UDN) in 2014. The UDN consists of multiple clinical sites, 2 sequencing cores, a metabolomics core and a model organism screening center, all aimed at investigating the biologic characteristics of undiagnosed diseases.[127] Multidisciplinary programs such as the UDN are an essential part of bridging the gap between identifying a mutation through genome sequencing, understanding the underlying pathophysiology, and developing therapies for patients using a precision medicine approach.[128,129] These targeted treatments have already been implemented in a subset of monogenic epilepsies such as pyridoxine-dependent epilepsy, GLUT1 deficiency, and Dravet syndrome in a truly bedside-to-bench-to-bedside fashion.[5] Identifying the genetic basis for specific epilepsies, particularly in cases of monogenic diseases, also introduces the potential for the development of gene therapies such as gene replacement, antisense oligonucleotide therapy, or RNA interference.[130] These therapies have already been implemented successfully in neuromuscular disorders such as spinal muscular atrophy (SMA), and have demonstrated strong potential in animal models of neurodevelopmental disorders with epilepsy such as Rett syndrome, Fragile X, and Angelman syndrome.[131–133]

Tissue banking

Shared tissue repositories have significantly expanded our ability to carry out research on the molecular mechanisms and pathologic condition of rare disease.[132] The European Epilepsy Brain Bank (EEBB), established in 2006, has accumulated approximately 10,000 brain tissue samples from patients who had undergone epilepsy surgery.[134] A recent analysis of these samples identified hippocampal sclerosis and focal cortical dysplasias as the most common underlying etiology of DRE in adults and children, respectively.[134,135] These tissue repositories can be expanded to include biospecimen collection for molecular studies that can help identify somatic mutations, DNA methylation profiles, and additional information to stratify epilepsy subtypes. The University of Saskatchewan's Epilepsy Brain Bank established in 2014 has a repository for both formaldehyde-fixed brain tissue and frozen tissue and patient blood samples that can be used for further research into pathophysiological mechanisms of epilepsy with technologies such as RNA sequencing, proteomic, and transcriptomic studies.[136] Understanding these underlying causes of epileptogenicity could significantly contribute to ongoing AED development and patient-specific therapeutic approaches.

CLINICS CARE POINTS

- The updated epilepsy syndrome classification encompasses clinical elements like seizure types, EEG and imaging characteristics and genetics with an emphasis on underlying etiology.

- The syndromic classification approach helps establish the clinical framework of understanding epilepsy with respect to clinical evaluation, underlying etiology, pathophysiology, amenable treatments and disease outcomes.

- The initial classification framework categorizes seizures with respect to focal, generalized, or of unknown onset. The most prominent motor or nonmotor aspect of the semiology are used for further sub classification.

- Etiologic categories include structural, genetic, infectious, metabolic, immune, unknown) have been defined that may impact clinical evaluation and treatment.

DISCLOSURE

The authors have nothing to disclose.

REFERENCES

1. Fiest KM, Sauro KM, Wiebe S, et al. Prevalence and incidence of epilepsy: a systematic review and meta-analysis of international studies. Neurology 2017;88(3):296–303.

2. Fisher RS, Cross JH, French JA, et al. Operational classification of seizure types by the International League Against Epilepsy: position paper of the ILAE Commission for Classification and Terminology. Epilepsia 2017;58(4):522–30.

3. Berg AT, Berkovic SF, Brodie MJ, et al. Revised terminology and concepts for organization of seizures and epilepsies: report of the ILAE Commission on Classification and Terminology, 2005-2009. Epilepsia 2010;51(4):676–85.

4. Beghi E. The concept of the epilepsy syndrome: how useful is it in clinical practice? Epilepsia 2009;50(SUPPL. 5):4–10.

5. Striano P, Minassian BA. From genetic testing to precision medicine in epilepsy. Neurotherapeutics 2020;17(2):609–15.

6. Reif PS, Tsai M-H, Helbig I, et al. Precision medicine in genetic epilepsies: break of dawn? Expert Rev Neurother 2017;17(4):381–92.

7. Walker LE, Mirza N, Yip VLM, et al. Personalized medicine approaches in epilepsy. J Intern Med 2015;277(2):218–34.

8. Pack AM. Epilepsy overview and revised classification of seizures and epilepsies. Continuum (Minneap Minn) 2019;25(2):306–21.

9. Wirrell E. Infantile, childhood, and adolescent epilepsies. Contin Lifelong Learn Neurol 2016;22(1):60–93.

10. El Kosseifi C, Cornet MC, Cilio MR. Neonatal developmental and epileptic encephalopathies. Semin Pediatr Neurol 2019;32:100770.

11. Ohtahara S, Yamatogi Y. Epileptic encephalopathies in early infancy with suppression-burst. J Clin Neurophysiol 2003;20(6):398–407.

12. Auvin S, Cilio MR, Vezzani A. Current understanding and neurobiology of epileptic encephalopathies. Neurobiol Dis 2016;92(Part A):72–89.

13. Ishii A, Kang JQ, Schornak CC, et al. A de novo missense mutation of GABRB2 causes early myoclonic encephalopathy. J Med Genet 2017;54(3):202–11.

14. Kato M, Yamagata T, Kubota M, et al. Clinical spectrum of early onset epileptic encephalopathies caused by KCNQ2 mutation. Epilepsia 2013;54(7):1282–7.

15. Pavone P, Polizzi A, Marino SD, et al. West syndrome: a comprehensive review. Neurol Sci 2020;41(12):3547–62.

16. Panayiotopolous C. Epileptic encephalopathies in infancy and early childhood in which the epileptiform abnormalities may contribute to progressive dysfunction. In: The epilepsies: seizures, syndromes and management. Bladon Medical Publishing; 2005. Available at: https://www.ncbi.nlm.nih.gov/books/NBK2611/.

17. O'Callaghan FJK, Edwards SW, Alber FD, et al. Safety and effectiveness of hormonal treatment versus hormonal treatment with vigabatrin for infantile spasms (ICISS): a randomised, multicentre, open-label trial. Lancet Neurol 2017;16(1):33–42.

18. Kossoff EH. Infantile spasms. Neurologist 2010;16(2):69–75.

19. Gul Mert G, Herguner MO, Incecik F, et al. Risk factors affecting prognosis in infantile spasm. Int J Neurosci 2017;127(11):1012–8.

20. Pearl PL. Epilepsy syndromes in childhood. Contin Lifelong Learn Neurol 2018;24(1):186–209.

21. Wu YW, Sullivan J, McDaniel SS, et al. Incidence of dravet syndrome in a US population. Pediatrics 2015;136(5):e1310–5.

22. McTague A, Appleton R, Avula S, et al. Migrating partial seizures of infancy: expansion of the electroclinical, radiological and pathological disease spectrum. Brain 2013;136(Pt 5):1578–91.

23. Guerrini R, Pellacani S. Benign childhood focal epilepsies. Epilepsia 2012;53:9–18.

24. Hughes JR. Benign epilepsy of childhood with centrotemporal spikes (BECTS): To treat or not to treat, that is the question. Epilepsy Behav 2010;19(3):197–203.

25. Vannest J, Tenney JR, Gelineau-Morel R, et al. Cognitive and behavioral outcomes in benign childhood epilepsy with centrotemporal spikes. Epilepsy Behav 2015;45:85–91.

26. Camfield CS, Camfield PR, Gordon K, et al. Incidence of epilepsy in childhood and adolescence: a population-based study in Nova Scotia from 1977 to 1985. Epilepsia 1996;37(1):19–23.

27. Berkovic SF. In: Engel JJ, Pedley TA, editors. Epilepsy: a comprehensive textbook. Lippincott-Raven; 1998. p. 217–24.

28. Glauser TA, Cnaan A, Shinnar S, et al. Ethosuximide, valproic acid, and lamotrigine in childhood absence epilepsy. N Engl J Med 2010;362(9):790–9.

29. Asadi-pooya AA. Lennox-Gastaut syndrome : a comprehensive review. Published online 2018;403–14.

30. Trevathan E, Murphy CC, Yeargin-Allsopp M. Prevalence and descriptive epidemiology of Lennox-Gastaut syndrome among Atlanta children. Epilepsia 1997;38(12):1283–8.

31. Micholaus A, Farrell K. Medical management of Lennox-Gastaut syndrome. CNS Drugs 2010;24(5):363–74.

32. Caraballo RH, Fortini S, Fresler S, et al. Ketogenic diet in patients with Lennox–Gastaut syndrome. Seizure 2014;23(9):751–5.

33. Douglass LM, Salpekar J. Surgical options for patients with Lennox-Gastaut syndrome. Epilepsia 2014;55:21–8.

34. Wyllie E, Lachhwani DK, Gupta A, et al. Successful surgery for epilepsy due to early brain lesions despite generalized EEG findings. Neurology 2007;69(4):389–97.

35. Asadi-Pooya AA, Malekmohamadi Z, Kamgarpour A, et al. Corpus callosotomy is a valuable therapeutic option for patients with Lennox–Gastaut syndrome and medically refractory seizures. Epilepsy Behav 2013;29(2):285–8.

36. Asadi-Pooya AA, Sharan A, Nei M, et al. Corpus callosotomy. Epilepsy Behav 2008;13(2):271–8.

37. Amrutkar C, Riel-Romero RM. Juvenile myoclonic epilepsy. 2021 Aug 11. In: StatPearls [Internet]. Treasure Island (FL): StatPearls Publishing; 2021.

38. Delgado-Escueta AV, Koeleman BPC, Bailey JN, et al. The quest for Juvenile Myoclonic Epilepsy genes. Epilepsy Behav 2013;28(1):S52–7.

39. Baise-Zung C, Guilhoto LMFF, Grossmann RM. Juvenile myoclonic epilepsy: non-classic electroencephalographical presentation in adult patients. Eur J Neurol 2006;13(2):171–5.

40. Dhanuka AK, Jain BK, Daljit S, et al. Juvenile myoclonic epilepsy: a clinical and sleep EEG study. Seizure 2001;10(5):374–8.

41. Tomson T, Battino D, Perucca E. Valproic acid after five decades of use in epilepsy: time to reconsider the indications of a time-honoured drug. Lancet Neurol 2016;15(2):210–8.

42. Bodenstein-Sachar H, Gandelman-Marton R, Ben-Zeev B, et al. Outcome of lamotrigine treatment in juvenile myoclonic epilepsy. Acta Neurol Scand 2011;124(1):22–7.

43. Verrotti A, Cerminara C, Coppola G, et al. Levetiracetam in juvenile myoclonic epilepsy: long-term efficacy in newly diagnosed adolescents. Dev Med Child Neurol 2008;50(1):29–32.

44. Asadi-Pooya AA, Emami M, Sperling MR. A clinical study of syndromes of idiopathic (genetic) generalized epilepsy. J Neurol Sci 2013;324(1–2):113–7.

45. Panayiotopoulos C. A clinical guide to epileptic syndromes and their treatment. 2nd edition. Springer; 2010.

46. Asadi-Pooya AA, Farazdaghi M. Seizure outcome in patients with juvenile absence epilepsy. Neurol Sci 2016;37(2):289–92.

47. Sadleir LG, Scheffer IE, Smith S, et al. EEG features of absence seizures in idiopathic generalized epilepsy: Impact of syndrome, age, and state. Epilepsia 2009;50(6):1572–8.

48. Tovia E, Goldberg-Stern H, Shahar E, et al. Outcome of children with juvenile absence epilepsy. J Child Neurol 2006;21(9):766–8.

49. Danhofer P, Brázdil M, Ošlejšková H, et al. Long-term seizure outcome in patients with juvenile absence epilepsy; a retrospective study in a tertiary referral center. Seizure 2014;23(6):443–7.

50. Téllez-Zenteno JF, Hernández Ronquillo L, Moien-Afshari F, et al. Surgical outcomes in lesional and non-lesional epilepsy: a systematic review and meta-analysis. Epilepsy Res 2010;89(2–3):310–8.

51. Stafstrom CE, Staedtke V, Comi AM. Epilepsy mechanisms in neurocutaneous disorders: tuberous sclerosis complex, neurofibromatosis type 1, and Sturge–Weber Syndrome. Front Neurol 2017;8:87.

52. Chu-Shore CJ, Major P, Camposano S, et al. The natural history of epilepsy in tuberous sclerosis complex. Epilepsia 2009;51(7):1236–41.

53. Kwan P, Schachter SC, Brodie MJ. Drug-resistant epilepsy. N Engl J Med 2011;365(10):919–26.

54. Jülich K, Sahin M. Mechanism-based treatment in tuberous sclerosis complex. Pediatr Neurol 2014;50(4):290–6.

55. Zhang K, Hu W, Zhang C, et al. Predictors of seizure freedom after surgical management of tuberous sclerosis complex: a systematic review and meta-analysis. Epilepsy Res 2013;105(3):377–83.

56. Comi AM. Sturge–Weber syndrome. Handb Clin Neurol 2015;132:157–68.

57. Bebin EM, Gomez MR. Prognosis in sturge-weber disease: comparison of unihemispheric and bihemispheric involvement. J Child Neurol 1988;3(3):181–4.

58. Kossoff EH, Ferenc L, Comi AM. An infantile-onset, severe, yet sporadic seizure pattern is common in Sturge-Weber syndrome. Epilepsia 2009;50(9):2154–7.

59. Pinto A, Sahin M, Pearl PL. Epileptogenesis in neurocutaneous disorders with focus in Sturge Weber syndrome. F1000Res 2016;5:370.

60. Bianchi F, Auricchio AM, Battaglia DI, et al. Sturge-Weber syndrome: an update on the relevant issues for neurosurgeons. Childs Nerv Syst 2020;36(10):2553–70.

61. Bourgeois M, Crimmins DW, De Oliveira RS, et al. Surgical treatment of epilepsy in Sturge-Weber syndrome in children. J Neurosurg 2007;106(1 SUPPL):20–8.

62. Almeida AN do, Marino R, Marie SK, et al. Factors of morbidity in hemispherectomies: Surgical technique×pathology. Brain Dev 2006;28(4):215–22.

63. Harmon KA, Day AM, Hammill AM, et al. Quality of life in children with Sturge-Weber Syndrome. Pediatr Neurol 2019;101:26–32.

64. Nix JS, Blakeley J, Rodriguez FJ. An update on the central nervous system manifestations of neurofibromatosis type 1. Acta Neuropathol 2020;139(4):625–41.

65. Barba C, Jacques T, Kahane P, et al. Epilepsy surgery in Neurofibromatosis Type 1. Epilepsy Res 2013;105(3):384–95.

66. Bernardo P, Santoro C, Rubino A, et al. Epilepsy surgery in neurofibromatosis type 1: an overlooked therapeutic approach. Child's Nerv Syst 2020;36(12):2909–10.

67. Leventer RJ, Phelan EM, Coleman LT, et al. Clinical and imaging features of cortical malformations in childhood. Neurology 1999;53(4):715–22.

68. Pardoe HR, Mandelstam SA, Hiess RK, et al. Quantitative assessment of corpus callosum morphology in periventricular nodular heterotopia. Epilepsy Res 2015;109:40–7.

69. Fujiwara T. Clinical spectrum of mutations in SCN1A gene: severe myoclonic epilepsy in infancy and related epilepsies. Epilepsy Res 2006; 70(Suppl 1):S223–30.

70. Sisodiya SM. Surgery for malformations of cortical development causing epilepsy. Brain 2000; 123(6):1075–91.

71. Noh GJ, Jane Tavyev Asher Y, Graham JM. Clinical review of genetic epileptic encephalopathies. Eur J Med Genet 2012;55(5):281–98.

72. Kuzniecky R. Epilepsy and malformations of cortical development: new developments. Curr Opin Neurol 2015;28(2):151–7.

73. Leventer RJ, Guerrini R, Dobyns WB. Malformations of cortical development and epilepsy. Dialogues Clin Neurosci 2008;10(1):47–62.

74. Li LM, Dubeau F, Andermann F, et al. Periventricular nodular heterotopia and intractable temporal lobe epilepsy: poor outcome after temporal lobe resection. Ann Neurol 1997;41(5):662–8.

75. Kothare SV, VanLandingham K, Armon C, et al. Seizure onset from periventricular nodular heterotopias: depth-electrode study. Neurology 1998; 51(6):1723–7.

76. Whiting AC, Bingaman JR, Catapano JS, et al. Laser interstitial thermal therapy for epileptogenic periventricular nodular heterotopia. World Neurosurg 2020;138:e892–7.

77. Kabat J, Król P. Focal cortical dysplasia - review. Polish J Radiol 2012;77(2):35–43.

78. Blümcke I, Thom M, Aronica E, et al. The clinicopathologic spectrum of focal cortical dysplasias: a consensus classification proposed by an ad hoc Task Force of the ILAE Diagnostic Methods Commission. Epilepsia 2011;52(1):158–74.

79. Fauser S. Clinical characteristics in focal cortical dysplasia: a retrospective evaluation in a series of 120 patients. Brain 2006;129(7):1907–16.

80. Hader WJ, Mackay M, Otsubo H, et al. Cortical dysplastic lesions in children with intractable epilepsy: role of complete resection. J Neurosurg 2004;100(2 Suppl):110–7.

81. Chaturvedi J, Rao MB, Arivazhagan A, et al. Epilepsy surgery for focal cortical dysplasia: Seizure and quality of life (QOLIE-89) outcomes. Neurol India 2018;66(6):1655–66.

82. Colombo N, Tassi L, Galli C, et al. Focal cortical dysplasias: MR imaging, histopathologic, and clinical correlations in surgically treated patients with epilepsy. AJNR Am J Neuroradiol 2003;24(4):724–33.

83. Porter BE, Brooks-Kayal A, Golden JA. Disorders of cortical development and epilepsy. Arch Neurol 2002;59(3):361.

84. Trounce JQ, Rutter N, Mellor DH. Hemimegalencephaly: diagnosis and teatment. Dev Med Child Neurol 1991;33(3):261–6.

85. King M, Stephenson JB, Ziervogel M, et al. Hemimegalencephaly–a case for hemispherectomy? Neuropediatrics 1985;16(1):46–55.

86. Chand P, Manglani P, Abbas Q. Hemimegalencephaly: seizure outcome in an infant after hemispherectomy. J Pediatr Neurosci 2018;13(1):106–8.

87. Leventer RJ, Jansen A, Pilz DT, et al. Clinical and imaging heterogeneity of polymicrogyria: a study of 328 patients. Brain 2010;133(Pt 5):1415–27.

88. Stutterd CA, Leventer RJ. Polymicrogyria: a common and heterogeneous malformation of cortical development. Am J Med Genet C Semin Med Genet 2014;166C(2):227–39.

89. Iannetti P, Nigro G, Spalice A, et al. Cytomegalovirus infection and schizencephaly: case reports. Ann Neurol 1998;43(1):123–7.

90. Barkovich AJ, Hevner R, Guerrini R. Syndromes of bilateral symmetrical polymicrogyria. AJNR Am J Neuroradiol 1999;20(10):1814–21.

91. Maillard L, Ramantani G. Epilepsy surgery for polymicrogyria: a challenge to be undertaken. Epileptic Disord 2018;20(5):319–38.

92. Ramantani G, Koessler L, Colnat-Coulbois S, et al. Intracranial evaluation of the epileptogenic zone in regional infrasylvian polymicrogyria. Epilepsia 2013;54(2):296–304.

93. Cossu M, Pelliccia V, Gozzo F, et al. Surgical treatment of polymicrogyria-related epilepsy. Epilepsia 2016;57(12):2001–10.

94. Ollivier I, Cebula H, Todeschi J, et al. Predictive factors of epilepsy in arteriovenous malformation. Neurochirurgie 2020;66(3):144–9.

95. Ding D, Starke RM, Quigg M, et al. Cerebral arteriovenous malformations and epilepsy, part 1: predictors of seizure presentation. World Neurosurg 2015;84(3):645–52.

96. Turjman F, Massoud TF, Sayre JW, et al. Epilepsy associated with cerebral arteriovenous malformations: a multivariate analysis of angioarchitectural characteristics. AJNR Am J Neuroradiol 1995; 16(2):345–50.

97. Soldozy S, Norat P, Yağmurlu K, et al. Arteriovenous malformation presenting with epilepsy: a multimodal approach to diagnosis and treatment. Neurosurg Focus 2020;48(4):E17.

98. Kraemer DL, Awad IA. Vascular malformations and epilepsy: clinical considerations and basic mechanisms. Epilepsia 1994;35(s6):S30–43.

99. Stephen LJ, Kwan P, Brodie MJ. Does the cause of localisation-related epilepsy influence the response to antiepileptic drug treatment? Epilepsia 2001; 42(3):357–62.

100. Josephson CB, Leach J-P, Duncan R, et al. Seizure risk from cavernous or arteriovenous malformations:

prospective population-based study. Neurology 2011;76(18):1548–54.

101. Ding D, Quigg M, Starke RM, et al. Cerebral arteriovenous malformations and epilepsy, part 2: predictors of seizure outcomes following radiosurgery. World Neurosurg 2015;84(3):653–62.

102. Yeo SS, Jang SH. Delayed neural degeneration following gamma knife radiosurgery in a patient with an arteriovenous malformation: a diffusion tensor imaging study. NeuroRehabilitation 2012;31(2):131–5.

103. Lv X, Li Y, Jiiang C, et al. Brain arteriovenous malformations and endovascular treatment: effect on seizures. Interv Neuroradiol 2010;16(1):39–45.

104. Awad IA, Polster SP. Cavernous angiomas: deconstructing a neurosurgical disease. J Neurosurg 2019;131(1):1–13.

105. Akers A, Al-Shahi Salman R, Awad I, et al. Synopsis of guidelines for the clinical management of cerebral cavernous malformations: consensus recommendations based on systematic literature review by the angioma alliance scientific advisory board clinical experts panel. Neurosurgery 2017;80(5): 665–80.

106. Al-Shahi Salman R, Hall JM, Horne MA, et al. Untreated clinical course of cerebral cavernous malformations: a prospective, population-based cohort study. Lancet Neurol 2012;11(3):217–24.

107. Chang EF, Gabriel RA, Potts MB, et al. Seizure characteristics and control after microsurgical resection of supratentorial cerebral cavernous malformations. Neurosurgery 2009;65(1):31–7 [discussion 37–8].

108. Baumann CR, Schuknecht B, Lo Russo G, et al. Seizure outcome after resection of cavernous malformations is better when surrounding hemosiderin-stained brain also is removed. Epilepsia 2006;47(3):563–6.

109. Englot DJ, Han SJ, Lawton MT, et al. Predictors of seizure freedom in the surgical treatment of supratentorial cavernous malformations. J Neurosurg 2011;115(6):1169–74.

110. Wong BKY, Sutton VR. Aicardi syndrome, an unsolved mystery: review of diagnostic features, previous attempts, and future opportunities for genetic examination. Am J Med Genet C Semin Med Genet 2018;178(4):423–31.

111. Aicardi J. Aicardi syndrome. Brain Dev 2005;27(3): 164–71.

112. Yamagata T, Momoi M, Miyamoto S, et al. Multiinstitutional survey of the Aicardi syndrome in Japan. Brain Dev 1990;12(6):760–5.

113. Rosser TL, Acosta MT, Packer RJ. Aicardi syndrome: spectrum of disease and long-term prognosis in 77 females. Pediatr Neurol 2002;27(5): 343–6.

114. Podkorytova I, Gupta A, Wyllie E, et al. Aicardi syndrome: epilepsy surgery as a palliative treatment

option for selected patients and pathological findings. Epileptic Disord 2016;18(4):431–9.

115. Proposal for revised clinical and electroencephalographic classification of epileptic seizures. From the Commission on Classification and Terminology of the International League Against Epilepsy. Epilepsia 1981;22(4):489–501.

116. Proposal for revised classification of epilepsies and epileptic syndromes. Commission on Classification and Terminology of the International League Against Epilepsy. Epilepsia 1989;30(4):389–99.

117. Koutroumanidis M, Arzimanoglou A, Caraballo R, et al. The role of EEG in the diagnosis and classification of the epilepsy syndromes: a tool for clinical practice by the ILAE Neurophysiology Task Force (Part 2). Epileptic Disord 2017;19(4):385–437.

118. Reddy S, Younus I, Sridhar V, et al. Neuroimaging biomarkers of experimental epileptogenesis and refractory epilepsy. Int J Mol Sci 2019;20(1):220.

119. Abela E, Rummel C, Hauf M, et al. Neuroimaging of epilepsy: lesions, networks, oscillations. Clin Neuroradiol 2014;24(1):5–15.

120. Scheffer IE, Berkovic S, Capovilla G, et al. ILAE classification of the epilepsies: position paper of the ILAE Commission for Classification and Terminology. Epilepsia 2017;58(4):512–21.

121. Møller RS, Dahl HA, Helbig I. The contribution of next generation sequencing to epilepsy genetics. Expert Rev Mol Diagn 2015;15(12):1531–8.

122. Dunn P, Albury CL, Maksemous N, et al. Next Generation Sequencing methods for diagnosis of epilepsy syndromes. Front Genet 2018;9:20.

123. Orsini A, Zara F, Striano P. Recent advances in epilepsy genetics. Neurosci Lett 2018;667:4–9.

124. Symonds JD, McTague A. Epilepsy and developmental disorders: next generation sequencing in the clinic. Eur J Paediatr Neurol 2020;24:15–23.

125. Tumienò B, Maver A, Writzl K, et al. Diagnostic exome sequencing of syndromic epilepsy patients in clinical practice. Clin Genet 2018;93(5):1057–62.

126. Elnady HG, Abdelmoneam N, Eissa E, et al. MicroRNAs as potential biomarkers for childhood epilepsy. Open Access Maced J Med Sci 2019; 7(23):3965–9.

127. Gahl WA, Markello TC, Toro C, et al. The National Institutes of Health Undiagnosed Diseases Program: insights into rare diseases. Genet Med 2012;14(1):51–9.

128. Wangler MF, Yamamoto S, Chao H-T, et al. Model organisms facilitate rare disease diagnosis and therapeutic research members of the undiagnosed diseases network (UDN), 2. Genetics 2017;207: 9–27.

129. Splinter K, Adams DR, Bacino CA, et al. Effect of genetic diagnosis on patients with previously undiagnosed disease. N Engl J Med 2018;379(22): 2131–9.

130. Turner TJ, Zourray C, Schorge S, et al. Recent advances in gene therapy for neurodevelopmental disorders with epilepsy. J Neurochem 2020; 157(2):229–62.

131. Aguti S, Malerba A, Zhou H. The progress of AAV-mediated gene therapy in neuromuscular disorders. Expert Opin Biol Ther 2018;18(6):681–93.

132. Cross JH. Epilepsy in 2020-a new dawn. Lancet Neurol 2021;20(1):8–10.

133. Meng L, Ward AJ, Chun S, et al. Towards a therapy for Angelman syndrome by targeting a long noncoding RNA. Nature 2015;518(7539):409–12.

134. Blumcke I, Spreafico R, Haaker G, et al. Histopathological findings in brain tissue obtained during epilepsy surgery. N Engl J Med 2017;377(17): 1648–56.

135. Lee JW. Histopathology of ~10,000 (Yes, That's TEN THOUSAND) brain tissue samples from epilepsy surgery. Epilepsy Curr 2018;18(2):101–3.

136. Hernandez-Ronquillo L, Miranzadeh Mahabadi H, Moien-Afshari F, et al. The Concept of an Epilepsy Brain Bank. Front Neurol 2020;11:1–11.

137. Gürsoy S, Erçal D. Diagnostic approach to genetic causes of early-onset epileptic encephalopathy. J Child Neurol 2016;31(4):523–32.

138. Anwar A, Saleem S, Patel UK, et al. Dravet syndrome: an overview. Cureus 2019;11(6):e5006.

139. Mastrangelo M. Lennox-gastaut syndrome: a state of the art review. Neuropediatrics 2017;48(3): 143–51.

140. Turnbull J, Tiberia E, Striano P, et al. Lafora disease. Epileptic Disord 2016;18(S2):38–62.

141. International League Against Epilepsy. Diagnostic manual. 2020. Available at: https://www. epilepsydiagnosis.org.

142. Epilepsy Foundation. Available at: https://www. epilepsy.com/learn/types-epilepsy-syndromes/.

143. Maraña Pérez AI, Ruiz-Falcó Rojas ML, Puertas Martín V, et al. Analysis of Sturge-Weber syndrome: a retrospective study of multiple associated variables. Neurologia 2017;32(6):363–70.

144. Wang DD, Knox R, Rolston JD, et al. Surgical management of medically refractory epilepsy in patients with polymicrogyria. Epilepsia 2016;57(1): 151–61.

145. Herbst SM, Proepper CR, Geis T, et al. LIS1-associated classic lissencephaly: a retrospective, multicenter survey of the epileptogenic phenotype and response to antiepileptic drugs. Brain Dev 2016; 38(4):399–406.

146. Hehr U, Uyanik G, Aigner L, et al. DCX-related disorders. 2007. In: Adam MP, Ardinger HH, Pagon RA, et al, editors. GeneReviews® [Internet]. Seattle (WA): University of Washington, Seattle; 1993–2021.

147. Bernasconi A, Martinez V, Rosa-Neto P, et al. Surgical resection for intractable epilepsy in "Double Cortex" syndrome yields inadequate results. Epilepsia 2002;42(9):1124–9.

148. Harvey AS, Freeman JL. Epilepsy in hypothalamic hamartoma: clinical and EEG features. Semin Pediatr Neurol 2007;14(2):60–4.

149. Scholly J, Staack AM, Kahane P, et al. Hypothalamic hamartoma: epileptogenesis beyond the lesion? Epilepsia 2017;58(Suppl 2):32–40.

150. Humbertclaude VT, Coubes PA, Robain O, et al. Early hemispherectomy in a case of hemimegalencephaly. Pediatr Neurosurg 1997;27(5):268–71.

151. Glass HC, Hong KJ, Rogers EE, et al. Risk factors for epilepsy in children with neonatal encephalopathy. Pediatr Res 2011;70(5):535–40.

Neurovascular Syndromes

Kristin A. Keith, DO, Laura K. Reed, MD, Anthony Nguyen, MD,
Rabia Qaiser, MD*

KEYWORDS

- Syndrome • Stroke • Cavernoma • Aneurysm • Cerebrovascular

KEY POINTS

- Patients with cerebrovascular syndromes are at risk for additional concerns associated with their syndrome.
- Multidisciplinary care is helpful to ensure comprehensive evaluation and management.
- Precise diagnosis and appreciation for the underlying syndrome is critical for effective cerebrovascular and broader care.

INTRODUCTION

A wide variety of syndromes are associated with cerebrovascular diseases (**Table 1**). This text focuses on these conditions with a focus on underlying pathophysiology and associated genetics, presentation, diagnosis, and management of each disease.

AUTOSOMAL DOMINANT

Hereditary hemorrhagic telangiectasia (HHT), also known as Osler-Weber-Rendu disease, is a heterogeneous autosomal dominant disorder characterized by mutations involved in the transforming growth factor-beta signaling pathway, endoglin (*ENG*), activin A receptor type II-like 1 (*ACVRL1*), and Mothers against decapentaplegic homolog 4 (*SMAD4*), which have been implicated in up to 85% of cases of HHT.[1,2]

HHT is characterized by recurrent epistaxis, telangiectasias of the hands, face, and oral cavity; and arteriovenous malformations (AVMs) involving select organs.[2,3] Most common presenting symptom in patients with HHT is epistaxis, with approximately 50% of patients reporting nosebleeds by the age of 10 years and 80% to 90% of patients reporting nosebleeds by the age of 21 years. Approximately 25% of patients with HHT develop gastrointestinal (GI) bleeding due to mucosal telangiectasia within the upper GI tract. Right-to-left shunting produced by pulmonary AVMs leads to development of paradoxic emboli, resulting in transient ischemic attack, stroke, and brain abscesses. Patients with HHT are at an increased risk of developing AVMs (**Fig. 1**), dural arteriovenous fistulas, cavernous malformations (CMs), or intracranial aneurysms, which may lead to either intracranial hemorrhage or seizurelike activity.[4]

The diagnosis of HHT is defined by the Curacao Criteria:

- Recurrent, spontaneous epistaxis
- Multiple mucocutaneous telangiectasias localized to the hands, face, nasal cavity, or oral cavity
- AVMs or telangiectasis localized to one or more of the following: lungs, liver, brain, stomach, spinal cord
- First-degree relative meeting definitive Curacao criteria for HHT or genetic diagnosis of HHT[5]

Management of HHT is supportive care based on symptoms. Epistaxis is typically managed conservatively unless unresponsive to medical management, thus requiring surgery. Use of tamoxifen, combined oral contraceptives, or tranexamic acid has been shown to decrease the frequency and/or severity of epistaxis.[6] Pulmonary AVMs with a feeding artery greater than 1 to 3 mm should be considered for treatment.

Baylor Scott & White Health/Texas A&M Neurosurgery Department, 2401 South 31st Street, MS-01-610A, Temple, TX 76508, USA
* Corresponding author.
E-mail addresses: Rabia.Qaiser@BSWHealth.org; rabiahq@gmail.com

neurosurgery.theclinics.com

Table 1
Cerebrovascular disease associated with syndromes

Hereditary Pattern	Syndrome	Associated Cerebrovascular Anomaly
Autosomal dominant	Hereditary hemorrhagic telangiectasia (HHT)/ Rendu-Osler-Weber syndrome	Aneurysm
	Vascular Ehlers-Danlos syndrome (vEDS)	Aneurysm
	Alagille syndrome (ALGS)	Aneurysm
	Marfan syndrome (MFS)	Aneurysm
	Loeys-Dietz syndrome (LDS)	Aneurysm
	Autosomal dominant polycystic kidney disease (ADPKD)	Aneurysm
	Neurofibromatosis type 1 (NF1)	Aneurysm
	Hutchinson-Gilford progeria syndrome (HGPS)	Stroke
	Familial cavernomatosis (FC)	Cavernoma
	Von Hippel-Lindau disease (VHL)	Hemangioblastoma
	Retinal vasculopathy with cerebral leukoencephalopathy (RVCL)	Stroke
	Cerebral autosomal dominant arteriopathy with subcortical infarcts and leukoencephalopathy (CADASIL)	Stroke
Autosomal recessive	Pseudoxanthoma elasticum (PXE)	Aneurysm
	Sickle cell disease (SCD)	Stroke
	Cerebral autosomal recessive arteriopathy with Subcortical Infarcts and Leukoencephalopathy (CARASIL)	Stroke
Sporadic	Sturge-Weber syndrome (SWS)	Seizures
	Klippel-Trénaunay-Weber syndrome (KTS)	Aneurysm
	Moyamoya disease (MMD)	Stroke
X-linked	Fabry disease	Stroke
Mitochondrial	Mitochondrial encephalopathy, lactic acidosis, and strokelike episodes (MELAS)	Stroke

Cerebral AVMs may typically require treatment via surgery, embolization, and/or stereotactic radiosurgery.[2]

Vascular Ehlers-Danlos syndrome (vEDS), previously known as Ehlers-Danlos type IV, is an autosomal dominant disorder involving type III collagen due to a mutation in the COL3A1 procollagen gene on chromosome 2.[7] The defect in type III collagen results in thin vessel walls, irregular elastic fibrils, and reduced cross-sectional area, leading to aneurysms, dissections, fistula formation, and ruptures.[8]

Significant allelic heterogeneity allows for varying degrees of symptoms.[7] The facial features include large eyes, sunken cheeks, thin nose and lips, micrognathia, and lobeless ears.[8] The disorder should be suspected in children if they bruise easily or have translucent skin with visible vasculature or acrogeria.[7] The neurovascular manifestations relevant to this text include spontaneous hemorrhage, internal carotid artery (ICA) aneurysms or others in the circle of Willis, carotid-cavernous fistulas (CCF), ischemic stroke, ectasia of blood vessels, vertebral artery aneurysms, dissections in extra- and intracranial arteries, and postarteriographic vascular blowouts. CCFs seem to be the most common complication[8] presenting with progressive chemosis, proptosis, ophthalmoplegia, and diminished visual acuity.[9]

Analysis by Sanger sequencing, exome sequence analysis, or genome sequence analysis are effective in revealing the gene mutation in 98% of patients. If a mutation is not found but the patient seems to have all the clinical features of vEDS, genome sequence analysis and examination of messenger RNA from cultured fibroblasts can aid in the identification of splicing variants in the introns.[7] Diagnostic procedures for neurovascular manifestations should remain noninvasive. Diagnostic angiography can have up to a 36% morbidity and 12% mortality according to one study.[8] Another study stated a 22% complication and a 5.6% death rate with angiography.[10] For these reasons, ultrasound Doppler, computed

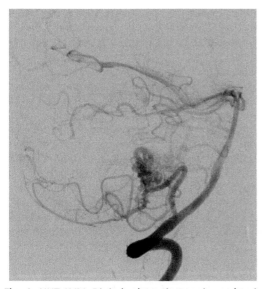

Fig. 1. HHT AVM. Digital subtraction angiography via the vertebral artery demonstrates an arteriovenous malformation arising from the posterior inferior cerebellar artery in a patient with hereditary hemorrhagic telangiectasia also known as Osler-Weber-Rendu disease.

tomography angiography, and MR angiography are preferred. Asymptomatic screening for intracranial vascular anomalies is not recommended at this point.[8]

Medical management is focused on avoiding adverse events associated with vEDS, for example, contact sports and activities resulting in rapid and frequent blood pressure elevations.[7] During neurovascular treatments, the mortality can be up to 40% due to the fragility of the blood vessels. Even with successful treatment, the disease recurrence rate is high and outcomes are poor.[8]

Endovascular management is preferred to open surgery if the anatomy is favorable. Because of the frailty of vasculature, puncture sites often have subsequent blowouts, fistulae development, and rupture. Aortic dissections/ruptures occur, and the death rate is high. Surgery may be the safer option for aneurysm treatment.[8]

Unruptured aneurysm treatment should be considered early, as delaying could allow development of a large, complicated, untreatable aneurysms. During aneurysm clipping, avulsion of any arterial branches or the aneurysm itself is common. Sharp dissection is recommended over blunt dissection. Proximal control is imperative and may be required in multiple locations. Minimal use of temporary clips can avoid future aneurysms or blowouts. Occasionally, temporary clips with less forceful closures can be preferred over permanent clips to decrease the risk of avulsion at the aneurysm neck. Treating all possible aneurysms in one surgery is preferred, with wrapping or clipping of any damaged arteries or infundibulums.[8]

CCF develop spontaneously and can be de novo or secondary to a cavernous ICA aneurysm rupture. An endovascular venous approach seems safer in order to avoid damage to major vessels in the transarterial approach.[8] Coils are preferred to permanent detachable balloons, as they are more easily controlled and cause less vascular disruption.[9]

Alagille Syndrome (ALGS) is an autosomal dominant disorder caused by defects of the Notch signaling pathway with most of the cases being due to JAG1 Notch ligand mutations. The second most common cause is mutations in the NOTCH2 receptor.[11,12]

The main organs/structures affected are the heart, liver, kidneys, skeletal system, eyes, face, and vasculature. The most common presenting signs and symptoms are cardiac murmurs, complications of pulmonic stenosis, and jaundice due to bile duct paucity. However, presentation varies widely among patients with ALGS.[11,12]

ALGS exhibits incomplete penetrance and variable expressivity. The classic criteria require that patients meet 3 of 5 criteria, which include neonatal conjugated hyperbilirubinemia, specific facial features, congenital heart disease, butterfly vertebrae or other particular vertebral abnormalities, and posterior embryotoxon. The advent of genetic testing has allowed for incorporation of JAG1 and NOTCH2 testing into diagnostic algorithms, but there are still yet patients with other gene mutations that cause ALGS.

The treatment of ALGS varies greatly from patient to patient due to the variability in phenotype. The management of cardiac, hepatic, renal, skeletal, facial, and ocular abnormalities is beyond the scope of this text.

Vascular complications have been described to account for 34% of mortality in patients with ALGS in one series described by a pediatric hospital.[13] It included patients who carried ALGS-associated mutations but did not necessarily exhibit signs/symptoms; 4% (11/268) of these patients were found to have intracerebral arterial abnormalities. Most of these patients (10/11) had aneurysms, and one was found to have Moyamoya syndrome (MMS). Two other series involving patients evaluated at pediatric hospitals detected cerebrovascular abnormalities in approximately one-third of patients. Most of these patients were asymptomatic and were undergoing screening. Arterial stenoses, dolichoectasia, aneurysms, and Moyamoya were the most commonly identified abnormalities. The treatment of patients with ALGS with Moyamoya is the same as those of patients with Moyamoya without ALGS. Aneurysms can be treated in a standard fashion. Screening of cerebrovascular disease in patients with ALGS is advocated for by some, although it is unclear whether early identification and treatment provides positive prognostic value.[14,15]

Marfan Syndrome (MFS) is an autosomal dominant disorder and is the most common connective tissue disorder. Up to 25% may be acquired through sporadic de novo mutations. The most frequent mutation is in the fibrillin 1 (*FBN1*) gene on chromosome 15, which is a regulator in the TGF-β signaling pathway.[16,17] The medial layer of the aortic root can demonstrate lamellae fragmentation, cystic necrosis, fibrosis, and loss of smooth muscle cells.[18]

MFS presents with aortic root dilation/dissection, mitral valve prolapse (MVP), long bones and joint laxity, pectus excavatum arachnodactyly, and ectopia lentis. Intracranial aneurysms in these patients are often found in the proximal intracranial ICA.[18,19] The prevalence can be up to 14%.[16] Patients with MFS can also develop ICA dissections. The risk of dissection is compounded by the severely tortuous carotid arteries that are present due to the mutations in collagen and elastic fibers.[17] Some literature also reports development of CCFs. Presentation of neurovascular abnormalities include ischemic stroke, transient ischemic attacks, subarachnoid hemorrhage, and so forth.[18] There is conflicting literature regarding the prevalence of aneurysms in MFS but the most recent study by Kim and colleagues demonstrated a prevalence of 11.9% in adults.[17,20]

MFS is diagnosed using the Ghent criteria that evaluate the aortic diameter, ectopia lentis, fibrillin-1 mutation, MVP, and family history of related connective tissue disorder. There is also a 20-point checklist that goes over the systemic features including skeletal and skin findings.[19]

The management of MFS focuses on identifying and preventing the main cause of death-aortic dissection and rupture. Screening for carotid tortuosity and risk of dissection or aneurysms is not currently recommended.[17]

Loeys-Dietz syndrome (LDS) is an autosomal dominant connective tissue disorder caused by mutations of the TGF-β signaling pathway. Several gene mutations have been identified, including TGFB2, TGFB3, TGFBR1, TGFBR2, SMAD2, and SMAD3.[21]

LDS presents somewhat similarly to Marfan syndrome but can be distinguished by thin, translucent skin with visible veins and easy bruisability.

Lens dislocation is not seen in LDS.[22] Aortic dilatation, pectus deformity, craniosynostosis, severe allergies, and blue sclerae are seen in patients with LDS.

LDS exhibits incomplete penetrance and variable expressivity, making diagnosis difficult. Diagnosis is made when an individual is found to be heterozygous for any of the 6 aforementioned gene mutations with either aortic root enlargement, type A aortic dissection, or typical cutaneous, craniofacial, vascular, and skeletal findings in combination.[21]

Given the multisystem involvement of LDS, the treatment involves multidisciplinary care. The median life expectancy in a series by Loeys and colleagues was 37 years.[23] Screening for intracerebral abnormalities, typically aneurysms or severe tortuosity, is recommended as death from intracerebral hemorrhage occurred at as young as 3 years of age.[24] Head and neck aneurysms have a reported prevalence of 10% to 56% of patients with LDS.[23,25,26] Patients should be appropriately screened. Both clipping and coiling have been successfully carried out.[27,28]

Autosomal dominant polycystic kidney disease (ADPKD) is the most common inherited renal disease; however it also results in multisystem extrarenal manifestations. ADPKD results from a mutation in 1 of 2 genes, PKD1 (chromosome 16) or PKD2 (chromosome 4); however, the presentation of the disease is highly variable and attributed to the "two-hit model" characterized by a germline mutation and a somatic mutation that inactivate PKD alleles independently.[29] There have been rare instances of severe disease presenting in infancy or early childhood, which have been hypothesized to be secondary to a contiguous gene syndrome involving the simultaneous deletion of PKD1 and TSC2 (tuberous sclerosis) genes, located on chromosome 16[30].

Presentation of ADPKD is highly variable within the population; however, studies have indicated that mutations in PKD1 gene are associated with earlier onset ESRD than that of mutations in PKD2 gene.[31] Clinical manifestations include hypertension, back and/or abdominal pain, urinary tract infections, hematuria, chronic kidney disease, and liver cysts. Vascular abnormalities include endothelial dysfunction, left ventricular hypertrophy, abnormal ventricular relaxation, dilated cardiomyopathy, and intracranial aneurysms.[32]

A positive family history of ruptured intracranial aneurysms in patients with ADPKD remains higher than that of the general population. In addition, studies have indicated a 3- to 5-fold higher incidence rate of intracranial aneurysms as compared with the general population with 8% to 9% in patients with ADPKD versus 2% to 3% in the general population. The mechanism behind this remains unclear; however, Sanchez Munoz reports that the mutations of ADPKD genes resulting in the loss of polycystic protein within the vasculature may lead to increased formation of intracranial aneurysms in the setting of known risk factors including smoking, hypertension, and chronic kidney disease.[32]

Diagnosis is based most commonly on renal ultrasonography, which demonstrates kidney enlargement with multiple middle-sized cysts and increased total kidney volume of more than 1 L.[33] In cases with an atypical presentation, ultrasonography and molecular genetic testing can be performed via either linkage analysis or direct mutation analysis.[34]

Management of intracranial aneurysms in ADPKD with or without subarachnoid hemorrhage should be managed similarly to non-ADPKD patients via endovascular versus open surgical procedures.[35] One of the main considerations in endovascular management of intracranial aneurysms in ADPKD is the concern for contrast-induced nephropathy, a known associated risk of angiography, particularly in patients with baseline chronic kidney disease stage 5 or high serum creatinine level (serum creatinine >2.0 mg/dL), both of which were associated with an increased risk of developing acute renal impairment.[36]

Neurofibromatosis-1 (NF1), also known as Von Recklinghausen disease, is an autosomal dominant disorder caused by a mutation in the NF1 gene found on chromosome 17q11.2, which encodes for the tumor suppressor protein neurofibromin. Loss of neurofibromin leads to dysregulation of the cell cycle and unregulated proliferation.

Signs/symptoms typically include cutaneous and subcutaneous neurofibromas, café au lait spots, hamartomas of the iris (Lisch nodules), axillary/inguinal freckling, or sphenoid bone dysplasia or leg bowing. Cutaneous neurofibromas can be numerous and can be extremely disfiguring.[37] Neurologic deficits can be seen in those with optic gliomas or intracerebral aneurysms.

The National Institutes of Health has published criteria for establishing the diagnosis of NF1. These criteria require that patients exhibit any 2 of the following at minimum: a first-degree relative with NF1, greater than 6 café au lait spots measuring either greater than 5 mm in prepubertal persons or greater than 15 mm in postpubertal persons, 2 neurofibromas or 1 plexiform neurofibroma, 2 Lisch nodules, axillary/inguinal freckling, sphenoid dysplasia or tibial pseudoarthrosis, or an optic glioma. Children with only one of the diagnostic criteria, if severe, may benefit from genetic testing to establish the diagnosis of NF1 at an earlier age.[37] Treatment of NF1 is targeted at an individual's particular symptoms but typically involves optimizing quality of life by addressing psychosocial factors, treating pain, and surgical intervention for amenable masses.[38]

NF1 is associated with an increased risk of intracranial aneurysms.[39] In addition, there have been reports of NF1 patients with AVMs and MMS.[40–42] Aneurysm treatment with microsurgical clipping and endovascular techniques has been described.[40,43,44] However, it has been reported that vessel walls are more fragile in patients with NF1; thus, vessel sacrifice may be a reasonable option in selected patients.[40,45,46] Noniatrogenic MMS has been identified in numerous children with NF1 as young as 8 months of age and has been successfully managed with surgical revascularization.[41,42,47]

Hutchinson-Gilford Progeria syndrome (HGPS), also known as progeria, is a sporadic autosomal dominant disorder caused by mutations in the LMNA gene, which encodes prelamin-A/C; this leads to truncation and persistent farnesylation of prelamin-A/C, which is known as progerin, and accumulation in the inner nuclear membrane, resulting in cell damage and early senescence.[48] Although the mutation demonstrates autosomal dominant patterns of expression, almost all individuals diagnosed with HGPS develop the condition as a result of a de novo mutation.

Neonates born with HGPS seem phenotypically normal; the median age of diagnosis is 19 months. Presenting symptoms are failure to thrive, skin atrophy, alopecia, osteolysis, and joint issues such as decreased range of motion.[48–50] Patients may experience seizures, strokes, and myocardial infarctions later on.

It is based on the aforementioned symptoms as well as typical physical characteristics such as prominent scalp veins, retrognathia, micrognathia, circumoral cyanosis, dystrophic nails, or low-frequency conductive hearing loss. On genetic testing the diagnosis of classic HGPS is then made if a c.1824C>T mutation in an allele of the LMNA gene is found. Nonclassic HGPS is confirmed with a pathogenic mutation in exon 11 splice junction or intron 11 of an allele of the LMNA gene, resulting in progerin production.[48,50]

Currently there is only one Federal Drug Administration–approved drug—Lonafarnib, which is a farnesyltransferase inhibitor and has demonstrated a mortality benefit in clinical trials.[51–54] It significantly lowered rates of transient ischemic attacks, strokes, and seizures. Although atherosclerosis and intracranial stenosis (distinct from Moyamoya) likely contribute to stroke, statins have not been demonstrated to provide a reduction in stroke burden or a mortality benefit.

Familial cavernomatosis (FC) is a highly penetrant autosomal dominant or sporadic disorder generally resulting in multiple CMs. Mutations have been found in CCM1/KRIT1, CCM2/MGC4607, and CCM3/PDCD10. These patients have a higher risk of intracranial hemorrhages. CCM3/PDCD10 mutations also have associated cutaneous and spinal lesions, cognitive delay, and brain tumors.[55]

The patients most often present with seizures, intracranial hemorrhage, or new neurologic deficit at an average age of 10 years. After one seizure, there is up to a 94% risk of developing epilepsy within 5 years.[55] The most common locations reported in children have been the brain stem, spinal cord, and basal ganglia.[56] Spinal CM can cause hemorrhage or edema in the spinal cord and present with paraplegia.[57]

Computed tomography (CT) scans may be used to identify hemorrhagic CMs or those causing hydrocephalus. MRI, specifically susceptibility-weighted imaging, is the recommended modality to identify suspected CMs (**Fig. 2**). MRI should be used when there is suspicion of familial disease or in children with newly diagnosed epilepsy with unknown cause.[55] The diagnosis of FC is officially diagnosed when there are multiple CMs; one CM plus another family member with CMs; and/or mutations in KRIT1, CCM2, or PDCD10.

Conservative management is preferred in asymptomatic lesions or in patients with well-controlled epilepsy. If a hemorrhage occurs or if seizures are uncontrolled, surgery or gamma-knife radiation can be considered. Radiation is favored for deep lesions or those in the brainstem to reduce the risk of future hemorrhage. Superficial lesions or those causing a large hemorrhage are more amenable to surgery but must be resected completely to reduce postoperative bleeding.[55] Before epilepsy surgery, a prolonged electroencephalogram is recommended to ensure the CM is the seizure focus. It is recommended that the surrounding gold-tinged margin also be resected to ensure the entire seizure focus has been removed. Postoperatively, seizure freedom is achieved in up to 60% of patients.[56]

Von Hippel-Lindau disease (VHL) is an autosomal dominant syndrome, with complete penetrance, due to mutations in the VHL tumor suppressor gene on chromosome 3. Hypoxia-inducible factors (HIFs) accumulate due to the lack of suppression from the VHL complex. They cause an increase in expression of tumorigenic factors such as vascular endothelial growth factor and platelet-derived growth factor, resulting in numerous vascular lesions. VHL has 2 types: type 1 involves an alteration in protein folding and has a low risk of pheochromocytoma, and type 2 is a missense mutation and is associated with renal cell carcinoma and pheochromocytoma. Neurovascularly, patients develop hemangioblastomas in the cerebellum, retina, brainstem, and spinal cord.[58] Currently, there are studies that show a possible association between intracranial aneurysms and VHL but the results have not been statistically significant.[59]

Cerebellar hemangioblastomas (**Figs. 3** and **4**) in pediatrics can present with headaches, nausea, vomiting, and hydrocephalus as also seen in other common pediatric posterior fossa tumors.[58] Spinal hemangioblastomas seem similar to AVMs, as they develop large arteries and veins entering and exiting the lesion. These tumors can involve the nerve root and present with syrinx, myelopathy, and/or radiculopathy.[2]

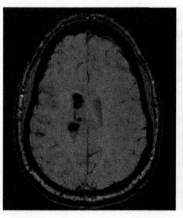 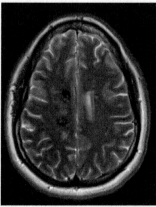

Fig. 2. Cavernomas. MRI of a patient with multiple cavernomas as demonstrated on susceptibility weighted imaging (SWI) (*left*) and T2-weighted imaging (*right*). Cavernomas demonstrate a blooming artifact on SWI and have a hypointense rim with heterogenous internal signal on T2-weighted imaging due to varying age of blood products.

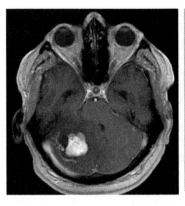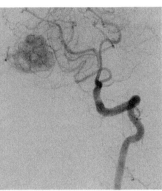

Fig. 3. Hemangioblastoma. T1-weighted MRI (*left*) demonstrating a contrast-enhancing cerebellar lesion consistent with hemangioblastoma. A blood vessel in close proximity is visualized. Digital subtraction angiography via the vertebral artery again demonstrates this hemangioblastoma, which seems as a highly vascular lesion (*right*).

Surveillance of children with a family history should begin at 1 year of age. Screening for neurologic changes, vision problems, hearing difficulties, and having an annual ophthalmologic examination is recommended. By age 5 years, urine metanephrines and audiology tests are standard. If the patient has frequent ear infections, MRI is recommended. By age 16 years, annual abdominal, brain, and spine MRI are recommended.[60] Without family history, diagnosis is made when children present with hemangioblastomas and the aforementioned testing with genetic screening ensues.[58]

Surgery with complete resection of hemangioblastomas can be curative.[58] Preoperative embolization during conventional angiography can aid in surgical preparation.[2]

Retinal vasculopathy with cerebral leukoencephalopathy (RVCL) is a rare autosomal dominant disorder that affects highly vascularized tissues including the retina, brain, liver, and kidneys that results due to C-terminal frameshift mutation within TREX1 gene.[61,62]

The most common presenting symptoms of RVCL are related to retinal vasculopathy including decreased visual acuity or visual field deficits. Neurologic symptoms, impaired hepatic and renal functions, and subclinical hypothyroidism are common.[62]

RCVL should be suspected in patients with vascular retinopathy, focal or global neurologic symptoms associated with MRI brain abnormalities restricted to the white matter, and a positive family history, although absence of positive family history does not preclude a diagnosis. The diagnosis is confirmed with TREX1 variant identified by genetic testing.[61–63] Treatment is supportive with treatment of the underlying symptoms.[62]

Cerebral autosomal dominant arteriopathy with subcortical infarcts and leukoencephalopathy (CADASIL) is an autosomal dominant disorder characterized by small vessel cerebrovascular arteriopathy that results from mutation in NOTCH3.[64,65] The most common presenting symptom is recurrent ischemic stroke with significant cognitive decline progressing to dementia.[64]

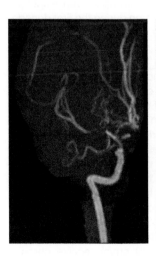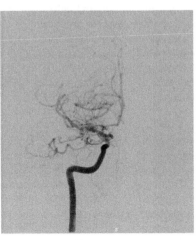

Fig. 4. Moyamoya. Magnetic resonance angiography demonstrates high-grade stenosis of the right middle cerebral artery with collateralization (*left*) consistent with Moyamoya disease. Digital subtraction angiography again demonstrates stenosis and extensive collateralization (*right*).

There is no consensus on criteria or characteristics needed for the diagnosis of CADASIL, and the findings are fairly nonspecific; however, it has been suggested that CADASIL should be suspected with the following findings:

- Unexplained white matter hyperintensity on MRI brain
- Positive family history of stroke and/or vascular dementia (although absence of positive family history does not preclude diagnosis)

In addition, diagnosis is confirmed with mutation in NOTCH3 determined via genetic testing.[64] Treatment is supportive for underlying symptoms.[64]

AUTOSOMAL RECESSIVE

Pseudoxanthoma elasticum (PXE) is an autosomal recessive metabolic disorder caused by ABCC6 gene mutations. ABCC6 is hypothesized to maintain systemic circulation of inorganic pyrophosphate, an antimineralization factor. As a result, individuals with PXE develop ectopic mineralization of their vasculature, skin, and eyes.[66]

PXE presents in childhood or adolescence with oculocutaneous manifestations such as retinal angioid streaks, retinal hemorrhage, or characteristic yellow papules in the lateral neck, nape, or flexural creases. Later on in the course of the disease, patients develop vascular signs and complications such as claudication, transient ischemic attack, stroke, or GI bleed.[66,67]

Diagnosis involves fundoscopy, skin biopsy, and ABCC6 gene testing. Genetic testing diagnostically classifies results as not PXE, probably not or possible PXE, probable PXE, and definite PXE.[68,69]

The treatment of PXE depends on the patient's manifestations. Vascular manifestations are managed in a standard fashion such as risk factor modification (diet, exercise, weight loss) for general cardiovascular health or bypass for high-grade stenosis. The blood vessels of a patient with PXE are not brittle despite calcification of the intima and media.[70] Although antiplatelet therapy is relatively contraindicated in PXE due to the increased risk of GI bleed, the benefits of lowering stroke risk with antiplatelet therapy may outweigh the risks of GI bleed in certain patients.[68,71,72] Future options may include gene editing; however, currently there is no cure currently for PXE.[66]

Sickle cell disease (SCD) results from a single base-pair point mutation within the β-globulin gene resulting in substitution of valine for glutamic acid within the sixth position of the β-chain of the hemoglobin molecule, leading to the formation of hemoglobin S (HbS). Red blood cells (RBCs) containing the HbS molecule when exposed to deoxygenated environments undergo polymerization of the HbS molecules, resulting in sickling and the formation of a rigid structure. Because of the rigid structure of the RBCs, hemolysis and vaso-occlusion with resulting tissue ischemia and infarction and altered blood flow mechanics are common.[73]

Patient presentation highly depends on the percentage of fetal hemoglobin (HbF) present. SCD typically manifests after 6 months of age—when the HbF levels begin to naturally decrease.[74] Findings include hemolytic anemia, vaso-occlusive pain crisis, frequent infection with encapsulated organisms (frequently *Streptococcus pneumoniae*, *Staphylococcus aureus*, *Haemophilus influenzae type B*, *Neisseria meningitidis*) due to functional asplenia or splenic infarcts resulting from vaso-occlusion and aplastic crisis related to bone marrow failure.[74]

Vaso-occlusive pain crisis results in severe pain related to stimulation of nociceptive pain fibers caused by microvascular occlusion, leading to restricted blood flow, ischemia, pain, and if prolonged, necrosis and organ damage. Vaso-occlusive pain crisis may occur as early as infancy and tends to result in "regression" tendencies (during infancy).[73]

Acute stroke or chronic cerebrovascular ischemia is one of the more severe consequences of SCD.[75] Internal carotid arteries and the circle of Willis are particularly vulnerable,[76] leading to the development of Moyamoya syndrome. Risk of stroke in patients with SCD is highest within the first decade of life at approximately 1.02% per year with a particularly high recurrence rate of stroke (approximately 66%); however, the stroke subtype seems to vary with age—with ischemic infarct being more common during the first decade of life and after age 30 years. Hemorrhagic stroke has been seen to be more common during the 20s.[77] In addition, the STOP1 trial demonstrated that children with abnormal transcranial Doppler (TCD) velocities (>200 cm/s) in large cerebral vessels had a 40% risk of stroke within 3 years.[77]

Mandatory newborn screening in the United States for SCD includes a test for HbS. Initial screening test includes a complete blood count with peripheral smear, which is followed by hemoglobin electrophoresis to confirm the diagnosis.[74]

Based off of findings from the STOP 1 trial, it was recommended that children ages 2 to 16 years with Sickle Cell Disease (HbSS) or Sickle ß-thalassemia without prior stroke history however with presence of abnormal TCDs (>200 cm/s) receive chronic blood transfusions with goal HbS 30 for prevention of ischemic stroke.[77,78] Use of hydroxyurea has been shown to increase HbF levels, and immunization against encapsulated organisms is recommended in patients with SCD due to functional asplenia.[79]

Cerebral autosomal recessive arteriopathy with subcortical infarcts and leukoencephalopathy (CARASIL) is an autosomal recessive disorder affecting cerebral small vessels that results from mutation in HTRA1. CARASIL is characterized as a "ischemic, non-hypertensive, small vessel cerebrovascular disease."[80] The clinical presentation is similar to CADASIL, with cerebrovascular ischemia that typically has earlier onset in comparison, as well as presence of gait disturbance, low back pain, lower extremity muscular spasticity, and alopecia[80,81]

Diagnosis of CARASIL is based on the "classic CARASIL" phenotype and should be suspected in patients presenting before 55 years of age with slowly progressive dementia and gait disturbances with associated development of spasticity of the bilateral lower extremities. The diagnosis is confirmed with mutation in HTRA1 determined via genetic testing.[80,81] Treatment is supportive of underlying symptoms.[81]

SPORADIC

Sturge-Weber syndrome (SWS) is a rare neurocutaneous syndrome caused by a sporadic somatic mutation in the GNAQ gene, key in the regulation of blood vessels.

Patients often present with a characteristic port-wine nevus, which typically involves the V1 distribution of the trigeminal nerve; however, it can extend onto the trunk and extremities. Ophthalmologic disorders, most commonly glaucoma or diffuse choroidal hemangioma, may be present. Neurologic manifestations include seizures, mental retardation, headaches/migraines, and/or focal neurologic deficits (usually hemiparesis) and are highly variable.[2,82]

Patients with intracranial involvement most commonly present with seizurelike activity in infancy. Seizures develop in approximately 80% of patients with unilateral intracranial involvement and approximately 93% of patients with bihemispheric intracranial involvement. Cognitive impairment frequently occurs; however, the degree of this varies significantly. Onset of seizures before age 2 years as well as bilateral brain involvement and severity or uncontrolled seizures increases the likelihood of severe cognitive impairment. There is an increased prevalence of endocrinology abnormalities, including growth hormone deficiency and central hypothyroidism. It has been postulated that the central hypothyroidism is related to long-term antiepileptic drug (AED) usage.[2,83]

SWS should be suspected in any newborn presenting with a port-wine nevus involving the V1 distribution of the trigeminal nerve. The risk of brain involvement in the setting of a port-wine nevus of any size within the V1 distribution is approximately 10% to 20%, which increases with size and/or presence of bilateral port wine nevus. In the presence of facial cutaneous angioma, neuroimaging studies can determine the presence of intracranial involvement. Head CT demonstrates the classic "cortical and subcortical gyral calcification." Commonly described "tram-track" sign first described in radiographs is not frequently visualized. The gold-standard for diagnosis of intracranial involvement in SWS is by visualization of classic leptomeningeal vascular malformation seen on contrast-enhanced T1-weighted MR image with dilation and enhancement of abnormal intracranial vasculature. Cerebral angiography is not necessary, but it can be helpful in patients with an atypical presentation or before epilepsy surgery and is abnormal in approximately 82% of cases and demonstrates enlarged, tortuous subependymal and medullary veins with absent or sparse superficial cortical veins.[2,83]

Treatment is typically multidisciplinary and directed at treating the underlying symptoms. Seizures are treated with AEDs, although the effectiveness of AEDs in managing seizurelike activity is highly variable.[2] Focal surgical resection of the underlying vascular abnormality has been shown to be beneficial particularly in management of medically refractory seizure, especially when arising from a focal area. Hemispherectomy has shown encouraging outcomes, with 81% of patients becoming seizure free and more than half of the patients no longer requiring AED medication usage.[2,83]

Klippel-Trénaunay-Weber syndrome (KTS) is a sporadically occurring dysfunction of capillary, venous, and lymphatic formation caused by mutations of the PIK3CA gene. The pathophysiology of the disease is unclear, but it is thought to be related to dysregulation of embryonic angiogenesis. KTS is similar to Parkes-Weber syndrome (PWS), but in PWS, AVMs are high flow malformations, and the gene involved is RASA1.[84,85]

Classic signs and symptoms are nevus flammeus at birth, skin breakdown, pain, lymphedema, port-wine stains, varicosities, and soft tissue and bone hypertrophy in the affected limb.[84,86] KTS has been reported to be associated with intracranial aneurysms and should be worked up in patients who exhibit neurologic signs or symptoms.[87–90]

Diagnosis is clinical when at least 2 of the classic triad are present: hypertrophy of bony and soft tissues, venous abnormalities, and capillary malformations.[86]

The severity of symptoms influences KTS management. Although the treatment of vascular malformations, capillary malformations, and limb-length discrepancy are beyond the scope of this article, there is promising evidence for rapamycin, an mTOR inhibitor for preventing worsening vascular lesions.[91] It is not yet known if this has an impact on intracranial aneurysm formation.

Patients with KTS may harbor multiple aneurysms. The exact prevalence of intracranial aneurysms in patients with KTS is unknown but is estimated at less than 10%. Reported interventions have included conservative serial monitoring due to high surgical risk, vessel sacrifice, and open clipping (which was performed on an 8-year-old patient).[87–90] Patients with KTS would likely benefit from newer endovascular interventions. Given the significant association of KTS with intracranial aneurysms, some advocate for screening in these patients.[90]

Moyamoya disease (MMD) is a progressive steno-occlusive disease of ICA, middle cerebral artery (MCA), and anterior cerebral artery (ACA). This disease causes development of collateral vessels that appear at the base of the brain and look similar to a "puff of smoke" (Moyamoya in Japanese). There have been many studies yielding innumerable genetic associations with MMD that go beyond the scope of this text; however, it is clear that the disease is a result of environmental factors, ethnicity, and genetic predisposition. Moyamoya syndrome refers to an angiopathy that is associated with other manifestations in diseases that can be inherited or acquired.[92]

Pediatric patients mostly present with recurrent ischemic events. These can be triggered by hyperventilation episodes due to physical activity, dehydration, fever, or crying. MMC children may also have intellectual disability, seizures, headaches, epilepsy, or, rarely, choreic movement disorders from basal ganglia infarcts.[92]

Angiography (MR, CT, or conventional) with demonstration of stenosis of one or all of ICAs, ACAs, and/or MCAs is required for diagnosis. The "puff of smoke" can be seen in the basal ganglia and thalamic regions. MRI will often show ischemia of varying chronicity.[92] Severity of the disease is graded using the Suzuki classification system.[93]

There is no cure for MMD. Children are advised to avoid hypotension, dehydration, and hyperventilation. They should take aspirin to avoid thrombosis at the stenotic areas. Revascularization surgeries are the mainstay of treatment. Indirect bypass using external carotid branches superimposed on the brain surface to promote angiogenesis are generally used in pediatric population.[93] Indirect bypasses include encephalomyosynangiosis (EMS), where a piece of the temporal muscle flap is placed on the brain surface, and encephaloduroarteriosynangiosis (EDAS), where the posterior branch of the superficial temporal artery and its surrounding galea is placed on the brain. Up to 30% of these patients still do not develop sufficient collaterals. Combined indirect approaches such as the frontotemporoparietal approach use all 3 branches of the STA; an encephalomyoarteriosynangiosis over the frontal lobe and EDAS and EMS over the temporal and parietal lobes can increase the chances of collateral development.[2] Direct bypass where an STA branch is directly anastomosed to an MCA branch is generally reserved for older patients.

X-LINKED

Fabry disease is an X-linked lysosomal storage disease with a deficiency in alpha-galactosidase A. Classic Fabry disease with minimal or no enzyme activity will present early in childhood. More commonly, there is residual enzyme function and those individuals present later in life. Cardiomyopathy and cerebrovascular disease present in mid- to late adulthood and are not found in the pediatric population.[94]

Children can present with angiokeratomas, acroparesthesias, and hypo-/hyperhidrosis. As globotriaosylceramide accumulates in the kidneys, cardiac tissue, and cerebrovascular system, multisystem organ failure develops.[95] Angiokeratomas appear as blue-black lesions. Facial dysmorphism may be present and include periorbital fullness, full eyebrows, recessed forehead, pronounced nose, bulbous nasal tip, prominent supraorbital rim, shallow midface, full lips, posteriorly rotated ears, and prognathism.[95] Other symptoms include GI changes, tinnitus, vertigo, and fatigue. Women tend to present later than men.[96] Patients can also present with pain caused by deposits in the dorsal root ganglia or by neuropathy.[97]

Children with family history of Fabry disease can be screened during newborn genetic testing. Tests include enzyme activity measurement, glycosphingolipid accumulation measurements, and genetic analyses. In men, the alpha-galactosidase A activity can be detected in plasma or leukocytes; women generally have normal levels of enzyme activity.[94]

Enzyme replacement therapy is the primary treatment regimen. The available recombinant alpha-galactosidase A include agalsidase alfa and agalsidase beta.[94,97]

MITOCHONDRIAL

Mitochondrial encephalomyopathy, lactic acidosis, and stroke-like episodes is a maternally inherited mitochondrial disorder that occurs due to an adenine to guanine transition in mitochondrial DNA.[98] Strokelike episodes are often the primary debilitating symptom. Up to 76% present before 20 years of age, and up to 99% have strokelike episodes as their primary symptom. Usually these do not follow a typical vascular distribution.[98]

Diagnostic criteria include strokelike episodes before age 40 years, encephalopathy with seizures and/or dementia, mitochondrial myopathy with lactic acidosis, or ragged-red fibers with at least 2 of the following: normal early psychomotor development, recurrent headaches, and recurrent vomiting.[98,99]

Patients are generally treated symptomatically. In some studies L-arginine is thought to increase vasodilation and blood flow through an increase in nitrous oxide synthesis.[100,101]

CLINICS CARE POINTS

- A multidisciplinary approach is recommended in patients with neurovascular disorders for optimal treatment.

- Genetic testing should be performed in any pediatric patient with an intracranial aneurysm to screen for possible syndromes. Additionally, certain syndromes may affect the standard-of-care for the patients' aneurysm(s), as some mutations result in more fragile vessel walls.

- Pediatric patients with Moyamoya disease (MMD) typically present with recurrent ischemic events and thus MMD should be suspected in those with multiple stroke-like episode.

REFERENCES

1. McDonald J, Wooderchak-Donahue W, VanSant Webb C, et al. Hereditary hemorrhagic telangiectasia: genetics and molecular diagnostics in a new era. Front Genet 2015;6. https://doi.org/10.3389/fgene.2015.00001.

2. Alexander MJ, Spetzler RF. Pediatric neurovascular disease: surgical, endovascular, and medical management. New York: Thieme; 2006.

3. Sadick H, Sadick M, Götte K, et al. Hereditary hemorrhagic telangiectasia: an update on clinical manifestations and diagnostic measures. Wien Klin Wochenschr 2006;118(3–4):72–80.

4. Maher CO, Piepgras DG, Brown RD, et al. Cerebrovascular Manifestations in 321 Cases of Hereditary Hemorrhagic Telangiectasia. Stroke 2001;32(4):877–82.

5. Shovlin CL, Guttmacher AE, Buscarini E, et al. Diagnostic criteria for hereditary hemorrhagic telangiectasia (Rendu-Osler-Weber syndrome). Am J Med Genet 2000;91(1):66–7.

6. Grigg C, Anderson D, Earnshaw J. Diagnosis and Treatment of Hereditary Hemorrhagic Telangiectasia. Ochsner J 2017;17(2):157–61.

7. Byers PH, Belmont J, Black J, et al. Diagnosis, natural history, and management in vascular Ehlers-Danlos syndrome. Am J Med Genet C Semin Med Genet 2017;175(1):40–7.

8. Olubajo F, Kaliaperumal C, Choudhari KA. Vascular Ehlers-Danlos Syndrome: Literature review and surgical management of intracranial vascular complications. Clin Neurol Neurosurg 2020;193:105775. https://doi.org/10.1016/j.clineuro.2020.105775.

9. Hollands JK, Santarius T, Kirkpatrick PJ, et al. Treatment of a direct carotid-cavernous fistula in a patient with type IV Ehlers-Danlos syndrome: a novel approach. Neuroradiology 2006;48(7):491–4.

10. Freeman RK, Swegle J, Sise MJ. The surgical complications of Ehlers-Danlos syndrome. Am Surg 1996;62(10):869–73.

11. Turnpenny PD, Ellard S. Alagille syndrome: pathogenesis, diagnosis and management. Eur J Hum Genet EJHG 2012;20(3):251–7.

12. Diaz-Frias J, Kondamudi NP. Alagille Syndrome. In: StatPearls. StatPearls Publishing. 2021. Available at: http://www.ncbi.nlm.nih.gov/books/NBK507827/. Accessed February 26, 2021.

13. Kamath BM, Spinner NB, Emerick KM, et al. Vascular anomalies in Alagille syndrome: a significant cause of morbidity and mortality. Circulation 2004;109(11):1354–8.

14. Emerick KM, Krantz ID, Kamath BM, et al. Intracranial vascular abnormalities in patients with Alagille syndrome. J Pediatr Gastroenterol Nutr 2005;41(1):99–107.

15. Carpenter CD, Linscott LL, Leach JL, et al. Spectrum of cerebral arterial and venous abnormalities in Alagille syndrome. Pediatr Radiol 2018;48(4):602–8.

16. Maleszewski JJ, Miller DV, Lu J, et al. Histopathologic findings in ascending aortas from individuals

with Loeys-Dietz syndrome (LDS). Am J Surg Pathol 2009;33(2):194–201.

17. Parlapiano G, Di Lorenzo F, Salehi LB, et al. Neurovascular manifestations in connective tissue diseases: The case of Marfan Syndrome. Mech Ageing Dev 2020;191:111346. https://doi.org/10.1016/j.mad.2020.111346.

18. Kim ST, Brinjikji W, Lanzino G, et al. Neurovascular manifestations of connective-tissue diseases: A review. Interv Neuroradiol 2016;22(6):624–37.

19. Radke RM, Baumgartner H. Diagnosis and treatment of Marfan syndrome: an update. Heart 2014;100(17):1382–91.

20. Kim JH, Kim JW, Song S-W, et al. Intracranial Aneurysms Are Associated With Marfan Syndrome: Single Cohort Retrospective Study in 118 Patients Using Brain Imaging. Stroke 2021;52(1):331–4.

21. Loeys BL, Dietz HC. Loeys-Dietz Syndrome. In: Adam MP, Ardinger HH, Pagon RA, et al, editors. GeneReviews®. Seattle (WA): University of Washington, Seattle; 1993. Available at: http://www.ncbi.nlm.nih.gov/books/NBK1133/. Accessed February 26, 2021.

22. MacCarrick G, Black JH, Bowdin S, et al. Loeys-Dietz syndrome: a primer for diagnosis and management. Genet Med 2014;16(8):576–87.

23. Loeys BL, Schwarze U, Holm T, et al. Aneurysm syndromes caused by mutations in the TGF-beta receptor. N Engl J Med 2006;355(8):788–98.

24. Williams JA, Loeys BL, Nwakanma LU, et al. Early surgical experience with Loeys-Dietz: a new syndrome of aggressive thoracic aortic aneurysm disease. Ann Thorac Surg 2007;83(2):S757–63.

25. van der Linde D, van de Laar IMBH, Bertoli-Avella AM, et al. Aggressive cardiovascular phenotype of aneurysms-osteoarthritis syndrome caused by pathogenic SMAD3 variants. J Am Coll Cardiol 2012;60(5):397–403.

26. van de Laar IMBH, van der Linde D, Oei EHG, et al. Phenotypic spectrum of the SMAD3-related aneurysms-osteoarthritis syndrome. J Med Genet 2012;49(1):47–57.

27. Carr SB, Imbarrato G, Breeze RE, et al. Clip ligation for ruptured intracranial aneurysm in a child with Loeys-Dietz syndrome: case report. J Neurosurg Pediatr 2018;21(4):375–9.

28. Levitt MR, Morton RP, Mai JC, et al. Endovascular treatment of intracranial aneurysms in Loeys-Dietz syndrome. J Neurointerventional Surg 2012;4(6):e37.

29. Tan Y-C, Blumenfeld J, Rennert H. Autosomal dominant polycystic kidney disease: genetics, mutations and microRNAs. Biochim Biophys Acta 2011;1812(10):1202–12.

30. Pei Y, Obaji J, Dupuis A, et al. Unified criteria for ultrasonographic diagnosis of ADPKD. J Am Soc Nephrol JASN 2009;20(1):205–12.

31. Harris PC, Rossetti S. Molecular diagnostics for autosomal dominant polycystic kidney disease. Nat Rev Nephrol 2010;6(4):197–206.

32. Kuo IY, Chapman A. Intracranial Aneurysms in ADPKD: How Far Have We Come? Clin J Am Soc Nephrol 2019;14(8):1119–21.

33. Sommerer C, Zeier M. Clinical Manifestation and Management of ADPKD in Western Countries. Kidney Dis 2016;2(3):120–7.

34. Lee K-B. Genetic diagnosis of autosomal dominant polycystic kidney disease: linkage analysis versus direct mutation analysis. Kidney Res Clin Pract 2016;35(2):67–8.

35. Pirson Y, Chauveau D, Torres V. Management of cerebral aneurysms in autosomal dominant polycystic kidney disease. J Am Soc Nephrol 2002;13(1):269–76.

36. Jung SC, Kim C-H, Ahn JH, et al. Endovascular Treatment of Intracranial Aneurysms in Patients With Autosomal Dominant Polycystic Kidney Disease. Neurosurgery 2016;78(3):429–35.

37. Friedman JM. Neurofibromatosis 1. In: Adam MP, Ardinger HH, Pagon RA, et al, editors. GeneReviews®. University of Washington, Seattle; 1993. Available at: http://www.ncbi.nlm.nih.gov/books/NBK1109/. Accessed February 26, 2021.

38. Gutmann DH, Ferner RE, Listernick RH, et al. Neurofibromatosis type 1. Nat Rev Dis Primers 2017;3:17004. https://doi.org/10.1038/nrdp.2017.4.

39. Schievink WI, Riedinger M, Maya MM. Frequency of incidental intracranial aneurysms in neurofibromatosis type 1. Am J Med Genet A 2005;134A(1):45–8.

40. Oderich GS, Sullivan TM, Bower TC, et al. Vascular abnormalities in patients with neurofibromatosis syndrome type I: clinical spectrum, management, and results. J Vasc Surg 2007;46(3):475–84.

41. Vargiami E, Sapountzi E, Samakovitis D, et al. Moyamoya syndrome and neurofibromatosis type 1. Ital J Pediatr 2014;40:59. https://doi.org/10.1186/1824-7288-40-59.

42. Serafini NB, Serafini CB, Vinhas AS, et al. Moyamoya syndrome associated with neurofibromatosis type 1 in a pediatric patient. An Bras Dermatol 2017;92(6):870–3.

43. Takeshima Y, Kaku Y, Nishi T, et al. Multiple Cerebral Aneurysms Associated With Neurofibromatosis Type 1. J Stroke Cerebrovasc Dis 2019;28(7):e83–91.

44. Baldauf J, Kiwit J, Synowitz M. Cerebral aneurysms associated with von Recklinghausen's neurofibromatosis: report of a case and review of the literature. Neurol India 2005;53(2):213–5.

45. Tatebe S, Asami F, Shinohara H, et al. Ruptured aneurysm of the subclavian artery in a patient with von Recklinghausen's disease. Circ J 2005;69(4):503–6.

46. Moratti C, Andersson T. Giant extracranial aneurysm of the internal carotid artery in neurofibromatosis type 1. A case report and review of the literature. Interv Neuroradiol J Peritherapeutic Neuroradiol Surg Proced Relat Neurosci 2012;18(3): 341–7.

47. Darrigo Júnior LG, Valera ET, Machado A de A, et al. Moyamoya syndrome associated with neurofibromatosis type I in a pediatric patient. Sao Paulo Med J 2011;129(2):110–2.

48. Sinha JK, Ghosh S, Raghunath M. Progeria: a rare genetic premature ageing disorder. Indian J Med Res 2014;139(5):667–74.

49. Gordon LB, Brown WT, Collins FS. Hutchinson-Gilford Progeria Syndrome. In: Adam MP, Ardinger HH, Pagon RA, et al, editors. GeneReviews®. University of Washington, Seattle; 1993. Available at: http://www.ncbi.nlm.nih.gov/books/NBK1121/. Accessed February 26, 2021.

50. Merideth MA, Gordon LB, Clauss S, et al. Phenotype and course of Hutchinson-Gilford progeria syndrome. N Engl J Med 2008;358(6):592–604.

51. Gordon LB, Kleinman ME, Massaro J, et al. Clinical Trial of the Protein Farnesylation Inhibitors Lonafarnib, Pravastatin, and Zoledronic Acid in Children With Hutchinson-Gilford Progeria Syndrome. Circulation 2016;134(2):114–25.

52. Gordon LB, Shappell H, Massaro J, et al. Association of Lonafarnib Treatment vs No Treatment With Mortality Rate in Patients With Hutchinson-Gilford Progeria Syndrome. JAMA 2018;319(16):1687–95.

53. Ullrich NJ, Kieran MW, Miller DT, et al. Neurologic features of Hutchinson-Gilford progeria syndrome after lonafarnib treatment. Neurology 2013;81(5): 427–30.

54. Gordon LB, Kleinman ME, Miller DT, et al. Clinical trial of a farnesyltransferase inhibitor in children with Hutchinson-Gilford progeria syndrome. Proc Natl Acad Sci U S A 2012;109(41):16666–71.

55. Paddock M, Lanham S, Gill K, et al. Pediatric Cerebral Cavernous Malformations. Pediatr Neurol 2021;116:74–83.

56. Zafar A, Quadri SA, Farooqui M, et al. Familial Cerebral Cavernous Malformations. Stroke 2019; 50(5):1294–301.

57. Xia C, Zhang R, Mao Y, et al. Pediatric cavernous malformation in the central nervous system: report of 66 cases. Pediatr Neurosurg 2009;45(2):105–13.

58. Findeis-Hosey JJ, McMahon KQ, Findeis SK. Von Hippel-Lindau Disease. J Pediatr Genet 2016; 5(2):116–23.

59. Klingler J-H, Krüger MT, Lemke JR, et al. Sequence variations in the von Hippel-Lindau tumor suppressor gene in patients with intracranial aneurysms. J Stroke Cerebrovasc Dis Off J Natl Stroke Assoc 2013;22(4):437–43.

60. van Leeuwaarde RS, Ahmad S, Links TP, et al. Von Hippel-Lindau Syndrome. In: Adam MP, Ardinger HH, Pagon RA, et al, editors. GeneReviews®. University of Washington, Seattle; 1993. Available at: http://www.ncbi.nlm.nih.gov/books/NBK1463/. Accessed February 26, 2021.

61. Stam AH, Kothari PH, Shaikh A, et al. Retinal vasculopathy with cerebral leukoencephalopathy and systemic manifestations. Brain 2016;139(11): 2909–22.

62. de Boer I, Pelzer N, Terwindt G. Retinal Vasculopathy with Cerebral Leukoencephalopathy and Systemic Manifestations. In: Adam MP, Ardinger HH, Pagon RA, et al, editors. GeneReviews®. University of Washington, Seattle; 1993. Available at: http://www.ncbi.nlm.nih.gov/books/NBK546576/. Accessed February 26, 2021.

63. Pelzer N, Hoogeveen ES, Haan J, et al. Systemic features of retinal vasculopathy with cerebral leukoencephalopathy and systemic manifestations: a monogenic small vessel disease. J Intern Med 2019;285(3):317–32.

64. Hack R, Rutten J, Lesnik Oberstein SA. CADASIL. In: Adam MP, Ardinger HH, Pagon RA, et al, editors. GeneReviews®. University of Washington, Seattle; 1993. Available at: http://www.ncbi.nlm.nih.gov/books/NBK1500/. Accessed February 26, 2021.

65. Joutel A, François A, Chabriat H, et al. [CADASIL: genetics and physiopathology]. Bull Acad Natl Med 2000;184(7):1535–42.

66. Germain DP. Pseudoxanthoma elasticum. Orphanet J Rare Dis 2017;12(1):85.

67. Terry SF, Uitto J. Pseudoxanthoma Elasticum. In: Adam MP, Ardinger HH, Pagon RA, et al, editors. GeneReviews®. University of Washington, Seattle; 1993. Available at: http://www.ncbi.nlm.nih.gov/books/NBK1113/. Accessed February 26, 2021.

68. Vanakker OM, Leroy BP, Coucke P, et al. Novel clinico-molecular insights in pseudoxanthoma elasticum provide an efficient molecular screening method and a comprehensive diagnostic flowchart. Hum Mutat 2008;29(1):205.

69. Plomp AS, Toonstra J, Bergen AAB, et al. Proposal for updating the pseudoxanthoma elasticum classification system and a review of the clinical findings. Am J Med Genet A 2010;152A(4):1049–58.

70. Chassaing N, Martin L, Calvas P, et al. Pseudoxanthoma elasticum: a clinical, pathophysiological and genetic update including 11 novel ABCC6 mutations. J Med Genet 2005;42(12):881–92.

71. van den Berg JS, Hennekam RC, Cruysberg JR, et al. Prevalence of symptomatic intracranial aneurysm and ischaemic stroke in pseudoxanthoma elasticum. Cerebrovasc Dis 2000;10(4): 315–9.

72. Sunmonu NA. Multiple Cerebrovascular Insults in Pseudoxanthoma Elasticum. J Stroke Cerebrovasc Dis Off J Natl Stroke Assoc 2021;30(3):105524.

73. Inusa B, Hsu L, Kohli N, et al. Sickle Cell Disease—Genetics, Pathophysiology, Clinical Presentation and Treatment. Int J Neonatal Screen 2019;5(2):20.

74. Mangla A, Ehsan M, Maruvada S. Sickle Cell Anemia. In: *StatPearls*. StatPearls Publishing. 2021. Available at: http://www.ncbi.nlm.nih.gov/books/NBK482164/. Accessed February 26, 2021.

75. Sydenstricked VP, Mulherin WA, Houseal RW. The AJDC archives. August 1923. Sickle cell anemia. Report of two cases in children, with necropsy in one case. By V. P. Sydenstricked [sic], W. A. Mulherin and R. W. Houseal. Am J Dis Child 1987; 141(6):612–5.

76. Stockman JA, Nigro MA, Mishkin MM, et al. Occlusion of large cerebral vessels in sickle-cell anemia. N Engl J Med 1972;287(17):846–9.

77. Verduzco LA, Nathan DG. Sickle cell disease and stroke. Blood 2009;114(25):5117–25.

78. Fullerton HJ, Adams RJ, Zhao S, et al. Declining stroke rates in Californian children with sickle cell disease. Blood 2004;104(2):336–9.

79. Pearson HA. Sickle cell anemia and severe infections due to encapsulated bacteria. J Infect Dis 1977;136(Suppl):S25–30.

80. Fukutake T. Cerebral autosomal recessive arteriopathy with subcortical infarcts and leukoencephalopathy (CARASIL): from discovery to gene identification. J Stroke Cerebrovasc Dis Off J Natl Stroke Assoc 2011;20(2):85–93.

81. Onodera O, Nozaki H, Fukutake T. HTRA1 Disorder. In: Adam MP, Ardinger HH, Pagon RA, et al, editors. GeneReviews®. University of Washington, Seattle; 1993. Available at: http://www.ncbi.nlm.nih.gov/books/NBK32533/. Accessed February 26, 2021.

82. Higueros E, Roe E, Granell E, et al. Sturge-Weber Syndrome: A Review. Actas Dermosifiliogr 2017; 108(5):407–17.

83. Comi AM. Presentation, diagnosis, pathophysiology, and treatment of the neurological features of Sturge-Weber syndrome. Neurologist 2011; 17(4):179–84.

84. Naganathan S, Tadi P. Klippel Trenaunay Weber Syndrome. In: StatPearls. StatPearls Publishing. 2021. Available at: http://www.ncbi.nlm.nih.gov/books/NBK558989/. Accessed February 26, 2021.

85. Banzic I, Brankovic M, Ž Maksimović, et al. Parkes Weber syndrome-Diagnostic and management paradigms: A systematic review. Phlebology 2017;32(6):371–83.

86. Billington AR, Shah J, Elston JB, et al. Klippel-trenaunay syndrome. Eplasty 2013;13:ic64.

87. De Blasi R, Zenzola A, Lanzilotti CM, et al. An unusual association of intracranial aneurysms and oesophageal duplication in a case of Klippel-Trenaunay syndrome. Neuroradiology 2000; 42(12):930–2.

88. Star A, Fuller CE, Landas SK. Intracranial aneurysms in klippel-trenaunay/weber syndromes: case report. Neurosurgery 2010;66(5):E1027–8.

89. Kim YW, Kim N, Hwang J-M, et al. Teaching Neuro-Images: Multiple giant intracranial aneurysms in Klippel-Trenaunay syndrome. Neurology 2013; 81(3):e17–8.

90. Smitherman AD, Woodall MN, Alleyne CH, et al. Open surgical management of a ruptured intracranial aneurysm in Klippel-Trenaunay-Weber (KTW) syndrome. BMJ Case Rep 2013;2013. https://doi.org/10.1136/bcr-2012-006857.

91. Hammer J, Seront E, Duez S, et al. Sirolimus is efficacious in treatment for extensive and/or complex slow-flow vascular malformations: a monocentric prospective phase II study. Orphanet J Rare Dis 2018;13(1):191.

92. Guey S, Tournier-Lasserve E, Hervé D, et al. Moyamoya disease and syndromes: from genetics to clinical management. Appl Clin Genet 2015;8: 49–68.

93. Suzuki J, Takaku A. Cerebrovascular "moyamoya" disease. Disease showing abnormal net-like vessels in base of brain. Arch Neurol 1969;20(3): 288–99.

94. Hsu T-R, Niu D-M. Fabry disease: Review and experience during newborn screening. Trends Cardiovasc Med 2018;28(4):274–81.

95. Namazova-Baranova LS, Baranov AA, Pushkov AA, et al. Fabry disease in children: a federal screening programme in Russia. Eur J Pediatr 2017;176(10):1385–91.

96. Ramaswami U, Whybra C, Parini R, et al. Clinical manifestations of Fabry disease in children: data from the Fabry Outcome Survey. Acta Paediatr 2006;95(1):86–92.

97. Chan B, Adam DN. A Review of Fabry Disease. Skin Therapy Lett 2018;23(2):4–6.

98. El-Hattab AW, Adesina AM, Jones J, et al. MELAS syndrome: Clinical manifestations, pathogenesis, and treatment options. Mol Genet Metab 2015; 116(1–2):4–12.

99. Pavlakis SG, Phillips PC, DiMauro S, et al. Mitochondrial myopathy, encephalopathy, lactic acidosis, and strokelike episodes: a distinctive clinical syndrome. Ann Neurol 1984;16(4):481–8.

100. Koga Y, Akita Y, Nishioka J, et al. L-arginine improves the symptoms of strokelike episodes in MELAS. Neurology 2005;64(4):710–2.

101. Kubota M, Sakakihara Y, Mori M, et al. Beneficial effect of L-arginine for stroke-like episode in MELAS. Brain Dev 2004;26(7):481–3.

Moving?

Make sure your subscription moves with you!

To notify us of your new address, find your **Clinics Account Number** (located on your mailing label above your name), and contact customer service at:

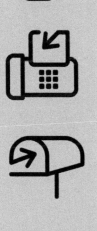

Email: journalscustomerservice-usa@elsevier.com

800-654-2452 (subscribers in the U.S. & Canada)
314-447-8871 (subscribers outside of the U.S. & Canada)

Fax number: 314-447-8029

Elsevier Health Sciences Division
Subscription Customer Service
3251 Riverport Lane
Maryland Heights, MO 63043

*To ensure uninterrupted delivery of your subscription, please notify us at least 4 weeks in advance of move.

Printed and bound by CPI Group (UK) Ltd, Croydon, CR0 4YY

08/05/2025

01864700-0015